ANIMAL SCIENCE, ISSUES AND RESEARCH

# LABORATORY ANIMALS AND NEUROSCIENCES

# Animal Science, Issues and Research

Additional books and e-books in this series can be found on Nova's website under the Series tab.

ANIMAL SCIENCE, ISSUES AND RESEARCH

# LABORATORY ANIMALS AND NEUROSCIENCES

BRAULIO HERNANDEZ GODINEZ
MARTIN GARCIA SERVIN
AND
ALEJANDRA IBAÑEZ CONTRERAS
EDITORS

nova
Medicine & Health
New York

## Library of Congress Cataloging-in-Publication Data

Names: Ibáñez Contreras, Alejandra, editor. | Hernández Godínez, Braulio, editor. | Garcia Servin, Martin, editor.
Title: Laboratory animals and neurosciences / Alejandra Ibañez Contreras, Non Human Unit of APREXBIO S.A.S. de C.V. Ciudad de México, México, Braulio Hernandez Godinez, 1Non Human Unit of APREXBIO S.A.S. de C.V. Ciudad de México, México, and Martin Garcia Servin, Instituto de Neurobiología, Universidad Nacional Autónoma de México, Campus Juriquilla, Queretaro, México. Description: New York: Nova Science Publishers, [2020] | Series: Animal science, issues and research | Includes bibliographical references and index. | Summary: "Laboratory animals are fundamental in learning and teaching within the various areas of neuroscience research. This from its proper management, animal welfare, standardization of protocols, use of the best biomodel in exprimentation. There are many different areas of study within neurosciences today. However, any use of any biomodel must be based on the context of the three Rs (Refinement, Reduction and Replacement). The objective of this book is to make known through different chapters the use of different laboratory animals in standardized research lines applied to neurosciences in different contexts and applications in basic research"-- Provided by publisher.
Identifiers: LCCN 2020038440 (print) | LCCN 2020038441 (ebook) | ISBN 9781536184624 (hardcover) | ISBN 9781536185881 (adobe pdf)
Subjects: LCSH: Mental illness--Animal models. | Nervous system--Diseases--Animal models. | Laboratory animals. | Neurosciences. | Animal experimentation.
Classification: LCC RC455.4.A54 L33 2020 (print) | LCC RC455.4.A54 (ebook) | DDC 616.8002/73--dc23
LC record available at https://lccn.loc.gov/2020038440
LC ebook record available at https://lccn.loc.gov/2020038441

*Published by Nova Science Publishers, Inc. † New York*

# CONTENTS

# PREFACE

The use of laboratory animals as models of experimentation for research in neuroscience in Mexico has acquired a progressive importance and concurrence in the scientific field. Currently these biomodels are not only the object of research, but are used in various areas of research as models to understand phenomena of scientific interest in areas as diverse as Veterinary Medicine, Chemistry, Ethology, Psychology and Biomedical Science. The proposal of this book arises from the need to update, link and disseminate scientific advances and the application of management and use of laboratory animals for human application.

In: Laboratory Animals and Neurosciences ISBN: 978-1-53618-462-4
Editors: B. Hernandez Godinez et al.© 2020 Nova Science Publishers, Inc.

***Chapter 1***

# ANIMAL MODELS OF DEPRESSION: A REVIEW

***Maribel Estevez Cabrera*** [1], ***Tania Molina Jiménez*** [2], ***Ofelia Limón Morales***[2,3], ***Alfonso Alfaro Rodríguez***[4] ***and Herlinda Bonilla Jaime***[3,*]

[1] Doctorado en Ciencias Biológicas y de la Salud, Universidad Autónoma Metropolitana, Unidad Iztapalapa, Ciudad de México, México

[2] Instituto Interdisciplinario de Investigaciones, Universidad de Xalapa, Xalapa-Enríquez, Veracruz, México

[3]Departamento de Biología de la Reproducción. Universidad Autónoma Metropolitana, Unidad Iztapalapa, Ciudad de México, México

[4]Departamento de Neurociencias, Instituto Nacional de Rehabilitación LGII, Ciudad de México, México

[*] Corresponding Author's E-mail: bjh@xanum.uam.mx.

## ABSTRACT

Depression is a common, complex, life-threatening mental disorder that imposes a serious social and economic burden worldwide as a debilitating mental illness with significant morbidity and mortality. Despite a recent increase in research, the precise mechanisms that underlie depression are not fully understood. Numerous animal models have been established to elucidate the pathophysiology of depression and test new treatment strategies but, despite these substantial efforts, the animal models currently available have only limited utility for these purposes, likely because none can completely mimic this complex disorder. Animal models must fulfill three basic requirements: face validity (i.e., a phenotype similar to humans with the illness); construct validity (i.e., they replicate the processes that generate this pathology in humans); and predictive validity (i.e., sensitivity to pharmacological and non-pharmacological interventions that effectively treat the disease or condition in humans). This article reviews the most widely-used animal models of depression, discusses their advantages and limitations, and delineates the salient features of each one in terms of its behavioral and neurobiological outcomes

**Keywords**: depression, animal model, antidepressants, stress

## INTRODUCTION

Major depressive disorder (MDD) is a widespread mental illness whose main symptoms include loss of interest and enjoyment. Other symptoms may be weight variation, loss of appetite, sleep disturbances, psychomotor symptoms like restlessness or retardation, low self-esteem, feelings of hopelessness, little interest in sex, and suicidal thoughts, among others (American Psychiatric Association, 2013). Recently, the World Health Organization reported an 18.4% increase in the incidence of depression over the 10-year period, 2005-2015. Today, 322 million people worldwide are living with this illness (World Health Organization, 2017), which in several countries affects women twice as often as men (Kessler and Bromet, 2013).

Several brain structures (prefrontal cortex, hippocampus, amygdala, hypothalamus, *nucleus accumbens* and cingulate cortex, among others) participate in regulating emotional and mood functions, so alterations in these neural circuits can generate mental disorders like depression. The goal of pharmacological therapy with antidepressant drugs is to reverse the dysfunctional changes in these circuits, which comprise the limbic system (Lorenzetti et al., 2009). One early proposal for explaining the origins of depression was the monoamine hypothesis, which held that the cause was the depletion of neurotransmitters like serotonin (5-HT), noradrenaline (NA) and dopamine (DA) in brain circuits of the limbic system. It suggested using antidepressants to increase 5-HT or NA concentrations in the synaptic cleft by blocking 5-HT transport (SERT) or NA transport (NAT), which reuptake 5-HT or NA, respectively, or by inhibiting the monoaminoxidase enzyme (MAO), which breaks down these molecules (Willner, Scheel-Krüger and Belzung, 2013). However, because the therapeutic effects of such antidepressant treatments did not become apparent until after three or four weeks of treatment, it seemed that a dysfunction in the monoamine system was only one hallmark of depression.

Depressed patients also present dysregulation of the hypothalamic-pituitary-adrenal (HPA) axis characterized by high levels of corticotropin-releasing factor (CRF) and cortisol, but decreased suppression of cortisol in response to dexamethasone treatment (Pruessner et al., 2003; Sher et al., 2013). Moreover, alterations of the HPA axis are associated with inappropriate stress responses due to the negative effects of chronically-high cortisol levels in key brain structures like the prefrontal cortex, hippocampus and amygdala, which regulate cognitive and emotional processes (Dean and Keshavan, 2017). Moreover, cortisol is a regulator of the brain-derived neurotrophic factor (BDNF), which plays an important role in promoting survival, growth, differentiation and the synaptogenesis process. The increase in glucocorticoids reduces BDNF levels and the TkrB receptor. Also, animals subjected to diverse stressful situations have shown low BDNF levels in the hippocampus (Duman and Monteggia, 2006; Kunugi et al., 2010). Antidepressants and electroconvulsive treatment increase BDNF and TkrB levels (Chen et al., 2001; Altar et al., 2003). Also, bilateral infusion of BDNF into the hippocampus reverts depressive-like behavior, evaluated by the forced-swimming test, and learned helplessness (Shirayama et al., 2002). These data suggest that neurotrophins participate in the characteristic alterations of depression and, therefore, should be targets of antidepressant action as well.

Additionally, there is evidence of the participation of the immunological system in the pathophysiology of depression, since patients with major depressive disorder have increased levels of proinflammatory cytokines (interferon-α, tumor necrosis factor-α (TNF-α), IL-6 and IL-1β) (O'Brien, Scott and Dinan, 2004). Cytokines regulate neurotransmitter metabolism by breaking down tryptophan (a 5-HT synthesis precursor) through the activation of the indoleamine 2,3 dioxygenase enzyme (IDO) or the MAPK signaling pathway, thus increasing SERT, NAT and DA transport (DAT) expression; that is, reuptake transports. Both situations reduce levels of those neurotransmitters, which constitute the principal problem in depression (Miller and Raison, 2016; Liu et al., 2019).

## TREATING DEPRESSION

Today, antidepressants constitute the primary therapeutic treatment, so selective 5-HT reuptake inhibitors (SSRI) like fluoxetine have become the first choice for treating depression, followed by selective 5-HT or NA reuptake inhibitors and atypical antidepressants (Montgomery et al., 2007; Vermeiden et al., 2017). Tricyclic antidepressants like imipramine and clomipramine have proven to be highly-effective in attenuating depressive symptoms but, unlike SSRI, their therapeutic efficacy is accompanied by side effects that include dizziness, cardiac arrhythmia, blurred vision and drowsiness (Farach et al., 2012). Other antidepressants, like monoamine oxidase inhibitors (MAOIs) are considered safe and efficacious (Shulman, Herrmann and Walker, 2013). The acute action of all these agents consists in increasing neurotransmitter levels in the synaptic clefts, but their therapeutic effect only becomes apparent after several weeks of treatment. Recent pre-clinical and clinical studies show that ketamine (a non-selective NMDA receptor antagonist) produces rapid antidepressant action, and the FDA recently approved intranasal ketamine due to its efficacy and tolerability in patients with treatment-resistant depression without suicidal ideation. It appears that this drug's antidepressant activity modulates the monoamine system and increases glutamate, BDNF release, and the synaptic proteins involved in synaptogenesis, among other effects (Scheuing et al., 2015; Blackburn, 2019). Although monotherapy with antidepressants is efficacious, some reports suggest that combining psychological and pharmacological therapies provides greater effectiveness in preventing relapses and recurrences during treatment (Segal, Vincent and Levitt, 2002). Up to now, data from clinical studies have been important for increasing our knowledge of depression, but studies using animal models have also played a significant role in analyzing the pathophysiology of depression, elucidating the action mechanisms of antidepressant drugs, and screening new drugs with antidepressant activity.

## ANIMALS MODELS

Animal models are defined as experimental preparations with non-human organisms designed to study a phenomenon observed in other species. In other words, animal models are used to reproduce a human pathology process under criteria of predictive validity (Urani, Chourbaji and Gass, 2005; Yan et al., 2010). It is important to note that animal models and animal testing are distinct, though they are often deemed equivalent. Testing differs from animal models because its main objective is to measure behavioral and physiological parameters as a means of evaluating changes caused by genetic, pharmacological or environmental manipulation (Urani, Chourbaji and Gass, 2005), while animal models are important tools that improve our understanding of the neurophysiologic mechanisms of depression, help screen and develop new substances with antidepressant activity for future treatment, and isolate the antidepressant mechanisms of drugs (Valvassori et al., 2013). These models usually employ some kind of stressor (acute or chronic) to induce depressive-like behaviors, and then attempt to revert them by administering a clinically-effective antidepressant, though some models are based on long-term manipulations designed to foster a predisposition to developing depressive behavior, such as stress during early stages of life, or pharmacological and surgical manipulation (Willner and Mitchell, 2002).

Our starting point is the clinical definition of depression as a complex series of psychological, neuroendocrine and somatic symptoms that cannot be reproduced completely in animals. Therefore, only specific, objective, hereditary and measurable characteristics or behaviors associated with an illness that are not evident without using instruments (endophenotypes or intermediate phenotypes) can be demonstrated as being relevant to human depression (Holmes et al., 2003; Matthews et al., 2005; Wang et al., 2017). Measures may be neurophysiological, biochemical, endocrinological, neuroanatomical, neuropsychological or cognitive. Some general principals have been developed to categorize the various types of behavioral models, and this allows us to determine how a model can be analyzed in neuroscience, psychology and psychopharmacology. There are three types of behavioral models, each one corresponding to one of these disciplines: those that can be used to study cerebral functions, those employed in psychological research, and those designed to determine the action of drugs. These three types can be called behavioral bioassays, simulations, and screening tests (Willner, 1991).

Screening tests analyze new psychotropic agents to discern the action of drugs using one of two strategies. The first consists in developing drugs by identifying agents that exert some type of clinical action; examples include neuroleptics, antidepressants and anxiolytics. Tests of this kind can isolate clinically-effective drugs that vary in their chemical structure. The second strategy consists in identifying the biochemical action as a target for developing new drugs. Behavioral bioassays allow us to analyze the functional state of a physiological system. One key use of behavioral assays is to study the mechanisms responsible for changes in cerebral functions caused by administering drugs, brain lesions, or other experimental manipulations. Finally, animal models that reproduce biochemical, physiological or anatomical findings are tools used to analyze therapeutic options designed for use with humans. As their name suggests, these simulations of human behaviors may imitate a symptom, a group of symptoms, or the complete disorder. Various methods exist to reproduce a disorder: inducing brain damage, selecting isogenic or transgenic sub-lines, applying drugs, enforcing social separation, and others related to age (Willner and Mitchell, 2002).

To ensure the utility of animal models, some authors have proposed validity criteria. For instance, McKinney and Bunney, stipulate that an animal model of depression must have the same etiology, symptomatology, response to clinically-effective treatment and biochemistry, but their criteria were not well-defined and only explain the external similarities between animal models and mental disorders in humans (Willner, 1991). For Willner, validating animal models of psychopathology requires focusing not only on what he calls face validity, but on two additional aspects: predictive validity and construct validity (Willner, 1995). Face validity implies that the symptomatology is similar to what is observed in depressive patients, whereas predictive validity evaluates the effectiveness of antidepressant medicines, arguing that clinically-effective drugs should reverse the depression-like symptoms induced in animal models. Construct validity refers to pathophysiological similarities between the animal model and human depression.

Although animal models are important tools for studying psychopathologies, they have limits that cannot be ignored. MDD, for example, is considered a syndrome with numerous symptoms, some of which simply cannot be mimicked in animal models of depression. These include feelings of worthlessness, sadness or guilt, and suicidal ideation. It is for this reason that most animal models of depression have focused on the main symptoms of MDD – such as anhedonia – because this suffices to evaluate new therapeutic agents with antidepressant activity (Abelaira, Reus and Quevedo, 2013). Few animal models satisfy all three validity criteria, and most fit only one or two because they reproduce only one or two aspects of the disorder. We now know that the physiopathology of depression is more complex than previously thought because it involves alterations in multiple systems; namely, monoamine systems, neurotrophic factors (BDNF), cytokine levels (Interleucin 1$\beta$ (L-1$\beta$), Interleucin -6 (IL-6), tumor necrosis factor (TNF$\alpha$), hyperactivity in the HPA axis, and anatomical changes (Palazidou, 2012).

Despite their limitations, animal models are important tools that increase our knowledge of the neurobiological aspects of major depressive disorders, and screen new therapeutic substances administered in attempts to ameliorate this disorder. This chapter reviews animal models of depression cited in the literature, their validation criteria, and their advantages and disadvantages.

## THE FORCED-SWIMMING-TEST (FST)

One of the animal models most used to screen drugs with antidepressant activity and their possible action mechanisms is the FST, which was first used in 1977 when Roger Porsolt and cols. (1977) described "a new behavioral method for inducing a depressive state". This model (also known as the behavioral despair test or the Porsolt test) uses water and space restriction for inducing stress in rodents. In this aspect, rodents are subjected to a session of forced swimming in a container from which there is no escape. The container is a transparent Plexiglas cylinder 40 cm high ×18 cm in diameter, with 15 cm of water at 21-24°C. The model consists of two swimming sessions separated by 24 hours. The first test (or pre-test) is a 15 minutes-session, while the second test is a 5 minutes-session. The first session is designed to induce stress and despair; while the second test is when active (swimming and climbing) and passive behavior (immobility) were measured. In the first few minutes, rats display exploratory activity that includes jumping, inspecting the walls, and exploring the bottom of the cylinder looking for a means of escape, but this activity ceases after a few minutes and the rat adopts a characteristic position of immobility witch is defined as standing erect position on its hind paws and supported by its tail, leaning one or both forepaws on the cylinder wall to keep its head barely above the water's surface. Moreover, antidepressant drugs reduce the duration of immobility and increased the active behavior in the FST that is why this test has become the most widely-used predictive test to evaluate the behavioral effects of antidepressants in rats (Porsolt, Le Pichon and Jalfre, 1977; Porsolt, 1981; Borsini and Meli, 1988; Lucki, 1997).

However, false positives are common; for example, medications like amphetamines, which are not antidepressants, enhance locomotor activity and prevent the shift to immobility (Porsolt et al., 1978; Hawkins et al., 1978). In addition, the GABA-A agonist, muscimol, barbiturates, benzodiazepanes and anticholinergic agents have been found to generate false positives (De Pablo et al., 1991). Moreover, rats that perform physical exercise, considered an anti-stress activity in humans (Krogh et al., 2011), showed greater immobility accompanied by high levels of corticosterone, even so these rats are more resistant (Reul, 2014). Thus, physical exercise could be considered a false negative in this context. Also, experience could be an important factor, for instance, animals that are more familiar with the test remain more immobile (Borsini, Volterra and Meli, 1986). Even, temperature can modify the parameters in this test; rats exposed to water at 19°C swim more and immobility is more marked in the water used as the new test, which is at 25°C, 6 degrees higher than the original temperature (Reul, 2014). Moreover, rats move more quickly in cold water and more slowly at warmer temperatures (Jefferys and Funder, 1994), and it is important to taking in to account that prolonged immersion in water causes serious hypothermia in rodents (Jefferys and Funder, 1994; Taltavull et al., 2003; Arai et al., 2000). Also, some studies that measure the rats' body temperature during a pharmacological treatment showed that antidepressants do not alter the hypothermic effects of exposure to water and also reduced immobility (Porsolt, Deniel and Jalfre, 1979; David et al., 2001). Hence, it is unlikely that the thermoregulating effects of antidepressants play a crucial role in the behavioral effects of the FST.

Several modifications of the original methodology have been performed since the first proposal. For example, some studies have reported changes in the video-recording of immobility time, cylinders diameters or dimensions, variations on the depth of the water, reversing the light-dark cycle and using constant illumination, as well as different species of rodents and strains of rat or mouse. Moreover, psychological and physical stress play significant roles in the development of affective disorders in humans (Caspi et al., 2003; Post, 1992). Thus, the induction of a sensation of losing control makes it possible to generate a behavioral state analogous to depression (Vollmayr and Henn, 2003). In this regard, rats exposed to chronic physical or emotional stressors have greater immobility times on the FST which implies that these rats showed more despair or low motivation to solve the situation (Gutiérrez-García and Contreras, 2009; Hageman et al., 2009; Rygula et al., 2005).

The fact that the traditional form of the FST did not prove reliable in detecting the antidepressive properties of SSRIs was a significant disadvantage, given the demonstrated clinical efficacy of these compounds (Borsini, 1995). Nevertheless, some modifications were performed to the FST procedure, especially in the evaluations of active (swimming and climbing) and passive behaviors like immobility. For instance, climbing, defined like actively moves of the rat with hindlegs in or out of the water, usually against the walls or towards the entrance to the cylinder; swimming behavior is defined as horizontal movements made by the rat beyond those required to simply keep its head above the water; and immobility is a simply floating passively in the water in a erect position on its hind legs and tail, and resting one or both forepaws on the cylinder wall to keep its head just above the water's surface (Detke, Rickels and Lucki, 1995; Detke and Lucki, 1996; Lucki, 1997). Also, several conditions were change like the water depth, which increased from 15-18 to 30 cm (Detke, Rickels, and Lucki 1995; Detke and Lucki 1996).

It is important to mention that the videotaping of the procedure allows measure not only the time but also frequency of each behavior in 5-second intervals during test sessions. In this way, at the end of each 5-second period during the 5-minute test session, the observer identifies one of the three aforementioned behaviors. This sampling method generates a total of 60 behaviors or counts evaluated during the 5 minutes of the test. Using these conditions improves the FST's sensitivity to the effects of the antidepressant drugs tested, especially SSRIs.

Evaluating active behaviors (swimming, climbing) as well as the decrease in immobility behavior allows us to determine possible mechanisms that may allow different antidepressant compounds to produce their effect. Thus, drugs that increase noradrenergic activity, like selective NA reuptake inhibitors (desipramine, reboxetine, maprotiline), reduce immobility behavior by selectively increasing climbing, while drugs that increase serotoninergic activity, like the SSRIs (fluoxetine, sertraline, paroxetine), reduce immobility by selectively increasing swimming (Detke, Rickels and Lucki, 1995; Lucki, 1997). However, new antidepressants with dual effects on the 5-HT and NA systems have shown mixed response profiles on the FST.

## RELIABILITY: WHAT DOES THE FST REALLY MEASURE?

The FST was originally considered an animal model of depression (Porsolt, Le Pichon, and Jalfre 1977; Porsolt 1981) with a significant level of predictive validity, while immobility behavior was believed to reflect the psychomotor delay or anergia that many depressed patients show. This endowed the FST with a certain level of apparent validity; however, theoretical support is controversial. Porsolt and cols. (1977, 1978) argue that the fact that rats remain more immobile during the second immersion indicates a state of "hopelessness" since they have learned that escape is impossible. Because the predictive value of this test for developing drugs was significant, the importance of the concept of a state of hopelessness was emphasized in reports that anthropomorphically interpreted immobility as depression (de Kloet and Molendijk, 2016). However, this interpretation has been questioned, and several alternative interpretations of immobility measures have been proposed. For example, it is obvious that once an animal learns that escaping from deep water is impossible, it will likely maximize its possibilities for survival by conserving energy, and so remain immobile. The early versions of the FST with their low water levels soon revealed that rats are good at using their tails for support. In addition, immobility also tends to correlate with body weight, perhaps because it is easier for fatter rats to remain on the surface. In light of these findings, an alternative explanation for greater immobility proposed that learning was involved (De Pablo et al., 1989; Enginar et al., 2016), but this led to a rather inconvenient current of thought; namely, that antidepressants act by deteriorating learning. An easier concept to assimilate was that the FST actually measures a strategy for coping with stress (Commons et al., 2017).

More recent theoretical formulations give some theoretical support to the FST (Dixon, 1998; Dixon and Fisch, 1998; Gilbert and Allan, 1998; Gilbert, Gilbert and Irons, 2004). Some propose that the psychopathological symptoms of depression may be related to the activation of defense mechanisms to respond to a threat and loss of control like immobility behavior. These mechanisms can become pathological when easily-activated or prolonged and interrupted, but not expressed (arrested), and/or when ineffective (e.g., active swimming and climbing behaviors). Indeed, recent studies show that depressed individuals can feel intense anger (fight) and the desire to escape (flight), but these 'fight-or-flight' defense behaviors can be blocked, inhibited and interrupted (arrested), thus increasing stress (Gilbert, Gilbert and Irons, 2004). In this aspect, immobility behavior on the FST is interpreted as a defensive mechanism that frees the animal from the stress of forced swimming and allows it to alternate the immobility posture with active escape behaviors (swimming, climbing) as part of a strategy for coping with the stress caused by being forced to swim (coping mechanism).

Alternatively, it may reflect a specific state of mammals' defensive repertoire known as 'arrested flight', which entails suppressing exploratory behaviors – like swimming and climbing – that indicate that the animal is trying to escape from the stressful situation, and adopting cryptic static postures, like immobility, that protect them and allow them to maintain continuous vigilance of their environment. These behaviors have been correlated with the psychological construct called 'entrapment', which has recently been observed and evaluated in endogenous human depression (Dixon, 1998; Dixon and Fisch, 1998; Gilbert and Allan, 1998; Fullilove, 2002; Willner and Goldstein, 2001; Gilbert, Gilbert and Irons, 2004). In humans, interrupting escape behavior or eliminating the possibility of escape ('arrested flight') has been linked to suicide (Baumeister, 1990). Thus, the theoretical bases of immobility behavioral on the FST may be related to variations in behavioral depression induced by stress that reflect defensive behaviors like arrested flight and entrapment, which are seen in patients with depression. This gives the forced swimming model not only significant predictive value, but also important theoretical and appearance support, though the symptoms just described are not formally-recognized as symptoms of depression.

Immobility on the FST is also interpreted as passive confrontation (Warden et al., 2012). The appearance of increased immobility reflects the change from a predominantly active behavior to one that is predominantly passive in a stressful situation (Molendijk and de Kloet, 2015). Antidepressants may well foster active confrontation strategies, while a passive confrontation strategy would not be foreign to the depressed state, though it is not a synonym of the latter.

Simultaneous, *in vivo* electrophysiological recordings allow us to measure the transition between active and passive behavioral states in real time, and these techniques have revealed surprising correlations between the activity of dopaminergic circuits in the medial prefrontal cortex (mPFC) and mesolimbic system in the transition between active and passive behavioral states on the 24-h FST pre-test (Lammel, Tye and Warden, 2014; Warden et al., 2012; Tye et al., 2012). Also, optogenetic activation of the mPFC and specific dopaminergic sub-circuits in the midbrain (the former projected to the dorsal raphe nuclei) induces behavioral transitions towards immobility that suggest a causal relation (Warden et al., 2012). Specifically, the Ventral Tegmental Area-A9 (VTA-A9) dopaminergic circuit has received much attention because of its immediate role in stress responses and in the pathogenesis of depression related to stress and psychosis. In fact, the dopaminergic circuit of the mesoaccumbens is important for coping with the stressor of forced swimming. On the FST, transitions pass progressively from styles of active confrontation to passive ones, culminating in prolonged periods of immobility, which can be evoked through optogenetic stimulation of the dopaminergic neurons in the VTA.

Dopaminergic activity is controlled by afferences in limbic areas such as amygdala and hippocampus. All limbic areas in the front brain are targets of the corticosteroid hormones that are released under stress. Just as exposure to the stressor of forced swimming induces a response by the sympathetic nervous system, it also stimulates the HPA axis and several neural circuits (e.g., DA, 5-HT, GABA) in the brain (Linthorst, Flachskamm and Reul, 2008; Droste et al., 2008; de Groote and Linthorst, 2007). Glucocorticoid receptors (GR) are expressed abundantly in the mesolimbic dopaminergic projection and ascending cortical A9 that innervates the target fronto-cortical regions and nucleus accumbens, while the limbic structures, especially the CA1 and CA2 neurons in the hippocampus and neurons in the dentate gyrus, are richly-endowed with both mineralocorticoid receptors (MR) and GR. GR and MR seem to be involved in the acquisition and retention of the immobility response (Solomon et al., 2012), through pharmacological blocking or GR activation. However, blocking the GR in the limbic regions fosters a greater dominion of corticosterone action through the MR, which could participate in the evaluation and selection of responses and the capacity for immediate confrontation. This role of MR has been firmly-established in other behavioral paradigms (Harris et al., 2012).

## Tail Suspenssion Test (TST)

The TST is similar to the FST, but differs in that it is used only with mice. Today, the TST is one of the most widely-used models for assessing antidepressant-like activity in mice. It is based on the finding that animals subjected to short-term, inescapable stress by being suspended by the tail will adopt an immobile posture (Cryan, Mombereau and Vassout, 2005). In the TST, the mouse's tail is attached and suspended by adhesive tape. The time that it spends in the immobile state during a 6-minute test is interpreted as a measure of depressive-like behavior. Various antidepressant drugs reverse this immobility and trigger escape-related behaviors. Both the TST and FST are considered predictive models of antidepressant activity, *not* animal models of depression, because they lack face and construct validity (Abelaira, Reus and Quevedo, 2013).

## Model of Alterations in Neurodevelopment by SSRI

The objective of these manipulations is to alter the viability of monoaminergic neurotransmission systems during a sensitive stage of development to modify their long-term balance and behavioral disturbances. One early study (1980s) in this field was conducted by Mirmiran et al. (1983) to analyze the importance of active or rapid eye movement sleep (REM) for neurodevelopment, since a greater amount of REM sleep occurs in early stages of development than in adulthood. Those authors deprived rats of REM sleep in the second and third weeks of life by administering clomipramine, a REM sleep inhibitor, tricyclic and SSRIs antidepressant. As adults, those animals presented behavioral and physiological disturbances (Corner et al., 1980; Mirmiran et al., 1983). Later, was observed that adult animals treated neonatally with clomipramine had decreased male sexual behavior and intracranial stimulation, with abnormalities in REM sleep and greater motor activity in stressful situations; alterations that resemble symptoms in patients with MDD (Vogel, Neill, Hagler and Kors, 1990; Vogel, Neill, Kors, et al. 1990; Vogel and Vogel, 1982). Because these behavioral alterations in rats treated with clomipramine were reversed by antidepressants like imipramine, neonatal clomipramine treatment was proposed as an animal model of MDD with predictive and face validity (Vogel, Neill, Kors, et al. 1990). In recent decades, the effect of different SSRIs administered during the prenatal or early postnatal period has been reported. In rodents, perinatal exposure to various SSRIs produces such long-term behavioral disturbances as increased depression-like behaviors, anhedonia, perturbed sleep and diminished sexual activity, which resemble depression in humans and other subjects (Vogel, Neill, Hagler, Kors, et al., 1990; Vogel, Neill, Hagler and Kors, 1990; Popa et al., 2008; Bhagya et al., 2008; Kovács et al., 2012; Mirmiran et al., 1981; Drago et al., 1985; De Boer et al., 1989; Neill et al., 1990; Bonilla-Jaime, Retana-Marquez and Velazquez-Moctezuma, 1998; Gouvêa et al., 2008; Harris et al., 2012; Maciag, Coppinger and Paul, 2006; Rayen et al., 2013; Rodriguez-Porcel et al., 2011). Thus, SSRIs treatment in early stages shows appearance validity by reflecting a phenomenological similarity between the behavioral manifestations seen in the animal model and symptoms observed in humans (Willner and Mitchell, 2002).

One of the most important signs of depressive disorder apart from the decrease in mood, and one that is a key for diagnosing MDD, is anhedonia; that is, decreased interest in pleasurable activities (American Psychiatric Association, 2014). Rats exposed perinatally to SSRIs manifest behaviors that suggest hedonic states, motivation and pleasure. One such behavior is intracranial self-stimulation, as male rats treated neonatally with clomipramine show less hypothalamic intracranial self-stimulation than controls (Vogel, Neill, Hagler, Kors, et al. 1990). Also, SSRIs lower sucrose consumption, regardless of the concentration used (Vogel, Neill, Hagler, and Kors 1990; Popa et al. 2008) or the duration of food and water deprivation (Bhagya et al., 2008; Kovács et al., 2012). Another type of conduct analyzed as an indicator of anhedonia is sexual behavior, which may resemble the decreased libido seen in humans with depression. It has been widely reported that early postnatal exposure to SSRIs antidepressants leads to impaired sexual behavior in adult male and female rat offspring. In this regard, neonatal exposure to clomipramine, fluoxetine and citalopram diminishes sexual behavior in male rat offspring; described as a decrease in the number, but an increase in the latency, of mounts, intromissions and ejaculations, with longer post-ejaculatory intervals (Mirmiran et al., 1981; Drago et al., 1985; De Boer et al., 1989; Neill et al., 1990; Bonilla-Jaime, Retana-Marquez and Velazquez-Moctezuma, 1998; Gouvêa et al., 2008; Harris et al., 2012; Maciag, Coppinger and Paul, 2006; Rayen et al., 2013; Rodriguez-Porcel et al., 2011). These effects could be dose-dependent (Vogel et al., 1996).

Also, neonatal clomipramine treatment decreases the percentage of males that copulate, as only 40% perform intromissions and 10% ejaculate (Limón-Morales, Soria-Fregozo, Arteaga-Silva, Hernández González, et al. 2014). Moreover, postnatal exposure to SSRIs decreases sexual motivation (Gouvêa et al., 2008; Harris et al., 2012; Maciag, Coppinger and Paul 2006; Rayen et al., 2013; Rodriguez-Porcel et al., 2011; Harris et al., 2012;

Hilakivi and Hilakivi, 1987; Velazquez-Moctezuma and Diaz Ruiz, 1992; Hansen, Sánchez, and Meier 1997; Yang et al., 2008; Rebello et al., 2014; Sarkar, Chachra and Vaidya, 2014; Glover et al., 2015; Zohar, Shoham and Weinstock, 2016; Boulle et al., 2016; Bhagya et al., 2015), though prenatal exposition to SSRIs, in contrast, has no effect on male copulatory behavior (Cagiano et al., 2008; Olivier et al., 2011). More recent reports indicate that neonatal clomipramine treatment also impairs sexual behavior in females as they present fewer proceptive (hopping, darting) and receptive behaviors (lower lordosis coefficient) (Molina-Jiménez, Limón-Morales, and Bonilla-Jaime, 2018).

Also, reports indicate that neonatal exposure to SSRIs produces behavioral changes that resemble secondary symptoms of human depression, including altered motor activity (hyperactivity or hypoactivity) on open-field tests (Mirmiran et al., 1983; Lee and Lee, 2012; Ansorge, 2004), sleep abnormalities (Mirmiran et al., 1981; Popa et al., 2008), greater food intake and weight gain (Kummet et al., 2012; Harris et al., 2012), reduced conspecific interaction and juvenile play (Rodriguez-Porcel et al., 2011), and cognitive alterations in spatial learning (Bairy et al., 2007; Bhagya et al., 2008). Greater HPA hyperactivity may occur in rats treated with clomipramine during the neonatal period (Prathiba, Kumar and Karanth, 1998), though these manifestations could depend on the type of antidepressant administered.

Various reports have shown the effects of perinatal exposure to SSRIs on adult depression-like behavior using the FST to analyze behavioral despair in rodents, which may be manifested as immobility. There, perinatal SSRIs exposure increased adult immobility on the FST (Hilakivi and Hilakivi, 1987; Velazquez-Moctezuma and Diaz Ruiz, 1992; Hansen, Sánchez and Meier, 1997; Vázquez-Palacios, Bonilla-Jaime, and Velázquez-Moctezuma, 2005; Yang et al., 2008; Rebello et al., 2014; Sarkar, Chachra and Vaidya, 2014; Glover et al., 2015; Zohar, Shoham, and Weinstock, 2016; Boulle et al., 2016; Bhagya et al., 2015; Limón-Morales, Soria-Fregozo, Arteaga-Silva, Vázquez-Palacios, et al., 2014). It has been proposed that alterations in SSRI-treated rats occur because different windows of vulnerability open during neurodevelopment, so that if brain functioning is altered, systems and behaviors will also be modified with effects that may continue into adulthood. 5-HT participates in synaptogenesis, improves neuron survival, accelerates axon differentiation and myelination (Jacobs and Azmitia, 1992), and has an inhibitory effect that limits the growth of synaptic cones and axon-branching (Jacobs and Azmitia, 1992). Thus, manipulating 5-HT in the neonatal stage modifies neuronal growth, synaptogenesis, maturation of other neurotransmission systems and, finally, the behavior of adult rats (Whitaker-Azmitia and Azmitia, 1986; Whitaker-Azmitia, 1991).

On the other hand, there are some reports show that some behavioral abnormalities in rats (sexual and motor) treated neonatally with clomipramine they tend to normalize after antidepressant treatments (imipramine) or after REM sleep deprivation (Vogel, Neill, Hagler and Kors, 1990) and respond to the chronic administration of fluoxetine in FST (Vázquez-Palacios, Bonilla-Jaime and Velázquez-Moctezuma, 2005). So, it could present predictive validity, however, is no animal model of depression used for screening of antidepressive drugs, so more studies are required.

The degree of construct validity is generally low in current animal models of depression, mainly because the pathophysiological bases of this condition are not yet fully understood (Duman, 2010). One of the first theories on the origin of depressive illness is called the monoaminergic theory. It holds that depression results from the decreased function of monoaminergic systems (Schildkraut, Gordon and Durell, 1965). Hence, some reports indicate that postnatal SSRIs exposure could affect the functioning of monoaminergic systems. With respect to biochemistry and the molecular parameters related to the construct validity of this animal model (Abelaira, Reus and Quevedo, 2013), there are reports that early SSRIs exposure reduces 5-HT fiber density in the hippocampus (Weaver et al., 2010) and alters monoamine levels in various brain regions (Hilakivi and Hilakivi, 1987; Feenstra et al., 1996; Vijayakumar and Meti, 1999; Yannielli et al., 1999). Research using animal models also shows that early-life exposure to SSRIs (citalopram) reduces adult tryptophan hydroxylase isoform 2 (TPH2) and SERT expression in the dorsal and medial raphe (Maciag, Coppinger, and Paul 2006), as well as in the hippocampus and cortex in both juvenile and adult stages (Simpson et al., 2011; Weaver et al., 2010; Maciag, Coppinger and Paul, 2006). Perinatal sertraline exposure, meanwhile, increases 5-$HT_{1A}$, 5-$HT_{2A}$, 5-$HT_{2C}$, TPH2 and SERT mRNA levels in the cerebral cortex (Meyer et al., 2018), and neonatal exposure to clomipramine increased 5-$HT_{1A}$ mRNA expression in the adult hippocampus but decreased presynaptic 5-$HT_{1A}$ expression in the dorsal raphe (Limón-Morales, Soria-Fregozo, Arteaga-Silva, Vázquez-Palacios, et al. 2014).

## Flinders Sensitive Line (FSL) Rats

Some rodent models began by selecting strains with specific characteristics that are reproduced to obtain pure strains of individuals with certain physiological or behavioral anomalies. These pure lines can be used to analyze several aspects related to the etiology of the condition studied (Overstreet et al., 2005). Flinders Sensitive Line (FSL) rats were selectively breed from the Sprague-Dawley strain because of their sensitivity to diisopropyl fluorophosphate, a selective anticholinesterase inhibitor that produces hypothermia (Overstreet et al., 2005; Overstreet and Russell, 1982; Overstreet and Wegener, 2013). FSL rats show behavioral and neurochemical alterations that resemble depressive symptoms in human patients (Overstreet et al., 2005; Overstreet, 2012; Overstreet and Wegener, 2013), so it follows that this model has face validity.

Depressed patients often show changes in appetite and/or weight (American Psychiatric Association, 2013). FSL rats have lower body weight than the Flinders Resistant Line (FRL) (Overstreet, 1993; Overstreet et al., 2005; Segal, Vincent and Levitt, 2002) and consume less food on the operant conditioning test (Bushnell, Levin and Overstreet, 1995). Also, FSL rats show lower REM sleep latencies but longer intervals of this sleep phase (Benca, 1996; Shiromani, 1988). It is interesting to note that depressed people report increased REM sleep. However, FSL rats also show hypoactivity on open-field tests (Overstreet and Russell, 1982) similar to depressed humans who show psychomotor delay. Other symptoms often seen in depressed patients are cognitive despair, learning difficulties and problems in maintaining concentration (American Psychiatric Association, 2013). FSL rats exhibit cognitive deficits on some tests; for example, difficulty in performing a shock-motivated, active avoidance task (Overstreet, Rezvani, and Janowsky, 1990). They also show deficits in working and reference memory on operant delayed matching-to-position/visual discrimination tests and the radial-arm maze (Bushnell, Levin and Overstreet, 1995). Finally, they display deteriorated memory acquisition and consolidation when evaluated by the Double-H test and the Morris Water maze (Thiele et al., 2016).

Core symptoms of depression include feelings of despair and hopelessness, but these are difficult to model. The term 'behavioral despair' test (Porsolt, Deniel and Jalfre, 1979) was introduced to describe displays of immobility by rodents on the FST, based on the hypothesis that immobility (making only the movements necessary to stay afloat) reflected feelings of 'despair' given the impossibility of escaping (Porsolt, Deniel and Jalfre, 1979; Thiele et al., 2016). In this context, FSL rats show greater immobility behavior on the FST (Overstreet and Russell, 1982).

However, the FSL model cannot fully simulate the anhedonic behaviors that are other core symptoms of depression. FSL rats drink significantly less sucrose solution only after stressors, but not in basal conditions (Pucilowski and Overstreet, 1993; Willner, 2005) and do not show changes in the rate of bar-pressing under electrical brain stimulation (Matthews et al., 1996). This model also displays impairments of male sexual behavior, such as lower ejaculatory frequency (Ferreira-Nuño et al., 2002). Therefore, FSL rats simulate only some of the symptoms that depressed patients present, though this might seem similar to some sub-types of depression given that this is such a heterogeneous condition.

The FSL rat model of depression has high predictive validity and has been used to test antidepressant responses to drugs, including all medications that have antidepressant effects on humans: tricyclic antidepressants, SSRI and other experimental substances, such as nicotine and melatonin antagonists (Overstreet and Wegener, 2013). All of these drugs were found to decrease immobility behavior on the FST.

Regarding construct validity, FSL rats display sensitivity to cholinergic agonists (Overstreet and Russell, 1982; Overstreet et al., 1984) and have high levels of MR (Overstreet et al., 1984; Daws, 1999), effects that support the cholinergic hypothesis of depression, which emerged from the theory proposed by Janowsky et al. (1972). A later proposal held that depressed individuals exhibit hyperactivity or cholinergic super-sensitivity, which may be observed as exacerbated hormonal responses to cholinergic agonists (Janowsky, Overstreet and Nurnberger, 1994).

Finally, FSL rats display abnormalities in the serotonergic function (Overstreet et al., 1994; Wallis, Overstreet and Crocker, 1988; Zangen, Overstreet and Yadid, 1997) that are similar to the serotonergic disturbances seen in depressed individuals. FSL rats have high 5-HT levels in the limbic brain regions (Zangen, Overstreet and Yadid, 1997), but these alterations can be normalized with chronic antidepressant treatment (Zangen, Overstreet and Yadid, 1997). FSL rats also have lower densities of 5-$HT_{1A}$ receptors, but higher densities of 5-$HT_{1B}$ receptors in the dental gyrus and septal nucleus (Nishi, Kanemaru and Diksic, 2009).

## Early Life Stress Model

Early life stress model resembles the adverse events experienced in early life which impacts in the development of later psychiatric illnesses, including depression (Heim and Nemeroff, 2001). One of the common models is the maternal separation, a condition that has long-lasting effects on emotionality and stress responses (Anisman et al., 1998). The maternal separation model was developed to examine the consequences of early adverse experiences on behavior and neurobiology given that the developing nervous system shows considerable plasticity in the early postnatal period. For this reason, the early postnatal environment is of crucial importance for its capacity to influence adult behavior.

Maternal separation has been used with various species – primates, chickens, rats, hamsters, cats, dogs – (McKinney and Bunney, 1969) and different separation times, running from a few hours to several days. One of the best-known models involves primates. It has shown that after an initial period of protest characterized by agitation and crying, infant monkeys separated from their mothers present depression symptoms that include desperation, diminished appetite and reduced activity and social interaction (Rosenblum and Paully, 1987). Several variants of the separation model exist; the one that separates two- or three-week-old rats triggers hyperactivity (Sahakian et al., 1975), but when separation occurs at two months, the result is aggression (Valzelli and Bernasconi, 1971). Many studies of repeated maternal separation during the first 2 weeks of neonatal life have found that affected rats show depression- and anxiety-like behaviors in adulthood (Newport, Stowe and Nemeroff, 2002; Lee et al., 2007; Ryu et al., 2009).

In particular, maternal separation was proposed to represent an important animal model for investigation of the pathophysiology and treatment of major depression. For example, treatment with antidepressants was able to normalize anxiety-like behavior, endocrine stress response, and preference for ethanol in adult male rats subjected to maternal separation.

To respect, rats deprived of maternal care have also shown depressive-like behavior on the FST, manifested as an increase in glucocorticoid levels, but a decrease in neurotrophins such as BDNF and neurotrophin-3 (Rüedi-Bettschen et al., 2006; Réus et al., 2011). Treating animals deprived of maternal care with antidepressants succeeded in reversing depressive-type behaviors and raising neurotrophin levels and neurogenesis (Nestler and Hyman 2010). This model seems to respond to tricyclic antidepressants, MAOI´s, atypical antidepressants and the beta-receptor agonist salbutamol, but one disadvantage is that the separation effect can be abolished by handling the animal, so this model has limited value for drug-detection testing.

## Unpredictable Chronic Mild Stress Model

The unpredictable chronic mild stress model (CMS) developed out of the diathesis-stress concept of depression (Zhu et al., 2014). Elaborated initially in the 1960s to explain the causes of schizophrenia, this approach was adapted to the study of depression in the 1980s. It sustains that stress can activate a diathesis or predisposition that may be either inherited or acquired through environmental factors. As a result, it proposes a synergism between the diathesis and stress that produces a combined impact on depressive symptomatology that is greater than their individual effects (Colodro-Conde et al., 2018). In the CMS, the stress of adverse life experiences predisposes vulnerable individuals to states of depression (Harro, 2019).

Katz and Hersh (1981) developed the first model of chronic stress that employed electrical discharges as a form of severe stress. After a few weeks of exposure, subjects showed higher base corticosterone levels and a reduced preference for saccharose consumption, suggestive of a reduced sensitivity to reward and an anhedonic condition (Czéh et al., 2016). However, as exposure time was extended, observations showed that test animals became habituated to the stressor. Based on these findings, Willner et al. (1991) modified the model, mainly by using milder stress factors over longer time frames and using anhedonia as the standard of evaluation (Wang et al., 2017). To achieve more realistic induction conditions, they imitated stressors from human life that are important triggers of depression (Willner, 2005).

The CMS model involves exposing animals to mild stressors in an unpredictable order for various weeks or months (Willner, 2005). In this sense, it imitates the natural psychosocial stress that often perturbs people, though the stressors are unrelated to trauma (Zurawek et al., 2017). At least two weeks of exposure to stress are required to perceive an effect of the model, since an anhedonic state is induced gradually over 3-4 weeks. If exposure to the stressor is suspended, the animal will recover in a lapse of 4-5 weeks, though another anhedonic-type state can be induced by renewing exposure. Here, the strategy of inducing and then repeating episodes of stress closely imitates the natural conditions of human life and MDD. These features make the CMS model unique and give it etiological validity (Czéh et al., 2016).

This model also produces consistent results in relation to behavioral, neurochemical, neuroendocrine and neuroimmune alterations, even though no natural, exact sequence exists. Of course, the number of elements included, their unpredictability, and the mild nature of the stressors are deemed key elements in developing this model. The stressors most often used to implement the CMS model are as follows: food and water deprivation (12.3%), modifying the light cycle (11.4%), exposure to dirty bedding (11.0%), inclining the cage (10.4%), social stress (6.4%), forced swimming (6.0%) and restriction (5.6%). These stressors trigger distinct patterns at the molecular and behavioral levels. There are reports that exposure to cold temperatures and physical immobilization are – primarily – physiological stress factors because they induce changes in noradrenalin expression in the hypothalamus, brain GMPc, pituitary AMPc and circulating prolactin (Antoniuk et al., 2019). Also, changes in the light cycle significantly alter chronobiological rhythms that, in turn, modify the endocrine physiology and metabolism of experimental animals (D'Aquila, Newton and Willner, 1997). Some researchers recommend eliminating certain stress factors – e.g., white noise, new odors and foreign objects in the cage – because they are not sufficiently stressful; that is, they cannot cause significant reductions in saccharose consumption (Antoniuk et al., 2019).

The effectiveness of the CMS model is not limited to any particular strain of animal. Initial studies of this type used Lister Hooded rats, but they were replaced by Wistar rats, which have more stable patterns of saccharose ingestion (Willner, 2017). Sprague Dawley rats have also been used, as have strains with depressive phenotypes – like Flinders Sensitive – or that are resistant to pharmacological treatment (Wistar-Kyoto) (Willner et al., 2019). Later, this protocol was extended and applied to mice, where the BALB/c strain showed the highest levels of depressive-type behavior through hyperactivation of the HPA axis (Antoniuk et al., 2019), while the C57BL/6 strain proved to be more resistant to various stressors. The fact that substantial differences have been observed in the sensitivity of the CMS model in the same strains obtained from distinct suppliers suggests the possible involvement of genetic variability or variations in breeding procedures (Willner, 2017).

Genetic variability in strains of animals is revealed in the heterogeneity of susceptibility to stress that is seen in rat populations. The following operational cohort values are used to compare the extremes: rats with low saccharose consumption <10% are defined as stress-resistant, while those with a reduced ingestion ≥30% are defined as susceptible (Czéh et al., 2016). The CMS model has been used with other species as well, such as zebra fish (Dos Santos Sampaio et al., 2018) and hens (Gualtieri et al., 2019).

The fact that affective disorders like MDD occur twice as often in women as men is well-documented, and suggests that sex differences may have a crucial role in the physiopathology of this illness. Prevalence by itself is not a decisive argument, but diathesis-stress mechanisms do differ significantly at the molecular level. Although the role of hormones and peptides in stress and MDD is not yet fully understood, we do know that they can deeply impact mood and can act in opposite directions. For example, cortisol levels are significantly higher in men who fulfill the MDD criteria than in healthy controls, but this difference is not apparent in depressed women. This suggests that hyperactivity of the HPA axis may be more characteristic of depression in men. There are also reports that stress factors affect women less than men. It is interesting to note that similar behavior has been seen in rodents (Harro 2019; Antoniuk et al. 2019).

Another significant aspect is that the incidence of MDD is significantly higher in adolescence and old age, but most CMS studies have been performed with young or adult animals. Although age has not received much attention, we know that depression in later life differs from the condition that affects younger subjects in terms of etiology, treatment and results. Therefore, depressive syndromes must be seen in the context of the associated aging process and concomitant physical illness. Here, the fundamental problem resides in extrapolating results, because older patients may be taking several medicines, may take longer to respond to them, may be more vulnerable to the secondary effects of antidepressants, and may find it more difficult to tolerate the dosage required even if it is within therapeutic range (Parikh, 2001).

Yet another important point to consider in achieving better assessments of the results of CMS studies is the via for administering antidepressants. Whenever possible, oral administration is recommended because it offers various advantages: it imitates clinical conditions, minimizes uncontrollable effects of the acute stress caused by injections, and considers the production of metabolites and changes in the concentrations of the antidepressants compared to those that occur with intravenous or intraperitoneal administration (Czéh et al., 2016).

The main stress response system is the HPA axis. Here, the behavioral and physiological effects generated by CMS can be imitated by chronic corticosterone administration, but chronic exposure to glucocorticoids is neurotoxic and leads the hippocampus to lose its inhibitory effect on the activity of this axis (Willner, 2017). The principal effects of exposure to CMS in the hippocampus include:

1. Reduced neurogenesis (Antoniuk et al., 2019; Willner, 2017)
2. Activation of the microglia; that is, the distinctive marker of neuropathology which, *under mild chronic stress becomes increasingly dysfunctional*, over-expresses pro-inflammatory cytokines, modulates the production of neurotrophins, especially BDNF, increases tryptophan metabolism through the kynurenine pathway, and can act on the glutamate route, leading to excitotoxicity that, in turn, triggers depressive-type behaviors (Singhal and Baune, 2017; Stein et al., 2017).
3. Reduced hippocampal expression of the CREB nuclear transcription factor, which decreases the expression of BDNF and other neurotrophins. This loss of trophic support for the neuronal structure and function contracts the dendritic tree of neurons in the hippocampus and reduces their volume, which is *the major anomaly reported in imaging studies* (Willner, 2005; Czéh et al., 2016).

These phenomena are important not only in terms of mood regulation, but also because observations show that chronic stress deteriorates cognitive functions, affects memory processes and decision-making, and can play an important role in the development of systemic inflammation, type 2 diabetes, Alzheimer's and Parkinson's disease, gastric ulcers, and cancer (Fakhoury, 2015). In contrast to chronic stress, acute stress differentiates stem cells into new nerve cells that improve cognitive performance and increase neurogenesis in the dentate gyrus, thus producing beneficial effects (Antoniuk et al., 2019).

In addition to CMS's effects on the hippocampus, the PFC is also damaged due to neurotoxic effects because high glucocorticoid concentrations exert negative feedback on the HPA axis. Added to these effects, CMS causes atrophy of the dendritic cells and astrocytes (Czéh et al., 2016), sensitization of the serotoninergic system, excessive activation of the noradrenergic system, and reduced dopamine release in the nucleus accumbens in response to rewards. This effect is closely-related to the anhedonic effects (Antoniuk et al., 2019). Finally, it causes other symptoms of depression, such as reduced sexual behavior, decreased locomotor activity, weight loss, behavioral deficits, and changes in sleep patterns (Willner, 2017).

Although saccharose consumption is a valid test of anhedonic behavior, the experimental designs using this test vary among laboratories. Some perform only one test at the end of the procedure, others perform tests before and after CMS, while still others conduct weekly follow-up on the effects because repeat tests make it possible to analyze effect patterns, such as habituation to the application of the CMS or an unstable base line, and so decide if it is necessary to increase the intensity of the stressors, or modify the test regimen. If the level of stress seems to decrease saccharose ingestion in controls, it may be that those animals were stressed inadvertently. This can occur quite easily if the control and CMS animals are in the same room, a procedure that must be avoided at all costs (Wiborg, 2013; Willner, 2017). In relation to the choice of the hours for performing the saccharose consumption test, there is evidence of circadian effects. Some authors observe more intense effects of CMS when the test is conducted at the onset of the dark phase of the light-dark cycle (D'Aquila, Newton and Willner, 1997), but others recommend carrying out this test at the onset of the light phase (Papp, 2012), so there is no consensus as to the best time of day to conduct the saccharose consumption test. However, several important considerations must be kept in mind:

1. The typical saccharose concentration used is 1% because at this concentration unstressed animals will drink 10-17g of solution. If an animal drinks less, then the concentration should be increased gradually by 0.1% until this consumption range is reached. The solution must never exceed 2% (Papp, 2012), however, because higher concentrations (2-5%) consistently cause a major preference over water which means that the protocol loses reliability (Willner, 2017).
2. The order of presentation of the stressors is not standardized among different authors, but the usual procedure is to measure the preference for saccharose consumption after 24h of food and water deprivation (Harro, 2019). Some authors consider this food restriction a stressor and argue that what is really being induced is a response to hunger and not the principal criterion of depression or anhedonia (Harro, 2019). Others, however, report decreased saccharose consumption in animals without food and water deprivation, so we are not dealing with a physiological phenomenon but, rather, a mental one, which confirms that decreased saccharose consumption suggests reduced reward-sensitivity (Wiborg, 2013).
3. To improve the reliability of the saccharose consumption test, the animals can be selected and distributed into groups before applying the test. The recommendation is to exclude subjects with very low, very high, or highly-variable saccharose consumption (~20%) (Papp, 2012).
4. The evaluation of depressive behavior is calculated as:
    a. Preference for saccharose
    b. Relative measure of saccharose ingestion
5. After the test, the recommendation is to wait at least 1 hour before providing food and water to avoid creating an association between the test and the reappearance of food (Papp, 2012).

## Table 1. A Quick Guide to Understanding the CMS Model

| Factors | Cite | Description |
|---|---|---|
| History | Czéhet al., 2015<br>Wang et al., 2017<br>Willner, 2005 | Katz and Hersh (1981) developed the first chronic stress model of anhedonia using severe stress factors, observing an ↑ in basal corticosterone levels and a ↓ in the preference for saccharose consumption that suggests reduced reward sensitivity. After a time, test animals become habituated to the stress. |
| | | Willner and cols. (1991) modified this model by using milder stress factors over a longer time period and introducing anhedonia as the standard of evaluation. |
| Implementation | Zurawek et al., 2016 | These authors exposed animals to mild stress factors in an unpredictable order for various weeks, or months, to imitate the natural psychosocial stress that often perturbs people, though unrelated to trauma. |
| Exposure time | Czéh et al., 2015 | A minimum of 2 weeks of exposure to stress is required to begin to see an effect of the model, since the anhedonic state is induced gradually over a period of 3-4 weeks. If exposure is suspended, the animal will recover in a space of 4-5 weeks, but another anhedonic-type state can be induced by renewing exposure. |
| Stressors | Antoniuk et al., 2018<br>D'Aquila et al.,1997 | The stressors most often utilized are: food and water deprivation, modifying the light cycle, exposure to dirty bedding, inclining the cage, social stress, and forced swimming, etc. There are reports that exposure to cold temperature, physical immobilization, and changes in the light cycle significantly alter the endocrine physiology and metabolism of experimental animals. One recommendation is to eliminate some stressors, including white noise, new odors and foreign objects, because they cannot significantly decrease saccharose consumption. |
| Strains | Willner, 2017<br>Antoniuk et al., 2018<br>Dos Santos Sampaio, 2018<br>Gualtieri et al., 2018 | The effectiveness of this model is not limited to any particular strain. Lister Hooded and Wistar rats have more stable patterns of saccharose ingestion. Depressive phenotypes: Flinders Sensitive; Resistant to pharmacological treatment: Wistar-Kyoto rats. In mice, BALB/c are sensitive to depressive behavior, while C57BL/6 are more resistant. Zebra fish and hens have also been used. |
| Sex | Antoniuk, 2018 | MDD is twice as common in women as men. Though the role of hormones and peptides in stress is not well-understood, we know that they deeply affect mood and act in opposite directions. Cortisol levels are higher in depressed men than healthy ones, unlike the situation in depressed women. In contrast, stress factors affect women less than men. |
| Age | Parikh, 2000 | The incidence of depression is significantly higher in adolescence and old age; however, studies with the CMS model usually involve young or adult animals. The fundamental problem is extrapolating results, because older patients normally take several medicines, can take longer to react to antidepressants, are more prone to secondary effects, and have more difficulty in tolerating the dose even if it is within therapeutic range. |
| Route of administration | Czéh et al., 2015 | Oral administration should be used because it offers various advantages: it imitates the clinical situation, minimizes the effects of injections, and considers the production of metabolites and changes in concentrations of the antidepressants. |

**Table 1. (Continued)**

| Factors | Cite | Description |
|---|---|---|
| Effects of stress | Willner, 2017, 2005<br>Antoniuk et al., 2018<br>Singhal & Baune, 2017<br>Stein et al., 2017<br>Czéh et al., 2015 | The principal stress response system is the Hypothalamic-Pituitary-Adrenal axis:<br>*Hippocampus:* reduced neurogenesis, activation of microglia, contraction of the dendritic tree and loss of volume.<br>*Prefrontal cortex:* high concentration of glucocorticoids exerts negative feedback on the HHA axis. Atrophy of dendritic cells and astrocytes has a neurotoxic effect.<br>*Others:* Sensitization of the serotoninergic system, excessive activation of the noradrenergic system and decreased release of dopamine in the nucleus accumbens. Also, cognitive deterioration, damage to memory processes, reduced sexual behavior, decreased locomotor activity, weight loss, behavior deficits, and changes in sleep patterns. |
| Saccharose consumption | Papp, 2012;<br>Wiborg, 2013;<br>Willner, 2017;<br>Harro, 2018 | A valid test of anhedonic behavior. Some researchers conduct a test at the end of the procedure, others carry out follow-up on the effect that allows them to analyze a pattern of effects like habituation and decide whether it is necessary to increase the intensity of the stressors or vary the study regimen |
| | | Saccharose is administered in a range of 1-2%, without exceeding this percentage because higher concentrations consistently cause major preference over water, so the protocol loses reliability.<br>Food and water deprivation for 24 hours: some authors consider this a stress factor that evaluates the response to hunger, but others report reduced saccharose consumption even without deprivation, which confirms that this is a mental phenomenon suggestive of a reduced reward response.<br>Evaluations of depressive behavior are calculated as a percentage of the preference for saccharose or as a relative mean of saccharose ingestion. |
| Resistant animals | Czéh et al., 2015;<br>Wiborg, 2013 | The specific stressors are unpredictable, but the stress itself is not. Based on this, some animals can cope with the stressors applied and maintain homeostasis; but others appear to be much more vulnerable. If the exposure to stress is combined with chronic antidepressive treatment, most animals can recover from the anhedonic state, though a significant sub-fraction of ~50% cannot. This result is quite similar to the refraction rate seen in antidepressive treatment in humans. |

Other interesting aspects are the degree of variability that the CMS model allows, since exposure times to the stressors range from 5 minutes to 12 hours (Harro, 2019), and the fact that while the model is maintained the anhedonic state will remain for months, preventing the animals from becoming habituated. Although the specific stressors applied are unpredictable, stress in itself is not, so there are adaptive responses to CMS. Because of this, some animals are resistant; that is, they can cope with the stressors applied and maintain homeostasis. Others, in contrast, are much more vulnerable or susceptible to entering anhedonic-type states (Czéh et al., 2016). In fact, if exposure to stress is combined with chronic antidepressive treatment, the animals can recover from the anhedonic state, though a sub-fraction of approximately 50% will be refractory to treatment, a figure quite similar to the refraction rate to antidepressive treatment in humans (Wiborg, 2013). Research on resilient animal has expanded but no great advances have been made to date (Harro, 2019).

In conclusion, animal models offer unique means of analyzing experimentally the factors that contribute to the development of behaviors related to psychiatric disorders and the brain mechanisms that participate in them. Based on this, the CMS model has emerged as an especially robust and reliable experimental tool, one that is essential for studying the neurobiological bases of depression, and that has made substantial contributions to our understanding of the consequences of chronic stress while also allowing us to design and evaluate diverse antidepressant treatments.

## CONCLUSION

Despite the difficulties in translating human affective disorders into relevant tests in rodents, attempts have been made to establish animal models of depression, or at least the models with some core symptoms. There are many animal models of depression, however, the development of a model that represents most symptoms of depression and meets all criteria for animal model validity would be ideal. All these models or tests can induce anhedonia or identify the effect of antidepressants in rodents, but the main limitation is that the pathophysiological changes observed in these models might be the results of our manipulation (e.g., stress or pharmacological treatment), rather than the true manifestation of the depressive state of animals (Urani, Chourbaji, and Gass 2005). However, it is remarkable that all animal models of depression have contributed to a better understanding of the neurobiology of this disorder, and offer new pharmacological targets for treatment.

## References

Abelaira, Helena M., Gislaine Z. Reus, and Joao Quevedo. 2013. "Animal Models as Tools to Study the Pathophysiology of Depression." *Revista Brasileira de Psiquiatria* 35 (suppl 2): S112–20. https://doi.org/10.1590/1516-4446-2013-1098.

Altar, C. Anthony, Richard E. Whitehead, Ruoyan Chen, Gitta Wörtwein, and Torsten M. Madsen. 2003. "Effects of Electroconvulsive Seizures and Antidepressant Drugs on Brain-Derived Neurotrophic Factor Protein in Rat Brain." *Biological Psychiatry* 54 (7): 703–9.

American Psychiatric Association. 2013. *Diagnostic and Statistical Manual of Mental Disorders*. Fifth Edition. American Psychiatric Association. https://doi.org/10.1176/appi.books.9780890425596.

American Psychiatric Association. 2014. *Guía de consulta de los criterios diagnósticos del DSM-5*. 5 ed. Arlington, VA: American Psychiatric Publishing. [*Reference guide to the DSM-5 diagnostic criteria*.]

Anisman, Hymie, Marilee D. Zaharia, Michael J. Meaney, and Zul Merali. 1998. "Do Early-Life Events Permanently Alter Behavioral and Hormonal Responses to Stressors?" *International Journal of Developmental Neuroscience* 16 (3–4): 149–64. https://doi.org/10.1016/S0736-5748(98)00025-2.

Ansorge, M. S. 2004. "Early-Life Blockade of the 5-HT Transporter Alters Emotional Behavior in Adult Mice." *Science* 306 (5697): 879–81. https://doi.org/10.1126/science.1101678.

Antoniuk, Svitlana, Monika Bijata, Evgeni Ponimaskin, and Jakub Wlodarczyk. 2019. "Chronic Unpredictable Mild Stress for Modeling Depression in Rodents: Meta-Analysis of Model Reliability." *Neuroscience & Biobehavioral Reviews* 99 (April): 101–16. https://doi.org/10.1016/j.neubiorev.2018.12.002.

Arai, I., Y. Tsuyuki, H. Shiomoto, M. Satoh, and S. Otomo. 2000. "Decreased Body Temperature Dependent Appearance of Behavioral Despair in the Forced Swimming Test in Mice." *Pharmacological Research* 42 (2): 171–76. https://doi.org/10.1006/phrs.2000.0672.

Bairy, K. L., S. Madhyastha, K. P. Ashok, Indira Bairy, and S. Malini. 2007. "Developmental and Behavioral Consequences of Prenatal Fluoxetine." *Pharmacology* 79 (1): 1–11. https://doi.org/10.1159/000096645.

Baumeister, R. F. 1990. "Suicide as Escape from Self." *Psychological Review* 97 (1): 90–113.

Benca, R. 1996. "Increased Basal REM Sleep But No Difference in Dark Induction or Light Suppression of REM Sleep in Flinders Rats with Cholinergic Supersensitivity." *Neuropsychopharmacology* 15 (1): 45–51. https://doi.org/10.1016/0893-133X(95)00154-6.

Bhagya, V., B. N. Srikumar, T. R. Raju, and B. S. Shankaranarayana Rao. 2008. "Neonatal Clomipramine Induced Endogenous Depression in Rats Is Associated with Learning Impairment in Adulthood." *Behavioural Brain Research* 187 (1): 190–94. https://doi.org/10.1016/j.bbr.2007.08.020.

Bhagya V, Srikumar BN, Raju TR, Shankaranarayana Rao BS. 2015. "The Selective Noradrenergic Reuptake Inhibitor Reboxetine Restores Spatial Learning Deficits, Biochemical Changes, and Hippocampal Synaptic Plasticity in an Animal Model of Depression." *Journal of Neuroscience Research* 93 (1): 104–20. https://doi.org/10.1002/jnr.23473.

Blackburn, Thomas P. 2019. "Depressive Disorders: Treatment Failures and Poor Prognosis over the Last 50 Years." *Pharmacology Research & Perspectives* 7 (3): e00472. https://doi.org/10.1002/prp2.472.

Bonilla-Jaime, H., S. Retana-Marquez, and J. Velazquez-Moctezuma. 1998. "Pharmacological Features of Masculine Sexual Behavior in an Animal Model of Depression." *Pharmacology, Biochemistry, and Behavior* 60 (1): 39–45.

Borsini, F. 1995. "Role of the Serotonergic System in the Forced Swimming Test." *Neuroscience and Biobehavioral Reviews* 19 (3): 377–95.

Borsini, F., and A. Meli. 1988. "Is the Forced Swimming Test a Suitable Model for Revealing Antidepressant Activity?" *Psychopharmacology* 94 (2): 147–60.

Borsini, F., G. Volterra, and A. Meli. 1986. "Does the Behavioral 'despair' test Measure 'despair'?" *Physiology & Behavior* 38 (3): 385–86.

Boulle, Fabien, Jodi L. Pawluski, Judith R. Homberg, Barbie Machiels, Yvet Kroeze, Neha Kumar, Harry W. M. Steinbusch, Gunter Kenis, and Daniel L. A. van den Hove. 2016. "Developmental Fluoxetine Exposure Increases Behavioral Despair and Alters Epigenetic Regulation of the Hippocampal BDNF Gene in Adult Female Offspring." *Hormones and Behavior* 80 (April): 47–57. https://doi.org/10.1016/j.yhbeh.2016.01.017.

Bushnell, P. J., E. D. Levin, and D. H. Overstreet. 1995. "Spatial Working and Reference Memory in Rats Bred for Autonomic Sensitivity to Cholinergic Stimulation: Acquisition, Accuracy, Speed, and Effects of Cholinergic Drugs." *Neurobiology of Learning and Memory* 63 (2): 116–32. https://doi.org/10.1006/nlme.1995.1012.

Cagiano, R., P. Flace, I. Bera, L. Maries, G. Cioca, R. Sabatini, V. Benagiano, et al. 2008. "Neurofunctional Effects in Rats Prenatally Exposed to Fluoxetine." *European Review for Medical and Pharmacological Sciences* 12 (3): 137–48.

Caspi, Avshalom, Karen Sugden, Terrie E. Moffitt, Alan Taylor, Ian W. Craig, HonaLee Harrington, Joseph McClay, et al. 2003. "Influence of Life Stress on Depression: Moderation by a Polymorphism in the 5-HTT Gene." *Science (New York, N.Y.)* 301 (5631): 386–89. https://doi.org/10.1126/science.1083968.

Chen, B., D. Dowlatshahi, G. M. MacQueen, J. F. Wang, and L. T. Young. 2001. "Increased Hippocampal BDNF Immunoreactivity in Subjects Treated with Antidepressant Medication." *Biological Psychiatry* 50 (4): 260–65.

Colodro-Conde, L., B. Couvy-Duchesne, G. Zhu, W. L. Coventry, E. M. Byrne, S. Gordon, M. J. Wright, et al. 2018. "A Direct Test of the Diathesis-Stress Model for Depression." *Molecular Psychiatry* 23 (7): 1590–96. https://doi.org/10.1038/mp.2017.130.

Commons, Kathryn G., Aram B. Cholanians, Jessica A. Babb, and Daniel G. Ehlinger. 2017. "The Rodent Forced Swim Test Measures Stress-Coping Strategy, Not Depression-like Behavior." *ACS Chemical Neuroscience* 8 (5): 955–60. https://doi.org/10.1021/acschemneuro.7b00042.

Corner, M. A., M. Mirmiran, H. L. M. G. Bour, G. J. Boer, N. E. Van De Poll, H. G. Van Oyen, and H. B. M. Uylings. 1980. "Does Rapid-Eye-Movement Sleep Play a Role in Brain Development?" In *Progress in Brain Research*, 53:347–56. Elsevier. https://doi.org/10.1016/S0079-6123(08)60074-6.

Cryan, John F., Cedric Mombereau, and Annick Vassout. 2005. "The Tail Suspension Test as a Model for Assessing Antidepressant Activity: Review of Pharmacological and Genetic Studies in Mice." *Neuroscience and Biobehavioral Reviews* 29 (4–5): 571–625. https://doi.org/10.1016/j.neubiorev.2005.03.009.

Czéh, Boldizsár, Eberhard Fuchs, Ove Wiborg, and Mária Simon. 2016. "Animal Models of Major Depression and Their Clinical Implications." *Progress in Neuro-Psychopharmacology and Biological Psychiatry* 64 (January): 293–310. https://doi.org/10.1016/j.pnpbp.2015.04.004.

D'Aquila, P, J Newton, and P Willner. 1997. "Diurnal Variation in the Effect of Chronic Mild Stress on Sucrose Intake and Preference." *Physiology & Behavior* 62 (2): 421–26. https://doi.org/10.1016/S0031-9384(97)00042-5.

David, D. J., B. A. Nic Dhonnchadha, P. Jolliet, M. Hascoët, and M. Bourin. 2001. "Are There Gender Differences in the Temperature Profile of Mice after Acute Antidepressant Administration and Exposure to Two Animal Models of Depression?" *Behavioural Brain Research* 119 (2): 203–11.

Daws, L. 1999. "Ontogeny of Muscarinic Cholinergic Supersensitivity in the Flinders Sensitive Line Rat." *Pharmacology Biochemistry and Behavior* 62 (2): 367–80. https://doi.org/10.1016/S0091-3057(98)00174-9.

De Boer, S., M. Mirmiran, F. Van Haaren, A. Louwerse, and N. E. van de Poll. 1989. "Neurobehavioral Teratogenic Effects of Clomipramine and Alpha-Methyldopa." *Neurotoxicology and Teratology* 11 (1): 77–84.

De Pablo, J. M., J. Ortiz-Caro, F. Sanchez-Santed, and A. Guillamón. 1991. "Effects of Diazepam, Pentobarbital, Scopolamine and the Timing of Saline Injection on Learned Immobility in Rats." *Physiology & Behavior* 50 (5): 895–99.

De Pablo, J. M., A. Parra, S. Segovia, and A. Guillamón. 1989. "Learned Immobility Explains the Behavior of Rats in the Forced Swimming Test." *Physiology & Behavior* 46 (2): 229–37.

Dean, J., and M. Keshavan. 2017. "The Neurobiology of Depression: An Integrated View." *Asian Journal of Psychiatry* 27 (June): 101–11. https://doi.org/10.1016/j.ajp.2017.01.025.

de Kloet, E. R., and M. L. Molendijk. 2016. "Coping with the Forced Swim Stressor: Towards Understanding an Adaptive Mechanism." *Neural Plasticity* 2016: 1–13. https://doi.org/10.1155/2016/6503162.

Detke, M. J., and I. Lucki. 1996. "Detection of Serotonergic and Noradrenergic Antidepressants in the Rat Forced Swimming Test: The Effects of Water Depth." *Behavioural Brain Research* 73 (1–2): 43–46.

Detke, M. J., M. Rickels, and I. Lucki. 1995. "Active Behaviors in the Rat Forced Swimming Test Differentially Produced by Serotonergic and Noradrenergic Antidepressants." *Psychopharmacology* 121 (1): 66–72.

Dixon, A. K. 1998. "Ethological Strategies for Defence in Animals and Humans: Their Role in Some Psychiatric Disorders." *The British Journal of Medical Psychology* 71 (Pt 4) (December): 417–45.

Dixon, A. K., and H. U. Fisch. 1998. "Animal Models and Ethological Strategies for Early Drug-Testing in Humans." *Neuroscience and Biobehavioral Reviews* 23 (2): 345–58.

Dos Santos Sampaio, Tafnis Ingret, Nayara Costa de Melo, Bianca Thais de Freitas Paiva, Gerley Anatê da Silva Aleluia, Fernando Luiz Pinheiro da Silva Neto, Heitor Ribeiro da Silva, Hady Keita, et al. 2018. "Leaves of Spondias Mombin L. a Traditional Anxiolytic and Antidepressant: Pharmacological Evaluation on Zebrafish (Danio Rerio)." *Journal of Ethnopharmacology* 224 (October): 563–78. https://doi.org/10.1016/j.jep.2018.05.037.

Drago, F., G. Continella, M. C. Alloro, and U. Scapagnini. 1985. "Behavioral Effects of Perinatal Administration of Antidepressant Drugs in the Rat." *Neurobehavioral Toxicology and Teratology* 7 (5): 493–97.

Droste, Susanne K., Lotte de Groote, Helen C. Atkinson, Stafford L. Lightman, Johannes M. H. M. Reul, and Astrid C. E. Linthorst. 2008.

"Corticosterone Levels in the Brain Show a Distinct Ultradian Rhythm but a Delayed Response to Forced Swim Stress." *Endocrinology* 149 (7): 3244–53. https://doi.org/10.1210/en.2008-0103.

Duman, Catharine H. 2010. "Models of Depression." In *Vitamins & Hormones*, 82:1–21. Elsevier. https://doi.org/10.1016/S0083-6729(10)82001-1.

Duman, Ronald S., and Lisa M. Monteggia. 2006. "A Neurotrophic Model for Stress-Related Mood Disorders." *Biological Psychiatry* 59 (12): 1116–27. https://doi.org/10.1016/j.biopsych.2006.02.013.

Enginar, Nurhan, Pınar Yamantürk-Çelik, Asiye Nurten, and Dilvin Berrak Güney. 2016. "Learning and Memory in the Forced Swimming Test: Effects of Antidepressants Having Varying Degrees of Anticholinergic Activity." *Naunyn-Schmiedeberg's Archives of Pharmacology* 389 (7): 739–45. https://doi.org/10.1007/s00210-016-1236-4.

Fakhoury, Marc. 2015. "New Insights into the Neurobiological Mechanisms of Major Depressive Disorders." *General Hospital Psychiatry* 37 (2): 172–77. https://doi.org/10.1016/j.genhosppsych.2015.01.005.

Farach, Frank J., Larry D. Pruitt, Janie J. Jun, Alissa B. Jerud, Lori A. Zoellner, and Peter P. Roy-Byrne. 2012. "Pharmacological Treatment of Anxiety Disorders: Current Treatments and Future Directions." *Journal of Anxiety Disorders* 26 (8): 833–43. https://doi.org/10.1016/j.janxdis.2012.07.009.

Feenstra, M. G., H. van Galen, P. J. Te Riele, M. H. Botterblom, and M. Mirmiran. 1996. "Decreased Hypothalamic Serotonin Levels in Adult Rats Treated Neonatally with Clomipramine." *Pharmacology, Biochemistry, and Behavior* 55 (4): 647–52.

Ferreira-Nuño, A, D.H Overstreet, A Morales-Otal, and J Velázquez-Moctezuma. 2002. "Masculine Sexual Behavior Features in the Flinders Sensitive and Resistant Line Rats." *Behavioural Brain Research* 128 (2): 113–19. https://doi.org/10.1016/S0166-4328(01)00313-8.

Fullilove, Mindy Thompson. 2002. "Social and Economic Causes of Depression." *The Journal of Gender-Specific Medicine: JGSM: The Official Journal of the Partnership for Women's Health at Columbia* 5 (2): 38–41.

Gilbert, P., and S. Allan. 1998. "The Role of Defeat and Entrapment (Arrested Flight) in Depression: An Exploration of an Evolutionary View." *Psychological Medicine* 28 (3): 585–98.

Gilbert, Paul, Jean Gilbert, and Chris Irons. 2004. "Life Events, Entrapments and Arrested Anger in Depression." *Journal of Affective Disorders* 79 (1–3): 149–60. https://doi.org/10.1016/S0165-0327(02)00405-6.

Glover, M. E., P. C. Pugh, N. L. Jackson, J. L. Cohen, A. D. Fant, H. Akil, and S. M. Clinton. 2015. "Early-Life Exposure to the SSRI Paroxetine Exacerbates Depression-like Behavior in Anxiety/Depression-Prone Rats." *Neuroscience* 284 (January): 775–97. https://doi.org/10.1016/j.neuroscience.2014.10.044.

Gouvêa, Thiago Santos, Helena K. Morimoto, Maria José S. S. de Faria, Estefânia Gastaldello Moreira, and Daniela Cristina Ceccatto Gerardin. 2008. "Maternal Exposure to the Antidepressant Fluoxetine Impairs Sexual Motivation in Adult Male Mice." *Pharmacology Biochemistry and Behavior* 90 (3): 416–19. https://doi.org/10.1016/j.pbb.2008.03.025.

Groote, L. de, and A. C. E. Linthorst. 2007. "Exposure to Novelty and Forced Swimming Evoke Stressor-Dependent Changes in Extracellular GABA in the Rat Hippocampus." *Neuroscience* 148 (3): 794–805. https://doi.org/10.1016/j.neuroscience.2007.06.030.

Gualtieri, F., E. A. Armstrong, G. K. Longmoor, R. B. D'Eath, V. Sandilands, T. Boswell, and T. V. Smulders. 2019. "Unpredictable Chronic Mild Stress Suppresses the Incorporation of New Neurons at the Caudal Pole of the Chicken Hippocampal Formation." *Scientific Reports* 9 (1). https://doi.org/10.1038/s41598-019-43584-x.

Gutiérrez-García, Ana G., and Carlos M. Contreras. 2009. "Stressors Can Affect Immobility Time and Response to Imipramine in the Rat Forced Swim Test." *Pharmacology, Biochemistry, and Behavior* 91 (4): 542–48. https://doi.org/10.1016/j.pbb.2008.09.008.

Hageman, Ida, Marianne Nielsen, Gitta Wortwein, Nils Henrik Diemer, and Martin Balslev Jorgensen. 2009. "Electroconvulsive Stimulations Normalizes Stress-Induced Changes in the Glucocorticoid Receptor and

Behaviour." *Behavioural Brain Research* 196 (1): 71–77. https://doi.org/10.1016/j.bbr.2008.07.037.

Hansen, H. H., C. Sánchez, and E. Meier. 1997. "Neonatal Administration of the Selective Serotonin Reuptake Inhibitor Lu 10-134-C Increases Forced Swimming-Induced Immobility in Adult Rats: A Putative Animal Model of Depression?" *The Journal of Pharmacology and Experimental Therapeutics* 283 (3): 1333–41.

Harris, Sharonda S., Dorota Maciag, Kimberly L. Simpson, Rick C. S. Lin, and Ian A. Paul. 2012. "Dose-Dependent Effects of Neonatal SSRI Exposure on Adult Behavior in the Rat." *Brain Research* 1429 (January): 52–60. https://doi.org/10.1016/j.brainres.2011.10.025.

Harro, Jaanus. 2019. "Animal Models of Depression: Pros and Cons." *Cell and Tissue Research* 377 (1): 5–20. https://doi.org/10.1007/s00441-018-2973-0.

Hawkins, J., R. A. Hicks, N. Phillips, and J. D. Moore. 1978. "Swimming Rats and Human Depression." *Nature* 274 (5670): 512–13. https://doi.org/10.1038/274512a0.

Heim, Christine, and Charles B Nemeroff. 2001. "The Role of Childhood Trauma in the Neurobiology of Mood and Anxiety Disorders: Preclinical and Clinical Studies." *Biological Psychiatry* 49 (12): 1023–39. https://doi.org/10.1016/S0006-3223(01)01157-X.

Hilakivi, L. A., and I. Hilakivi. 1987. "Increased Adult Behavioral 'Despair' in Rats Neonatally Exposed to Desipramine or Zimeldine: An Animal Model of Depression?" *Pharmacology, Biochemistry, and Behavior* 28 (3): 367–69.

Holmes, Andrew, Markus Heilig, Nadia M. J. Rupniak, Thomas Steckler, and Guy Griebel. 2003. "Neuropeptide Systems as Novel Therapeutic Targets for Depression and Anxiety Disorders." *Trends in Pharmacological Sciences* 24 (11): 580–88. https://doi.org/10.1016/j.tips.2003.09.011.

Jacobs, B. L., and E. C. Azmitia. 1992. "Structure and Function of the Brain Serotonin System." *Physiological Reviews* 72 (1): 165–229. https://doi.org/10.1152/physrev.1992.72.1.165.

Janowsky, David S., David H. Overstreet, and John I. Nurnberger. 1994. "Is Cholinergic Sensitivity a Genetic Marker for the Affective Disorders?" *American Journal of Medical Genetics* 54 (4): 335–44. https://doi.org/10.1002/ajmg.1320540412.

Janowsky, DavidS, JohnM Davis, M.Khaled El-Yousef, and H.Joseph Sekerke. 1972. "A Cholinergic-Adrenergic Hypothesis Of Mania And Depression." *The Lancet* 300 (7778): 632–35. https://doi.org/10.1016/S0140-6736(72)93021-8.

Jefferys, D., and J. Funder. 1994. "The Effect of Water Temperature on Immobility in the Forced Swimming Test in Rats." *European Journal of Pharmacology* 253 (1–2): 91–94. https://doi.org/10.1016/0014-2999(94)90761-7.

Katz, R. J., and S. Hersh. 1981. "Amitriptyline and Scopolamine in an Animal Model of Depression." *Neuroscience and Biobehavioral Reviews* 5 (2): 265–71.

Kessler, Ronald C., and Evelyn J. Bromet. 2013. "The Epidemiology of Depression Across Cultures." *Annual Review of Public Health* 34 (1): 119–38. https://doi.org/10.1146/annurev-publhealth-031912-114409.

Kovács, Zsolt, András Czurkó, Katalin A. Kékesi, and Gábor Juhász. 2012. "Neonatal Tricyclic Antidepressant Clomipramine Treatment Reduces the Spike-Wave Discharge Activity of the Adult WAG/Rij Rat." *Brain Research Bulletin* 89 (3–4): 102–7. https://doi.org/10.1016/j.brainresbull.2012.07.010.

Krogh, Jesper, Merete Nordentoft, Jonathan A. C. Sterne, and Debbie A. Lawlor. 2011. "The Effect of Exercise in Clinically Depressed Adults: Systematic Review and Meta-Analysis of Randomized Controlled Trials." *The Journal of Clinical Psychiatry* 72 (4): 529–38. https://doi.org/10.4088/JCP.08r04913blu.

Kummet, Gary J., Sarah E. Haskell, Gregory M. Hermann, Charles Ni, Kenneth A. Volk, Areej K. Younes, Alise K. Miller, and Robert D. Roghair. 2012. "Neonatal SSRI Exposure Programs a Hypermetabolic State in Adult Mice." *Journal of Nutrition and Metabolism* 2012: 1–8. https://doi.org/10.1155/2012/431574.

Kunugi, Hiroshi, Hiroaki Hori, Naoki Adachi, and Tadahiro Numakawa. 2010. "Interface between Hypothalamic-Pituitary-Adrenal Axis and Brain-Derived Neurotrophic Factor in Depression: HPA, BDNF and Depression." *Psychiatry and Clinical Neurosciences* 64 (5): 447–59. https://doi.org/10.1111/j.1440-1819.2010.02135.x.

Lammel, S., K. M. Tye, and M. R. Warden. 2014. "Progress in Understanding Mood Disorders: Optogenetic Dissection of Neural Circuits." *Genes, Brain, and Behavior* 13 (1): 38–51. https://doi.org/10.1111/gbb.12049.

Lee, Jong-Ho, Hyung Jin Kim, Jae Goo Kim, Vitaly Ryu, Bom-Taeck Kim, Dong-Won Kang, and Jeong Won Jahng. 2007. "Depressive Behaviors and Decreased Expression of Serotonin Reuptake Transporter in Rats That Experienced Neonatal Maternal Separation." *Neuroscience Research* 58 (1): 32–39. https://doi.org/10.1016/j.neures.2007.01.008.

Lee, Li-Jen, and Lukas Jyuhn-Hsiarn Lee. 2012. "Neonatal Fluoxetine Exposure Alters Motor Performances of Adolescent Rats." *Developmental Neurobiology* 72 (8): 1122–32. https://doi.org/10.1002/dneu.20942.

Limón-Morales, Ofelia, Cesar Soria-Fregozo, Marcela Arteaga-Silva, Marisela Hernández González, Gonzalo Vázquez-Palacios, and Herlinda Bonilla-Jaime. 2014. "Hormone Replacement with 17β-Estradiol plus Dihydrotestosterone Restores Male Sexual Behavior in Rats Treated Neonatally with Clomipramine." *Hormones and Behavior* 66 (5): 820–27. https://doi.org/10.1016/j.yhbeh.2014.09.014.

Limón-Morales, Ofelia, Cesar Soria-Fregozo, Marcela Arteaga-Silva, Gonzalo Vázquez-Palacios, and Herlinda Bonilla-Jaime. 2014. "Altered Expression of 5-HT1A Receptors in Adult Rats Induced by Neonatal Treatment with Clomipramine." *Physiology & Behavior* 124 (January): 37–44. https://doi.org/10.1016/j.physbeh.2013.10.026.

Linthorst, Astrid C. E., Cornelia Flachskamm, and Johannes M. H. M. Reul. 2008. "Water Temperature Determines Neurochemical and Behavioural Responses to Forced Swim Stress: An in Vivo Microdialysis and Biotelemetry Study in Rats." *Stress (Amsterdam, Netherlands)* 11 (2): 88–100. https://doi.org/10.1080/10253890701533231.

Liu, Chun-Hong, Guang-Zhong Zhang, Bin Li, Meng Li, Marie Woelfer, Martin Walter, and Lihong Wang. 2019. "Role of Inflammation in Depression Relapse." *Journal of Neuroinflammation* 16 (1). https://doi.org/10.1186/s12974-019-1475-7.

Lorenzetti, Valentina, Nicholas B. Allen, Alex Fornito, and Murat Yücel. 2009. "Structural Brain Abnormalities in Major Depressive Disorder: A Selective Review of Recent MRI Studies." *Journal of Affective Disorders* 117 (1–2): 1–17. https://doi.org/10.1016/j.jad.2008.11.021.

Lucki, I. 1997. "The Forced Swimming Test as a Model for Core and Component Behavioral Effects of Antidepressant Drugs." *Behavioural Pharmacology* 8 (6–7): 523–32.

Maciag, Dorota, David Coppinger, and Ian A. Paul. 2006. "Evidence That the Deficit in Sexual Behavior in Adult Rats Neonatally Exposed to Citalopram Is a Consequence of 5-HT1 Receptor Stimulation during Development." *Brain Research* 1125 (1): 171–75. https://doi.org/10.1016/j.brainres.2006.10.009.

Matthews, Keith, Brian A. Baldo, Athina Markou, Olwen Lown, David H. Overstreet, and George F. Koob. 1996. "Rewarding Electrical Brain Stimulation: Similar Thresholds for Flinders Sensitve Line Hypercholinergic and Flinders Resistant Line Hypocholinergic Rats." *Physiology & Behavior* 59 (6): 1155–62. https://doi.org/10.1016/0031-9384(95)02212-0.

Matthews, Keith, David Christmas, John Swan, and Eleanor Sorrell. 2005. "Animal Models of Depression: Navigating through the Clinical Fog." *Neuroscience and Biobehavioral Reviews* 29 (4–5): 503–13. https://doi.org/10.1016/j.neubiorev.2005.03.005.

McKinney, W. T., and W. E. Bunney. 1969. "Animal Model of Depression. I. Review of Evidence: Implications for Research." *Archives of General Psychiatry* 21 (2): 240–48.

Meyer, Lauritz R., Benjamin Dexter, Cecilia Lo, Elizabeth Kenkel, Takahito Hirai, Robert D. Roghair, and Sarah E. Haskell. 2018. "Perinatal SSRI Exposure Permanently Alters Cerebral Serotonin Receptor mRNA in Mice but Does Not Impact Adult Behaviors." *The Journal of Maternal-*

*Fetal & Neonatal Medicine* 31 (11): 1393–1401. https://doi.org/10.1080/14767058.2017.1317342.

Miller, Andrew H., and Charles L. Raison. 2016. "The Role of Inflammation in Depression: From Evolutionary Imperative to Modern Treatment Target." *Nature Reviews Immunology* 16 (1): 22–34. https://doi.org/10.1038/nri.2015.5.

Mirmiran, M., N. E. van de Poll, M. A. Corner, H. G. van Oyen, and H. L. Bour. 1981. "Suppression of Active Sleep by Chronic Treatment with Chlorimipramine during Early Postnatal Development: Effects upon Adult Sleep and Behavior in the Rat." *Brain Research* 204 (1): 129–46.

Mirmiran, M., J. Scholtens, N. E. van de Poll, H. B. Uylings, J. van der Gugten, and G. J. Boer. 1983. "Effects of Experimental Suppression of Active (REM) Sleep during Early Development upon Adult Brain and Behavior in the Rat." *Brain Research* 283 (2–3): 277–86. https://doi.org/10.1016/0165-3806(83)90184-0.

Molendijk, Marc L., and E. Ronald de Kloet. 2015. "Immobility in the Forced Swim Test Is Adaptive and Does Not Reflect Depression." *Psychoneuroendocrinology* 62 (December): 389–91. https://doi.org/10.1016/j.psyneuen.2015.08.028.

Molina-Jiménez, Tania, Ofelia Limón-Morales, and Herlinda Bonilla-Jaime. 2018. "Early Postnatal Treatment with Clomipramine Induces Female Sexual Behavior and Estrous Cycle Impairment." *Pharmacology Biochemistry and Behavior* 166 (March): 27–34. https://doi.org/10.1016/j.pbb.2018.01.004.

Montgomery, Stuart A., David S. Baldwin, Pierre Blier, Naomi A. Fineberg, Siegfried Kasper, Malcolm Lader, Raymond W. Lam, et al. 2007. "Which Antidepressants Have Demonstrated Superior Efficacy? A Review of the Evidence:" *International Clinical Psychopharma-cology* 22 (6): 323–29. https://doi.org/10.1097/YIC.0b013e3282eff7e0.

Neill, D., G. Vogel, M. Hagler, D. Kors, and A. Hennessey. 1990. "Diminished Sexual Activity in a New Animal Model of Endogenous Depression." *Neuroscience and Biobehavioral Reviews* 14 (1): 73–76.

Nestler, Eric J., and Steven E. Hyman. 2010. "Animal Models of Neuropsychiatric Disorders." *Nature Neuroscience* 13 (10): 1161–69. https://doi.org/10.1038/nn.2647.

Newport, D. Jeffrey, Zachary N. Stowe, and Charles B. Nemeroff. 2002. "Parental Depression: Animal Models of an Adverse Life Event." *American Journal of Psychiatry* 159 (8): 1265–83. https://doi.org/10.1176/appi.ajp.159.8.1265.

Nishi, Kyoko, Kazuya Kanemaru, and Mirko Diksic. 2009. "A Genetic Rat Model of Depression, Flinders Sensitive Line, Has a Lower Density of 5-HT1A Receptors, but a Higher Density of 5-HT1B Receptors, Compared to Control Rats." *Neurochemistry International* 54 (5–6): 299–307. https://doi.org/10.1016/j.neuint.2008.12.011.

O'Brien, Sinead M., Lucinda V. Scott, and Timothy G. Dinan. 2004. "Cytokines: Abnormalities in Major Depression and Implications for Pharmacological Treatment." *Human Psychopharmacology: Clinical and Experimental* 19 (6): 397–403. https://doi.org/10.1002/hup.609.

Olivier, J. D. A., T. Blom, T. Arentsen, and J. R. Homberg. 2011. "The Age-Dependent Effects of Selective Serotonin Reuptake Inhibitors in Humans and Rodents: A Review." *Progress in Neuro-Psychopharmacology & Biological Psychiatry* 35 (6): 1400–1408. https://doi.org/10.1016/j.pnpbp.2010.09.013.

Overstreet, D. H. 1993. "The Flinders Sensitive Line Rats: A Genetic Animal Model of Depression." *Neuroscience and Biobehavioral Reviews* 17 (1): 51–68.

Overstreet, D. H., D. S. Janowsky, O. Pucilowski, and A. H. Rezvani. 1994. "Swim Test Immobility Co-Segregates with Serotonergic but Not Cholinergic Sensitivity in Cross-Breeds of Flinders Line Rats." *Psychiatric Genetics* 4 (2): 101–7.

Overstreet, D. H., and R. W. Russell. 1982. "Selective Breeding for Diisopropyl Fluorophosphate-Sensitivity: Behavioural Effects of Cholinergic Agonists and Antagonists." *Psychopharmacology* 78 (2): 150–55.

Overstreet, D. H., and G. Wegener. 2013. "The Flinders Sensitive Line Rat Model of Depression--25 Years and Still Producing." *Pharmacological Reviews* 65 (1): 143–55. https://doi.org/10.1124/pr.111.005397.

Overstreet, David H. 2012. "Modeling Depression in Animal Models." In *Psychiatric Disorders*, edited by Firas H. Kobeissy, 829:125–44. Totowa, NJ: Humana Press. https://doi.org/10.1007/978-1-61779-458-2_7.

Overstreet, David H., Elliot Friedman, Aleksander A. Mathé, and Gal Yadid. 2005. "The Flinders Sensitive Line Rat: A Selectively Bred Putative Animal Model of Depression." *Neuroscience & Biobehavioral Reviews* 29 (4–5): 739–59. https://doi.org/10.1016/j.neubiorev.2005.03.015.

Overstreet, David H., Amir H. Rezvani, and David S. Janowsky. 1990. "Impaired Active Avoidance Responding in Rats Selectively Bred for Increased Cholinergic Function." *Physiology & Behavior* 47 (4): 787–88. https://doi.org/10.1016/0031-9384(90)90097-N.

Overstreet, David H., Roger W. Russell, Ann D. Crocker, and Grant D. Schiller. 1984. "Selective Breeding for Differences in Cholinergic Function: Pre- and Postsynaptic Mechanisms Involved in Sensitivity to the Anticholinesterase, DFP." *Brain Research* 294 (2): 327–32. https://doi.org/10.1016/0006-8993(84)91044-8.

Palazidou, Eleni. 2012. "The Neurobiology of Depression." *British Medical Bulletin* 101: 127–45. https://doi.org/10.1093/bmb/lds004.

Papp, Mariusz. 2012. "Models of Affective Illness: Chronic Mild Stress in the Rat." In *Current Protocols in Pharmacology*, edited by S. J. Enna, Michael Williams, John F. Barret, John W. Ferkany, Terry Kenakin, and Roger D. Porsolt. Hoboken, NJ, USA: John Wiley & Sons, Inc. https://doi.org/10.1002/0471141755.ph0509s57.

Parikh, C. 2001. "Antidepressants in the Elderly: Challenges for Study Design and Their Interpretation: Antidepressants in the Elderly." *British Journal of Clinical Pharmacology* 49 (6): 539–47. https://doi.org/10.1046/j.1365-2125.2000.00201.x.

Popa, D., C. Lena, C. Alexandre, and J. Adrien. 2008. "Lasting Syndrome of Depression Produced by Reduction in Serotonin Uptake during Postnatal Development: Evidence from Sleep, Stress, and Behavior."

*Journal of Neuroscience* 28 (14): 3546–54. https://doi.org/10.1523/JNEUROSCI.4006-07.2008.

Porsolt, R. D. 1981. "Behavioral Despair." In *Antidepressants: Neurochemical, Behavioral and Clinical Persperctives*, 121–39. New York: Raven Press.

Porsolt, R. D., G. Anton, N. Blavet, and M. Jalfre. 1978. "Behavioural Despair in Rats: A New Model Sensitive to Antidepressant Treatments." *European Journal of Pharmacology* 47 (4): 379–91. https://doi.org/10.1016/0014-2999(78)90118-8.

Porsolt, R. D., M. Deniel, and M. Jalfre. 1979. "Forced Swimming in Rats: Hypothermia, Immobility and the Effects of Imipramine." *European Journal of Pharmacology* 57 (4): 431–36. https://doi.org/10.1016/0014-2999(79)90507-7.

Porsolt, R. D., M. Le Pichon, and M. Jalfre. 1977. "Depression: A New Animal Model Sensitive to Antidepressant Treatments." *Nature* 266 (5604): 730–32. https://doi.org/10.1038/266730a0.

Post, R. M. 1992. "Transduction of Psychosocial Stress into the Neurobiology of Recurrent Affective Disorder." *The American Journal of Psychiatry* 149 (8): 999–1010. https://doi.org/10.1176/ajp.149.8.999.

Prathiba, J., K. B. Kumar, and K. S. Karanth. 1998. "Hyperactivity of Hypothalamic Pituitary Axis in Neonatal Clomipramine Model of Depression." *Journal of Neural Transmission (Vienna, Austria: 1996)* 105 (10–12): 1335–39. https://doi.org/10.1007/s007020050135.

Pruessner, Marita, Dirk H. Hellhammer, Jens C. Pruessner, and Sonia J. Lupien. 2003. "Self-Reported Depressive Symptoms and Stress Levels in Healthy Young Men: Associations with the Cortisol Response to Awakening." *Psychosomatic Medicine* 65 (1): 92–99.

Pucilowski, O., and D. H. Overstreet. 1993. "Effect of Chronic Antidepressant Treatment on Responses to Apomorphine in Selectively Bred Rat Strains." *Brain Research Bulletin* 32 (5): 471–75.

Rayen, Ine, Harry W. M. Steinbusch, Thierry D. Charlier, and Jodi L. Pawluski. 2013. "Developmental Fluoxetine Exposure and Prenatal Stress Alter Sexual Differentiation of the Brain and Reproductive

Behavior in Male Rat Offspring." *Psychoneuroendocrinology* 38 (9): 1618–29. https://doi.org/10.1016/j.psyneuen.2013.01.007.

Rebello, T. J., Q. Yu, N. M. Goodfellow, M. K. Caffrey Cagliostro, A. Teissier, E. Morelli, E. Y. Demireva, et al. 2014. "Postnatal Day 2 to 11 Constitutes a 5-HT-Sensitive Period Impacting Adult mPFC Function." *Journal of Neuroscience* 34 (37): 12379–93. https://doi.org/10.1523/JNEUROSCI.1020-13.2014.

Reul, Johannes M. H. M. 2014. "Making Memories of Stressful Events: A Journey along Epigenetic, Gene Transcription, and Signaling Pathways." *Frontiers in Psychiatry* 5: 5. https://doi.org/10.3389/fpsyt.2014.00005.

Réus, Gislaine Z., Roberto B. Stringari, Karine F. Ribeiro, Andreza L. Cipriano, Bruna S. Panizzutti, Laura Stertz, Camila Lersch, Flávio Kapczinski, and João Quevedo. 2011. "Maternal Deprivation Induces Depressive-like Behaviour and Alters Neurotrophin Levels in the Rat Brain." *Neurochemical Research* 36 (3): 460–66. https://doi.org/10.1007/s11064-010-0364-3.

Rodriguez-Porcel, Federico, Donald Green, Nidhi Khatri, Sharonda Swilley Harris, Warren L. May, Rick C. S. Lin, and Ian A. Paul. 2011. "Neonatal Exposure of Rats to Antidepressants Affects Behavioral Reactions to Novelty and Social Interactions in a Manner Analogous to Autistic Spectrum Disorders." *The Anatomical Record: Advances in Integrative Anatomy and Evolutionary Biology* 294 (10): 1726–35. https://doi.org/10.1002/ar.21402.

Rosenblum, Leonard A., and Gayle S. Paully. 1987. "Primate Models of Separation-Induced Depression." *Psychiatric Clinics of North America* 10 (3): 437–47. https://doi.org/10.1016/S0193-953X(18)30553-7.

Rüedi-Bettschen, Daniela, Weining Zhang, Holger Russig, Boris Ferger, Anna Weston, Else-Marie Pedersen, Joram Feldon, and Christopher R. Pryce. 2006. "Early Deprivation Leads to Altered Behavioural, Autonomic and Endocrine Responses to Environmental Challenge in Adult Fischer Rats." *European Journal of Neuroscience* 24 (10): 2879–93. https://doi.org/10.1111/j.1460-9568.2006.05158.x.

Rygula, Rafal, Nashat Abumaria, Gabriele Flügge, Eberhard Fuchs, Eckart Rüther, and Ursula Havemann-Reinecke. 2005. "Anhedonia and Motivational Deficits in Rats: Impact of Chronic Social Stress." *Behavioural Brain Research* 162 (1): 127–34. https://doi.org/10.1016/j.bbr.2005.03.009.

Ryu, Vitaly, Sang Bae Yoo, Dong-Won Kang, Jong-Ho Lee, and Jeong Won Jahng. 2009. "Post-Weaning Isolation Promotes Food Intake and Body Weight Gain in Rats That Experienced Neonatal Maternal Separation." *Brain Research* 1295 (October): 127–34. https://doi.org/10.1016/j.brainres.2009.08.006.

Sahakian, B. J., T. W. Robbins, M. J. Morgan, and S. D. Iversen. 1975. "The Effects of Psychomotor Stimulants on Stereotypy and Locomotor Activity in Socially-Deprived and Control Rats." *Brain Research* 84 (2): 195–205. https://doi.org/10.1016/0006-8993(75)90975-0.

Sarkar, Ambalika, Parul Chachra, and Vidita A. Vaidya. 2014. "Postnatal Fluoxetine-Evoked Anxiety Is Prevented by Concomitant 5-HT2A/C Receptor Blockade and Mimicked by Postnatal 5-HT2A/C Receptor Stimulation." *Biological Psychiatry* 76 (11): 858–68. https://doi.org/10.1016/j.biopsych.2013.11.005.

Scheuing, Lisa, Chi-Tso Chiu, Hsiao-Mei Liao, and De-Maw Chuang. 2015. "Antidepressant Mechanism of Ketamine: Perspective from Preclinical Studies." *Frontiers in Neuroscience* 9: 249. https://doi.org/10.3389/fnins.2015.00249.

Schildkraut, J. J., E. K. Gordon, and J. Durell. 1965. "Catecholamine Metabolism in Affective Disorders. I. Normetanephrine and VMA Excretion in Depressed Patients Treated with Imipramine." *Journal of Psychiatric Research* 3 (4): 213–28.

Segal, Zindel, Pierre Vincent, and Anthony Levitt. 2002. "Efficacy of Combined, Sequential and Crossover Psychotherapy and Pharmacotherapy in Improving Outcomes in Depression." *Journal of Psychiatry & Neuroscience: JPN* 27 (4): 281–90.

Sher, Leo, Maria A. Oquendo, Ainsley K. Burke, Thomas B. Cooper, and J. John Mann. 2013. "Combined Dexamethasone Suppression–corticotrophin-Releasing Hormone Stimulation Test in Medication-Free

Major Depression and Healthy Volunteers." *Journal of Affective Disorders* 151 (3): 1108–12. https://doi.org/10.1016/j.jad.2013.06.049.

Shirayama, Yukihiko, Andrew C.-H. Chen, Shin Nakagawa, David S. Russell, and Ronald S. Duman. 2002. "Brain-Derived Neurotrophic Factor Produces Antidepressant Effects in Behavioral Models of Depression." *The Journal of Neuroscience: The Official Journal of the Society for Neuroscience* 22 (8): 3251–61. https://doi.org/20026292.

Shiromani, P. 1988. "Increased REM Sleep in Rats Selectively Bred for Cholinergic Hyperactivity." *Neuropsychopharmacology* 1 (2): 127–33. https://doi.org/10.1016/0893-133X(88)90004-8.

Shulman, Kenneth I., Nathan Herrmann, and Scott E. Walker. 2013. "Current Place of Monoamine Oxidase Inhibitors in the Treatment of Depression." *CNS Drugs* 27 (10): 789–97. https://doi.org/10.1007/s40263-013-0097-3.

Simpson, K. L., K. J. Weaver, E. de Villers-Sidani, J. Y.- F. Lu, Z. Cai, Y. Pang, F. Rodriguez-Porcel, I. A. Paul, M. Merzenich, and R. C. S. Lin. 2011. "Perinatal Antidepressant Exposure Alters Cortical Network Function in Rodents." *Proceedings of the National Academy of Sciences* 108 (45): 18465–70. https://doi.org/10.1073/pnas.1109353108.

Singhal, Gaurav, and Bernhard T. Baune. 2017. "Microglia: An Interface between the Loss of Neuroplasticity and Depression." *Frontiers in Cellular Neuroscience* 11 (September). https://doi.org/10.3389/fncel.2017.00270.

Solomon, M. B., A. R. Furay, K. Jones, A. E. B. Packard, B. A. Packard, A. C. Wulsin, and J. P. Herman. 2012. "Deletion of Forebrain Glucocorticoid Receptors Impairs Neuroendocrine Stress Responses and Induces Depression-like Behavior in Males but Not Females." *Neuroscience* 203 (February): 135–43. https://doi.org/10.1016/j.neuroscience.2011.12.014.

Stein, Dirson J., Mailton F. Vasconcelos, Lucas Albrechet-Souza, Keila M. M. Ceresér, and Rosa M. M. de Almeida. 2017. "Microglial Over-Activation by Social Defeat Stress Contributes to Anxiety- and Depressive-Like Behaviors." *Frontiers in Behavioral Neuroscience* 11 (October). https://doi.org/10.3389/fnbeh.2017.00207.

Taltavull, J. F., V. I. Chefer, T. S. Shippenberg, and E. A. Kiyatkin. 2003. "Severe Brain Hypothermia as a Factor Underlying Behavioral Immobility during Cold-Water Forced Swim." *Brain Research* 975 (1–2): 244–47. https://doi.org/10.1016/s0006-8993(03)02695-7.

Thiele, S., T. S. Spehl, L. Frings, F. Braun, M. Ferch, A. H. Rezvani, L. L. Furlanetti, P. T. Meyer, V. A. Coenen, and M. D. Döbrössy. 2016. "Long-Term Characterization of the Flinders Sensitive Line Rodent Model of Human Depression: Behavioral and PET Evidence of a Dysfunctional Entorhinal Cortex." *Behavioural Brain Research* 300 (March): 11–24. https://doi.org/10.1016/j.bbr.2015.11.026.

Tye, Kay M., Julie J. Mirzabekov, Melissa R. Warden, Emily A. Ferenczi, Hsing-Chen Tsai, Joel Finkelstein, Sung-Yon Kim, et al. 2012. "Dopamine Neurons Modulate Neural Encoding and Expression of Depression-Related Behaviour." *Nature* 493 (December): 537.

Urani, Alexandre, Sabine Chourbaji, and Peter Gass. 2005. "Mutant Mouse Models of Depression: Candidate Genes and Current Mouse Lines." *Neuroscience and Biobehavioral Reviews* 29 (4–5): 805–28. https://doi.org/10.1016/j.neubiorev.2005.03.020.

Valvassori, Samira S., Josiane Budni, Roger B. Varela, and Joao Quevedo. 2013. "Contributions of Animal Models to the Study of Mood Disorders." *Revista Brasileira de Psiquiatria* 35 (suppl 2): S121–31. https://doi.org/10.1590/1516-4446-2013-1168.

Valzelli, L., and S. Bernasconi. 1971. "Differential Activity of Some Psychotropic Drugs as a Function of Emotional Level in Animals." *Psychopharmacologia* 20 (1): 91–96.

Vázquez-Palacios, Gonzalo, Herlinda Bonilla-Jaime, and Javier Velázquez-Moctezuma. 2005. "Antidepressant Effects of Nicotine and Fluoxetine in an Animal Model of Depression Induced by Neonatal Treatment with Clomipramine." *Progress in Neuro-Psychopharma-cology & Biological Psychiatry* 29 (1): 39–46. https://doi.org/10.1016/j.pnpbp.2004.08.008.

Velazquez-Moctezuma, Javier, and Oscar Diaz Ruiz. 1992. "Neonatal Treatment with Clomipramine Increased Immobility in the Forced Swim Test: An Attribute of Animal Models of Depression."

*Pharmacology Biochemistry and Behavior* 42 (4): 737–39. https://doi.org/10.1016/0091-3057(92)90022-8.

Vermeiden, M., A. M. Kamperman, W. J. G. Hoogendijk, W. W. van den Broek, and T. K. Birkenhäger. 2017. "A Randomized Clinical Trial Comparing Two Two-Phase Treatment Strategies for in-Patients with Severe Depression." *Acta Psychiatrica Scandinavica* 136 (1): 118–28. https://doi.org/10.1111/acps.12743.

Vijayakumar, M., and B. L. Meti. 1999. "Alterations in the Levels of Monoamines in Discrete Brain Regions of Clomipramine-Induced Animal Model of Endogenous Depression." *Neurochemical Research* 24 (3): 345–49.

Vogel, G., M. Hagler, A. Hennessey, and C. Richard. 1996. "Dose-Dependent Decrements in Adult Male Rat Sexual Behavior after Neonatal Clorimipramine Treatment." *Pharmacology, Biochemistry, and Behavior* 54 (3): 605–9.

Vogel, G., D. Neill, M. Hagler, and D. Kors. 1990. "A New Animal Model of Endogenous Depression: A Summary of Present Findings." *Neuroscience and Biobehavioral Reviews* 14 (1): 85–91.

Vogel, G., D. Neill, M. Hagler, D. Kors, and P. Hartley. 1990. "Decreased Intracranial Self-Stimulation in a New Animal Model of Endogenous Depression." *Neuroscience and Biobehavioral Reviews* 14 (1): 65–68.

Vogel, G., D. Neill, D. Kors, and M. Hagler. 1990. "REM Sleep Abnormalities in a New Animal Model of Endogenous Depression." *Neuroscience and Biobehavioral Reviews* 14 (1): 77–83.

Vogel, G. W., and F. A. Vogel. 1982. "A New Animal Model of Human Endogenous Depression." *Sleep Research* 11: 222.

Vollmayr, Barbara, and Fritz A Henn. 2003. "Stress Models of Depression." *Clinical Neuroscience Research* 3 (4–5): 245–51. https://doi.org/10.1016/S1566-2772(03)00086-0.

Wallis, Elisabeth, David H. Overstreet, and Ann D. Crocker. 1988. "Selective Breeding for Increased Cholinergic Function: Increased Serotonergic Sensitivity." *Pharmacology Biochemistry and Behavior* 31 (2): 345–50. https://doi.org/10.1016/0091-3057(88)90356-5.

Wang, Qingzhong, Matthew A. Timberlake, Kevin Prall, and Yogesh Dwivedi. 2017. "The Recent Progress in Animal Models of Depression." *Progress in Neuro-Psychopharmacology and Biological Psychiatry* 77 (July): 99–109. https://doi.org/10.1016/j.pnpbp.2017.04.008.

Warden, Melissa R., Aslihan Selimbeyoglu, Julie J. Mirzabekov, Maisie Lo, Kimberly R. Thompson, Sung-Yon Kim, Avishek Adhikari, Kay M. Tye, Loren M. Frank, and Karl Deisseroth. 2012. "A Prefrontal Cortex-Brainstem Neuronal Projection That Controls Response to Behavioural Challenge." *Nature* 492 (7429): 428–32. https://doi.org/10.1038/nature11617.

Weaver, Kristin J., Ian A. Paul, Rick C. S. Lin, and Kimberly L. Simpson. 2010. "Neonatal Exposure to Citalopram Selectively Alters the Expression of the Serotonin Transporter in the Hippocampus: Dose-Dependent Effects." *Anatomical Record (Hoboken, N.J.: 2007)* 293 (11): 1920–32. https://doi.org/10.1002/ar.21245.

Whitaker-Azmitia, P. M. 1991. "Role of Serotonin and Other Neurotransmitter Receptors in Brain Development: Basis for Developmental Pharmacology." *Pharmacological Reviews* 43 (4): 553–61.

Whitaker-Azmitia, P. M., and E. C. Azmitia. 1986. "Autoregulation of Fetal Serotonergic Neuronal Development: Role of High Affinity Serotonin Receptors." *Neuroscience Letters* 67 (3): 307–12. https://doi.org/10.1016/0304-3940(86)90327-7.

Wiborg, Ove. 2013. "Chronic Mild Stress for Modeling Anhedonia." *Cell and Tissue Research* 354 (1): 155–69. https://doi.org/10.1007/s00441-013-1664-0.

Willner, P. 1991. "Animal Models as Simulations of Depression." *Trends in Pharmacological Sciences* 12 (4): 131–36.

Willner, P. 1995. "Animal Models of Depression: Validity and Applications." *Advances in Biochemical Psychopharmacology* 49: 19–41.

Willner, P., and R. C. Goldstein. 2001. "Mediation of Depression by Perceptions of Defeat and Entrapment in High-Stress Mothers." *The British Journal of Medical Psychology* 74 (Pt 4): 473–85.

Willner, P, K. Golembiowska, V. Klimek, and R Muscat. 1991. "Changes in Mesolimbic Dopamine May Explain Stress-Induced Anhedonia." *Psychobiology* 19 (1): 79–84.

Willner, P., and P. J. Mitchell. 2002. "The Validity of Animal Models of Predisposition to Depression." *Behavioural Pharmacology* 13 (3): 169–88.

Willner, Paul. 2005. "Chronic Mild Stress (CMS) Revisited: Consistency and Behavioural-Neurobiological Concordance in the Effects of CMS." *Neuropsychobiology* 52 (2): 90–110. https://doi.org/10.1159/000087097.

Willner, Paul. 2017. "The Chronic Mild Stress (CMS) Model of Depression: History, Evaluation and Usage." *Neurobiology of Stress* 6 (February): 78–93. https://doi.org/10.1016/j.ynstr.2016.08.002.

Willner, Paul, Piotr Gruca, Magdalena Lason, Katarzyna Tota-Glowczyk, Ewa Litwa, Monika Niemczyk, and Mariusz Papp. 2019. "Validation of Chronic Mild Stress in the Wistar-Kyoto Rat as an Animal Model of Treatment-Resistant Depression:" *Behavioural Pharmacology* 30 (April): 239–50. https://doi.org/10.1097/FBP.0000000000000431.

Willner, Paul, Jørgen Scheel-Krüger, and Catherine Belzung. 2013. "The Neurobiology of Depression and Antidepressant Action." *Neuroscience & Biobehavioral Reviews* 37 (10): 2331–71. https://doi.org/10.1016/j.neubiorev.2012.12.007.

World Health Organization. 2017. *World Health Statistics 2017: Monitoring Health for the SDGs, Sustainable Development Goals*. Geneve: World Health Organization.

Yan, Hua-Cheng, Xiong Cao, Manas Das, Xin-Hong Zhu, and Tian-Ming Gao. 2010. "Behavioral Animal Models of Depression." *Neuroscience Bulletin* 26 (4): 327–37. https://doi.org/10.1007/s12264-010-0323-7.

Yang, Li-Min, Bing Hu, Ying-Hong Xia, Bei-Lin Zhang, and Hua Zhao. 2008. "Lateral Habenula Lesions Improve the Behavioral Response in Depressed Rats via Increasing the Serotonin Level in Dorsal Raphe

Nucleus." *Behavioural Brain Research* 188 (1): 84–90. https://doi.org/10.1016/j.bbr.2007.10.022.

Yannielli, P. C., L. Kargieman, L. Gregoretti, and D. P. Cardinali. 1999. "Effects of Neonatal Clomipramine Treatment on Locomotor Activity, Anxiety-Related Behavior and Serotonin Turnover in Syrian Hamsters." *Neuropsychobiology* 39 (4): 200–206. https://doi.org/10.1159/000026584.

Zangen, A., D. H. Overstreet, and G. Yadid. 1997. "High Serotonin and 5-Hydroxyindoleacetic Acid Levels in Limbic Brain Regions in a Rat Model of Depression: Normalization by Chronic Antidepressant Treatment." *Journal of Neurochemistry* 69 (6): 2477–83. https://doi.org/10.1046/j.1471-4159.1997.69062477.x.

Zhu, Shenghua, Ruoyang Shi, Junhui Wang, Jun-Feng Wang, and Xin-Min Li. 2014. "Unpredictable Chronic Mild Stress Not Chronic Restraint Stress Induces Depressive Behaviours in Mice:" *NeuroReport* 25 (14): 1151–55. https://doi.org/10.1097/WNR.0000000000000243.

Zohar, Inbar, Shai Shoham, and Marta Weinstock. 2016. "Perinatal Citalopram Does Not Prevent the Effect of Prenatal Stress on Anxiety, Depressive-like Behaviour and Serotonergic Transmission in Adult Rat Offspring." Edited by James Herman. *European Journal of Neuroscience* 43 (4): 590–600. https://doi.org/10.1111/ejn.13150.

Zurawek, Dariusz, Maciej Kusmider, Agata Faron-Gorecka, Piotr Gruca, Paulina Pabian, Joanna Solich, Magdalena Kolasa, Mariusz Papp, and Marta Dziedzicka-Wasylewska. 2017. "Reciprocal MicroRNA Expression in Mesocortical Circuit and Its Interplay with Serotonin Transporter Define Resilient Rats in the Chronic Mild Stress." *Molecular Neurobiology* 54 (8): 5741–51. https://doi.org/10.1007/s12035-016-0107-9.

In: Laboratory Animals and Neurosciences ISBN: 978-1-53618-462-4
Editors: B. Hernandez Godinez et al.© 2020 Nova Science Publishers, Inc.

*Chapter 2*

# ANIMAL MODELS OF ANXIETY IN RODENTS

***Tania Molina Jiménez[1],***
***José Armando Sánchez-Salcedo[2],***
***Claudia Juárez-Portilla[3]***
***and Herlinda Bonilla Jaime[4,*]***
[1]Instituto Interdisciplinario de Investigaciones, Universidad de Xalapa, Xalapa-Enríquez, Veracruz, México
[2]Doctorado en Ciencias Biológicas y de la Salud, Universidad Autónoma Metropolitana, Unidad Iztapalapa, Ciudad de México, México
[3]Centro de Investigaciones Biomédicas, Universidad Veracruzana. Veracruz, México
[4]Departamento de Biología de la Reproducción, Universidad Autónoma Metropolitana, Unidad Iztapalapa, Ciudad de México, México

* Corresponding Author's E-mail: bjh@xanum.uam.mx.

## ABSTRACT

Anxiety disorders are the most common psychiatric disorders in the population; they are considered a cause of disability worldwide. These disorders included fear and anxiety, two highly conserved adaptive emotions with the main purpose of protecting the organism against every real danger. Nevertheless, those emotional states could become excessive in absence of real threat leading to high disability and burden illness. Etiologically, these disorders include several causes such as psychosocial factors, stress, traumatic events, genetic vulnerability which can leads to dysfunctional neurophysiological and behavioral manifestation. In this context, animal models are a useful tool to evaluate neurobiological circuits involved in the regulation of anxiety. Also, these models are important to the screening of new molecules with anxiolytic activity. The use of animal models of these disorders has been a challenge due to the complexity of the condition itself. For that reason, a large number of animal models has been developed. In this chapter we highligh some epidemiological data of anxiety disorders along with the description of some of the most relevant and widely animal models used for studying anxiety.

**Keywords**: fear, psychiatric disorders, animals, anxiolytics

## INTRODUCTION

Anxiety disorders include generalized anxiety disorder (GAD), panic disorder, specific phobias, social anxiety disorder, selective mutism and some others, which have in common the excessive fear and anxiety (American Psychiatric Association, 2013). Epidemiological data indicate that in many countries, these disorders are the most prevalent over population followed by mood, substance use disorder and impulsive control (Demyttenaere et al., 2004; Kessler et al., 2010). Moreover, it was estimated a 12-month prevalence ranging between 3.3% and 20.4% worldwide. Recently, the World Health Organization reported that there are approximately 264 millions of people living with anxiety disorders, being women more vulnerable than man to develop them (WHO, 2017).

Anxiety therapeutics is based in pharmacotherapy and psychobiological therapies. Recently, antidepressants have been used as the first line to treat these disorders, including selective serotonin reuptake inhibitors (SSRIs) and serotonin-norepinephrine reuptake inhibitors (SNRIs) which are efficacious and are well tolerate. Besides, the use of SSRIs and SNRIs shows low risk to develop drug dependences, and presents just few side effects. For instance, tricyclic antidepressants represents one of the first options for treating it, even when their efficacy is equal to SSRI in some disorders as panic and generalized anxiety disorders, they show more side effects (dizziness, cardiac arrhythmia, blurred vision, urinary retention, sedation) that interfere with the daily life of patients (Farach et al., 2012; Ravindran and Stein, 2010). On the other hand, benzodiazepines are considered a second choice for treating due to their short-term effects and rapid reduction of anxiety. Nevertheless, prolonged use of benzodiazepines is associated with pharmacologic dependence and impairment in psychomotor and cognitive functions (Otto et al., 2010). In addition, the azapirones, which bind at the $5HT_{1A}$ receptor, do not present problems in causing dependence as benzodiazepines, but they only have showed consisted efficacy for GAD, especially if is comorbid with depression (Silverstone and Salinas, 2001). Its true that the used of psychotherapy is also benefit for the patients but to date pharmacotherapy is more efficient. Thus, the more understanding we have about the neurobiological mechanism of this illnes the more we will have the probability to develop new molecules or substances with an anxiolytic action with minor side effects.

## Criteria for Validity of Animal Models

The use of animals as models to understand biological processes began in Greece, with two historical figures, Hippocrates and Aristoteles. Both performed several manipulations in different animal species in order to generate knowledge about anatomical structure and physiological processes of humans (Franco, 2013). Until now, animals are still being used as models in several disciplines of science, for this reason ethical guidelines have emerged over time to guarantee the well handle of experimental animals.

Therefore, an animal model is defined as an organism used to simulate a normal or abnormal biological process. In psychiatry, animal models reproduced a human psychopathology, such as anxiety or depression. Thus, animal models constitute an important tool to study the etiology, psychopathological process and the screening of new molecules with relevant biological activity of psychiatric disease such as anxiety disorders (Valvassori et al., 2013).

In this aspect, some validity criteria have been established in order to evaluate wether an animal model is adequate for studying a disease. The animal model validity requires similarity in many aspects between the model and the human pathology. Hence, Mckinney and Bunney (1969) proposed some criteria validity related to the similarity in symptoms observed and in the effectiveness of the pharmacology treatment, but also they establish that an animal model should has same etiology and same biochemistry as happens in human, but these criteria were not well defined.

On the other hand, Willner (1984) proposed three evaluation criteria, which include not only superficial similarities between the animal model and the human psychopathology (face validity), but also other paradigms related with the pharmacological treatment and the theoretical mechanism involved in the pathology, such as predictive and construct validity (Belzung and Lemoine, 2011; Bourin et al., 2015). See Table 1.

**Table 1. Validation criteria for an animal model**

| | |
|---|---|
| **Face validity** | Refers to the similarities in behavioral and physiological responses between the animal model and the human pathology. |
| **Predictive validity** | Is related to the treatment, clinical effective drugs must revert the symptoms mimic in the animal model. |
| **Construct validity** | Similarity between the theoretical rationale underlying the animal model and the human behavior. In this aspect, the construct validity requires that the etiology and physiopathological processes of the human illness must be similar in the animal. |

Even when the use of animal models constituted a useful tool for the study of psychiatric illness like anxiety disorders, they also have some limitations due to the incapability of observed subjective feelings such as excessive worry, lack of concentration or feeling as though the mind goes blank. Despite of these inconvenients, animal models are helpful for studying the neurobiological mechanism of anxiety by the evaluation of specific behavioral repertory and also by predicting the therapeutic effect of a drug clinically effective for it (Bourin, 2015).

In consistency, since the appearance of benzodiazepines and their efficacy on the clinical management, predictive criteria of animal models of anxiety were strongly related with the selective responsivity of $GABA_A$ agents such as diazepam. Nevertheless, there are other drugs with anxiolytic activity through different mechanisms of action. For instance, buspirone is an anxiolytic showing high affinity to $5HT_{1A}$ receptor, acting as a partial agonist to produce its clinical effects. However, the effectiveness is only for some anxiety disorders like GAD. Indeed, buspirone is used as a second line of agents with anxiolytic effect, when patient do not respond to selective serotonin reuptake inhibitors (Wilson and Tripp, 2019). Also, buspirone is not effective in some anxiety tests, but it had shown anxiolytic effect in light/dark test, burying behavior paradigm and elevated plus maze test (Griebel et al., 1995; Picazo and Fernández-Guasti, 1998; Shimada et al., 1995). It seems that the effectiveness of buspirone depends of the appropriated doses, the therapeutics schedule and the levels of anxiety (Castanheira et al., 2018). Besides, a strong interaction between levels of steroid hormones of female rats in different stages of its estrous cycle and the serotonergic components influence emotional states like anxiety (Picazo and Fernández-Guasti, 1998). This indicates that anxiety is regulated not only by GABAergic system but also by different neurochemical systems which is reflected in the heterogeneity of anxiety disorders. Thus, the development of several animal models implies the emulation of those differences which is a difficult goal to achieve.

## Classification of Animal Models of Anxiety

Animal models of anxiety evaluate the emotional reactivity (behavioral and physiological) of rodents induced by different stressful manipulations such as predator odor, foot shocks, bright light, new environments or even drugs. Based on the aversive stimulus (if it requires to be learned or wheter is part of the innate behavioral repertory of the animal) and the response elicited by those stimuli. Animal models can be classified in two main groups (Griebel, 1995; Rodgers, 1997): unconditioned response and conditioned response test. The first includes ethological paradigms which involves natural behavioral reaction to non-painful stimulus like predator odor, illuminates areas, novel places. On the other hand, conditioned response test includes an associative learning process which requires a precise training of the rodents and in some cases involves water or food deprivation along with the use of painful and unplessant events such as footshocks (Steimer, 2011).

Interestingly, animal models of anxiety emulate some aspects of the etiology, behavioral and physiological expression of fear and anxiety; some of them are more sensitive to some components with anxiolytic activity while in others the effect could be variable due to several factors including handling conditions, testing apparatus, sex, age, species and strain (Barrett and Vanover, 1993; Griebel, 1995; Prut and Belzung, 2003). Even though there is already a main classification of the anxiety animal models, there are other categories in which could be grouped, taking into account the stimulus inducing the anxiety state, like natural or non-natural aversive stimulus that spontaneously evoke anxiety-like behavior, conflict situation, stressful events during early life for emulating predisposition, physiological and genetic manipulation (Figure 1). In this aspect, all these models have contributed in the neurochemistry of anxiety disorders and the development of new drugs with anxiolytic effects and also in the identification of neuronal circuits affected by traumatic events during life (Kumar et al., 2013; Shekhar et al., 2001). Furthermore, is important to describe some of the relevant tests to evaluate anxiety in rodents.

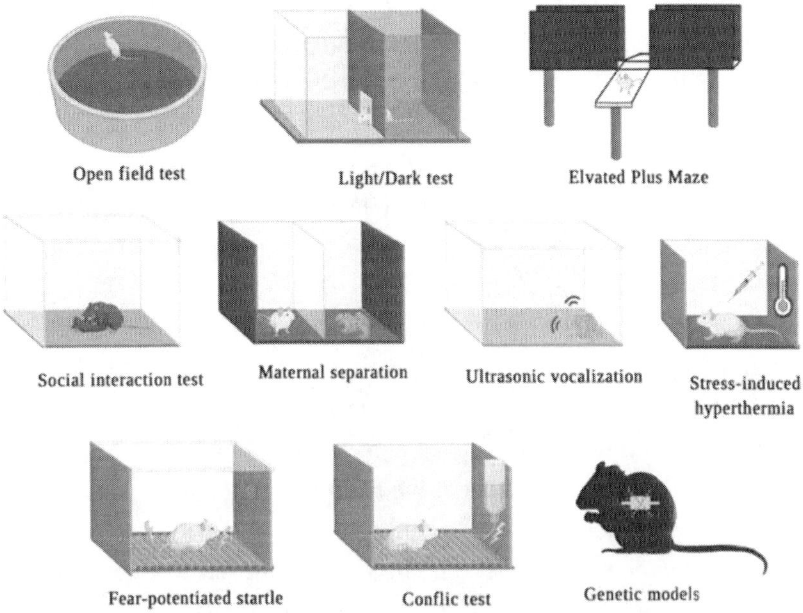


Figure 1. Schematic representation of the most commonly used animal models of anxiety. Some paradigms are based on conditioned operand conflict (fear potentiate startle, conflict test, burying), while others evaluate spontaneous fear reactions to external threats (elevated plus maze, light/dark test, social interaction, open field test, ultrasonic vocalization, stress-induced hyperthermia). Moreover, there are models which evaluate early time life stress and its long-lasting neurobiological effects (maternal separation) and genetic models providing relevant information about gen and proteins involved in anxiety disorders.

# ETHOLOGIC TEST

## Elevated Plus Maze Test

Elevated plus maze test (EPM) has been suggested to be an ethologically valid animal model of human anxiety standing as one of the most popular in vivo test, which is intensively used for the study of the neurobiological basis of anxiety, to define brain areas related to fear/anxiety and in the screening for anxiolytic/anxiogenic-like drugs and novel targets (Carobrez and Bertoglio, 2005; Ennaceur and Chazot, 2016). The EPM consists of four elevated arms forming a plus-shape; with two opposed open and two enclosed, where initially the experimental animal is released in the central area and left to explore the mazes for 5-10 min (Ennaceur and Chazot, 2016). Traditionally the EPM test has been performed with rodents, however there are other animal species used for the evaluation of anxiety-like behaviors such as pigs (Andersen et al., 2000) and larval and juvenile zebra fish (Varga et al., 2018).

Generally, when the EPM test is used for the screening of new therapeutic approaches, the new anxiogenic or anxiolytic drug is compared with diazepam. Normal exploratory behavior is in favor of the closed arms that can be enhanced by compounds that increase the aversion towards the anxiety-provoking open arms. In contrast, administration of anxiolytic compounds like diazepam reduces the natural aversion to the open arms and promotes the exploration thereof (Hoog, 1996). In addition, the total number of entries and/or the number of entries into the closed arms reflects a measure of locomotor activity (Korte and De Boer, 2003), which is a sing of the need for security, revealing anxiety traits (Padurariu et al., 2017). Additional anxiety-related behaviors are evaluated including head dipping in open arms, protected stretch-attend postures in the closed arms, and grooming (Padurariu et al., 2017).

Due to the potential side effects of benzodiazepines such as diazepam for the treatments of anxiety symptoms, several alternatives for reducing of anxiety has been explored. It is known that natural compounds such as flavonoid chrysin isolated from Passiflora caerulea produces anxiolytic-like activity similar to diazepam without the sedative effects in male mice and rats in the EPM at 2 and 4 mg/kg, increasing the time spent rearing and grooming, without altering the locomotor activity (Rodríguez-Landa et al., 2019). Similarly, ketamine best known as an anesthetic agent has the property to reduce locomotor activity when it is acutely administered to mice. In contrast, chronic ketamine treatment (7 days) has no significant effect on locomotor activity whereas decreased anxiety, as evidenced by increased time spent on open arms in the EPM test (Shin et al., 2019).

However, behavioral responses related to anxiety usually overlapped with emotional states like fear eliciting a range of defensive responses designed to protect the organism from harm (Lamontagne et al., 2016). Besides, the clinical heterogeneity of anxiety has made it more complex so for the understanding of the physiopathology the use of EPM is still relevant.

## Light/Dark Box

The light/dark box test is based on the innate aversion of rodents to brightly illuminated areas and on the spontaneous exploratory behaviour of rodents in response to mild stressors, that is, novel environment and light (Bourin and Hascoët, 2003). This test is one of the few paradigms originally developed for using mice. The advantages of this test include the quickness and ease to use without requiring prior mice training. (Kulesskaya and Voikar, 2014). However, many authors have modified it regarding to its size, the use of the light cycle (normal or inversed), length of the test and the used parameters. Nowadays, the utilization of this test has been expanded to other animal models like planarians due that this flatworm, like rodents, instinctively spend more time in darkness versus light environments (negative phototaxis) when given a choice, which may reveal defensive response related to an anxiety-like phenotype (Zewde et al., 2018).

In light/dark test there is a conflict between the exploratory behavior and the neophobia. The exploratory activity exposes the combined result of these tendencies in novel situations (Bourin and Hascoët, 2003). The conventional measures of anxiety-like behavior are the latency time for the first passage from the light compartment to the dark one, the number of transitions made between two compartments, the movement in each compartment and the time spent in brightly illuminated area (Bourin, 2015; Kulesskaya and Voikar, 2014).

After anxiolytic drug treatment the apparent apprehension of remaining in or moving to the light area is abolished (Bourin, 2015). Treatment with benzodiazepines increases the time spent in the lit compartment as well as the number of transitions between the two areas; yet, particular attention should be given to drug or genetic-induced changes in basal locomotor activity since they could produce false positive results (Campos et al., 2013).

However, the light/dark box test is still useful for discovering new targets in the field of anxiety-related disorders (Bourin, 2015).

### *Open Field Test*

The open field test (OFT) is the most classical method for assessing anxiety-like behavior in rodents. Originally, this test was developed by Calvin Hall in the 1930s to measure defecation as an index of timidity in mice. Nowadays, OFT is considered a conflict test based on the opposing drives to explore new environments and fearful avoidance of bright/exposed areas (Sturman et al., 2018). Even OFT is considered a standardized test, the arenas used by different laboratories differ in size, material, color and shape. Moreover, this test has been one of the methods showing idiosyncratic results after standardization (Kulesskaya and Voikar, 2014).

In the OFT the animals are allowed to freely explore an open arena surrounded by walls, where naturally, rodents show thigmotaxis, a tendency to avoid the central region of the arena and stay in the periphery. In addition, they show increases and decreases in center activity are indicative of anxiolysis and anxiogenesis, respectively (Kuniishi et al., 2017). A classic exploratory behavior recorded in the open field include grooming, behavior horizontal locomotion (number of floor line crossings) and frequency of vertical activity like rearing behavior (Belovicova et al., 2017), where wall leaning only loads onto a factor related to locomotion/activity. Rearing also loads onto a factor related to emotional behavior and is inversely correlated with defecation, a marker related to stress and anxiety (Sturman et al., 2018).

### *Social Interaction*

The social interaction test described by File and Hyde in 1978 consists in placing familiar or unfamiliar pairs of male or female rodents in a novel environment and monitoring their exploratory and social behavior for 5-15 min (Toth and Neumann, 2013). This test differs from the others as it involves the relevant component of eliminating the need to introduce aversive or appetitive conditions, and it does not require previous animal training (Campos et al., 2013).

The social interaction test emulates an ethologically natural interaction and allows for free interaction between rodents, but makes it difficult to distinguish the level of social approach or avoidance that each individual shows during the interaction (Toth and Neumann, 2013). However, such models have demonstrated central aspects of facing, predictive and construct validity whereby treatment with clinical antidepressants reversed behavioral and physiological effects induced by the model (Keenan et al., 2018).

The performance of the test in a novel environment decreases the level of aggressive behavior between rodents, and a decreased interaction with the same-sex conspecific indicates social avoidance (Toth and Neumann, 2013). Anxiolytic-like behavior is inferred by the increasing of social interaction. For example, a single administration of paroxetine at oral doses of 0.3, 1, 3 and 10 mg/kg had no effect on social interaction between pair of male rats. However, after 21 days of daily administration of paroxetine (3 mg/kg), the time spent in social interaction by pairs of rats tested under the same conditions has an anxiolytic-like effect without affecting the locomotor activity (Lightowler et al., 1994).

### *Ultrasonic Vocalization*

One of the major models of testing unlearned fear in developing rodents utilizes ultrasonic vocalizations, which can be likened to a form of separation anxiety (Ganella and Kim, 2014). Some rodents like rats emit two types of high-frequency vocalizations in different behavioral situations. These vocalizations involve two patterns: the alarm call (18-32 kHz) emitted in stressful and dangerous situations also known as the 22 kHz call, and 50 kHz call during non-aversive appetitive stimulation (Hamed et al., 2009).

The model that became commonly used to screen anxiolytic drugs is the foot shock conditioned 22-kHz ultrasonic vocalization. This frequency is produced when rats are confronted with a natural predator and has been also correlated with defensive behaviors such as conditioned freezing and staying in the closed arms of an elevated plus maze (Steele et al., 2017).

Anxiolytic drugs like diazepam significantly increased isolation-induce appetitive ultrasonic vocalization and decreased aversive context-evoked vocalization. The disinhibitory effects of diazepam indicated that

GABAergic-related mechanism might control high-frequency vocalization, whereas buspirone almost entirely blocked fear-related ultrasonic calls of rats in the same test (Hamed et al., 2009), on the other hand, haloperidol had no effect on the ultrasonic vocalizations, which supports the conclusion that dopamine receptor antagonism does not affect this anxiolytic measure; thus suppression of vocalization emission is believed to be an ethologically valid marker of anxiolytic drug efficacy (Ganella and Kim, 2014).

# CONFLICT TEST

## Vogel Test

The Vogel conflict test (VCT) is a well-established conflict model based in the approach-avoidance behaviors where water-deprived animals face the conflict of receiving a mild shock punishment when they drink water from a bottle (De Jesús-Burgos et al., 2016). This test may expose a type of anxiety associated with controllable aversive events (Bourin and Hascoët, 2003). Moreover, conflict behavior in animals has relevance to human anxiety disorders and the VCT has played a key role in the characterization of drugs acting on GABAergic, glutamatergic and monoaminergic neurotransmitter systems (Mathiasen and Mirza, 2005).

The VCT is responsive to benzodiazepines, which produces anti-conflict response by increasing the number of punished responses and/or shocks received by the animal in comparison to control animals (De Jesús-Burgos et al., 2016; Resstel et al., 2008). In contrast, several anxiogenic compounds that inhibit the GABAergic transmission like bicuculline, picrotoxin, and the β-carboline FG-7142, display proconflict effects in this test (Corda et al., 2018).

Even though this test has a good predictive value for benzodiazepines and barbiturates, the VCT also responds to some non-anxiolytic drugs, producing false-negative results, being susceptible to interference from several variables, such as hunger, thirst, pain, learning and memory (Campos et al., 2013).

### Geller-Seifter Test

The Geller-Seifter test is considered a conditioned operant paradigm. In this test, food-deprived rats learn to press a bar to obtained food, but this action is paired with an unpleasant stimulus like a footshock. Then, rats have to decide between satisfy a biological drive like hungry (even when they receive a punishment), or avoid the aversive stimulus and not receive the food reinforcement (Geller et al., 1962). Thus, in this paradigm, anxious rats diminished the food intake seeking and the administration of anxiolytics (benzodiazepines and agonist of $5HT_{1A}$ receptors) increased the punished responses in order to obtained the reward (Britton et al., 1985; Shimizu et al., 1992). The Geller-Seifter test is a good model with high predictive validity but requires a training, otherwise the model could be ineffective.

## Development Test

### Maternal Separation

Maternal care is essential for the adequate pup development, as well as for the health of the doe. Exposure to stress in early stages of life can disrupt this bond promoting altered neurobiological and behavioral phenotypes (Orso et al., 2018). In rats, the neonatal period between postnatal days 3-14 is known as the stress hyporesponsive period, that is a critical developmental stage for the hypothalamic-pituitary-adrenal axis (HPA) maturation (e.g., neurogenesis, migration, synaptogenesis and pruning), in which stimulation of corticosterone secretion is attenuated following mild stressors, which otherwise would elicit a marked response in adults (Trujillo et al., 2016).

Recent animal studies strongly suggest that adverse early life stress can have such an effect on some individuals and may explain how anxiety disorders become chronic (Ganella and Kim, 2014). Rodent maternal separation during early-development is a widely used model to mimic aspects of behaviors seen in human patients with anxiety disorders (McGregor et al., 2018). This test supports the idea that disturbance in the maternal care period generates alterations in the pups that can lead to structural cerebral changes and hyper-reactivity of the HPA axis in adulthood, accompanied by a propensity to develop anxious or depressive-like disorders and cognitive deficits, although that the circuits underlying emotional behaviour maintain certain degree of plasticity in adulthood (Koe et al., 2016; Trujillo et al., 2016). However, due to the variability in this model, only sometimes it can be found the same alterations that in early stressed humans. While maternal separation paradigms in rat models are relatively well established, behavioral effects upon this paradigms in mice are often inconsistent, where it seems that the length of the protocols and the species are the key to disentangle these controversial results (Banqueri et al., 2017; Tan et al., 2017).

A recent study has shown that chronic, but not acute, treatment using ketamine reverses the anxiety and aggressive-like behavior induced by maternal separation in mice (Shin et al., 2019). Also, tianeptine, an antidepressant with anxiolytic effects reversed the increased anxiety produced by chronic stress and maternal separation treatments in Wistar rats (Trujillo et al., 2016). Nevertheless, the maternal separation paradigm result contradictory, with studies showing no alterations, decreased or even increased social behaviors after similar maternal protocols in adulthood (Toth and Neumann, 2013).

## Aversive Test

### Defensive Burying Test

In 1950, Hudson termed an innate response of burying behavior in rodent as "defensive burying," where rats, mice, hamsters and even ground squirrels in response to an aversive stimulus displayed this behavior (Fucich and Morilak, 2018). Defensive burying refers to the rodent behavior of displacing bedding material as a defensive reaction with typical alternating forward-pushing movements of their forepaws directed at localized sources of aversive threat (De Boer and Koolhaas, 2003).

In this test, the rats attempt to bury an electrified probe, from which they have been shocked, by pushing the bedding material from the test chamber's floor towards and over the probe (Lamontagne et al., 2016); the behavioral repertoire evaluated is well delineated in rats and mice where the ambulation, rearing, immobility, burying, grooming, prod explore and pica behavior can be distinguished (De Boer and Koolhaas, 2003; Lapiz-Bluhm et al., 2008).

This test is an accepted and validated experimental model of anxiety in adults. However, may differ between infants, juveniles, and adults where the apparent absence of the detectable effects of anxiolytic drugs in very young animals may be attributable to the shape and size of the chamber used to test burying behavior (Cueto-Escobedo et al., 2013).

Additionally, it has also been suggested that the non-reactive nature of harmless stimuli such as glass marbles may elicit a form of anxiety in the animal and it remains arguable whether this form of burying is entirely devoid of a stress-related construct (de Brouwer and Wolmarans, 2018). However, the well documented finding that burying is also reduced by anxiolytic drugs that do not have anti-compulsive activity, such as diazepam and clonazepam undermines the predictive validity of marble burying (Albelda and Joel, 2012).

Anxious animals spend more time burying than animals treated with anxiolytic drugs, such as diazepam, which spend less time burying. This drug effect occurs in a clinically relevant dose-dependent manner and including benzodiazepines and serotonergic drugs (Lapiz-Bluhm et al., 2008; Rodriguez-Landa et al., 2013). In counterpart, the decreasing in defensive burying induced by these agents was blocked by benzodiazepine/GABA-receptor antagonist and $(5HT)_{1A}$-receptor antagonist, respectively (Lapiz-Bluhm et al., 2008) confirming the validity of the model.

### Predator Exposition

Nowadays, predator exposure is considered a useful animal model to analyze the behavioral, physiological and neural mechanisms involved in unconditioned fear, allowing to explore in detail the relationship among defensive behaviors, fear-relation disorders and anxiety state (Campos et al., 2013; Sampedro-Piqueiro et al., 2016). Freezing, which is operationally defined as the absence of movement other than breathing is typically used as the measure of anxiety response to predator odors (Ganella and Kim, 2014). This model was pharmacologically validated with the chronic, but not acute, administration of panicolytic drugs, which decrease the fight reactions induced by the predator, whereas benzodiazepines preferentially inhibit the avoidance behavior (Campos et al., 2013).

Traumatic stress in the form of predator exposure in adult rats causes long-lasting anxiety, and this anxiogenesis is dependent on the basolateral nucleus of the amygdala (BLA) and secretion of stress hormones (Koe et al., 2016). Moreover, it is known that acute predator exposure can produce Post-traumatic stress disorder-like sequale in rats, including a persistent traumatic memory, hypervigilance, heightened anxiety, and neurotransmitter and hormonal abnormalities (Seetharaman et al., 2016). However, predator odour-induced freezing appears more suitable to characterize the pharmacological mechanisms underlying unlearned fear across development, although future studies are needed to fully understand anxiety in early life (Ganella and Kim, 2014).

## CONDITIONING TEST

### Fear-Potentiated Startle

The fear-potentiated startle is a paradigm base on classical conditioning. In this paradigm, rats are trained to fear a stimulus that initially is neutral or with no emotional relevance (tone or light) but when is paired with a footshock, then acquires an emotional value (conditioned stimulus) and as a result of that association, the conditioned stimulus is capable to induce a fear responses like a freezing posture, a startle reflex and changes in autonomic (increased in heart rate, blood pressure, breathing) and endocrine (increased in corticosterone and adrenaline levels) responses (Davis et al., 1993; Rudy et al., 2004). The fear-potentiated startle is sensitive to drugs like benzodiazepines, barbituric, 5-$HT_{1A}$ receptor agonist and opioids, which are clinically effective as anxiolytics (Davis, 1986; 1990). Also, chronic administration of antidepressant (citalopram and tianeptine) with different mechanism of action, impairs the acquisition of fear response (Burghardt et al., 2004).

## Stress-Induced Hyperthermia

During stressful situation, organisms such as mammals express physiological changes related with the activation of the autonomic nervous system, for instance, an increased blood pressure, tachycardia and hyperthermina (Nakamura, 2015). Thus, stress-induced hyperthermia, or emotional fever, is a short-lasting elevation of the body temperature (±1.0 - 1.5°C) in response to stressful situations. The temperature elevation is related with the organism preparation to affront the stressor by fighting of flighting (Vinkers et al., 2008).

This test was proposed by Borsini et al. (1989). The paradigm consisted on measuring the temperature to 10 or 20 male mice housed in a cage. They measured the rectal temperature of all animals that sequentially were removed from the home cage, then they realized that the last mice that were removed showed higher levels of temperature than the first ones. They also observed that the administration of diazepam and nitrazepam prevented the hyperthermia (Borsini et al., 1989). Actually, some variation of the original model exists. For instance, hyperthermia stress-induced also can be detected by measuring the rectal temperature twice in the same single-animal housed, 60 minutes after an injection (Olivier et al., 2003). Moreover, several stressors can induce hyperthermia like footshocks (2 mA), immobilization, repeated manipulation, repeated temperature measure and injections, but the administration of diazepam and 5-$HT_{1A}$ receptor agonist reduced the hyperthermia to the baseline levels (Van der Heyden et a., 1997). These data indicate that in both model version is present the pharmacologic consistency.

# Genetic Test

## GAD65 Knockout

Along with the study of the neurobiology of anxiety, new knowledge about the target molecules involve in the anxiety process has emerged. In this sense, several genetical models such as GAD65 knockout have been developed. The main inhibitory neurotransmitter of the central nervous system is γ-amino butyryc acid (GABA). Glutamate is the amino acid precursor of GABA, which is decarboxylated by two isoenzymes of glutamic acid decarboxylase, GAD65 and GAD67 (Müller et al., 2015). Although these isoenzymes are co-expressed in GABAergic neurons, co-expression levels are differnt depending on the region in the brain and among cells. In fact, (GAD)65 is more related with the metabolic needs of the cells and also with GABA levels during postnatal stage (Kaufman et al., 1991). Then, mice with a disruption in (GAD)65 gene tend to show high levels of anxiety in open field test and elevated zero maze (Kash et al., 1999) and disrupt the conditioned stress response (Müller et al., 2015; Stork et al., 2003).

## 5-$HT_{1A}$ Knockout

Serotonergic system, especially the 5-$HT_{1A}$ receptor is implicated in anxiety. Partial agonist and full agonist of the 5-$HT_{1A}$ receptor have and anxiolytic effect (Celada et al., 2013). 5-$HT_{1A}$ receptor-mutant mice presented anxiety-like behaviors evaluated in open field test, elevated-zero maze, novel-object assays and novelty suppress feeding task (Gross et al.,

2000; Heisler et al., 1998; Ramboz et al., 1998). Also, these animals showed an increase of autonomic responses such as body temperature and heart rate (Gross et al., 2000; Oliviert et al., 2001). These data indicated that 5-$HT_{1A}$ receptor is involved in many of the core symptoms of anxiety becoming in a useful model with face and construct validity.

## Conclusion

Fear and anxiety are emotional mechanisms highly conserved to adapt and respond to dangerous situations. A disruption in this response could lead to an excessive fear and bad strategies to affronted aversive events that could interfere with daily life. Certainly, animal model is a useful tool to study the neurobiology of anxiety disorders and develop potencial new drugs with anxiolytic activity. Nevertheless, the interpretation of the preclinical data must be accompanied with psychiatric and psychological studies in order to have a hallmark of the neurophysiology dysfunction in anxiety disorders. Herein, we proved plenty grouped information of the basis to better undesrtand the neurochesmistry of this neuropsychopatology. It appears that new directions are focusing in studiying genetic and epigenetic factors, traumatic events during different stages of life that lead to be more vulnerable to suffer anxiety disorders, and this will be required refinement in the techniques and in the criteria validation.

## References

Albelda, Noa, and Daphna Joel. 2012. "Animal Models of Obsessive-Compulsive Disorder: Exploring Pharmacology and Neural Substrates." *Neuroscience & Biobehavioral Reviews* 36 (1): 47–63. https://doi.org/10.1016/j.neubiorev.2011.04.006.

American Psychiatric Association., 2013. *Diagnostic and statistical manual of mental disorders*, 5th ed. Arlington, Virginia.

Andersen, Inger Lise, Knut Egil Bøe, Gry Fœrevik, Andrew M Janczak, and Morten Bakken. 2000. "Behavioural Evaluation of Methods for Assessing Fear Responses in Weaned Pigs." *Applied Animal Behaviour Science* 69 (3): 227–40. https://doi.org/10.1016/S0168-1591(00)00133-7.

Bandelow, Borwin, and Sophie Michaelis. 2015. "Epidemiology of Anxiety Disorders in the 21st Century." *Dialogues in Clinical Neuroscience* 17 (3): 327–35.

Banqueri, María, Marta Méndez, and Jorge L. Arias. 2017. "Behavioral Effects in Adolescence and Early Adulthood in Two Length Models of Maternal Separation in Male Rats." *Behavioural Brain Research* 324 (May): 77–86. https://doi.org/10.1016/j.bbr.2017.02.006.

Belovicova, Kristina, Eszter Bogi, Kristina Csatlosova, and Michal Dubovicky. 2017. "Animal Tests for Anxiety-like and Depression-like Behavior in Rats." *Interdisciplinary Toxicology* 10 (1): 40–43. https://doi.org/10.1515/intox-2017-0006.

Barrett, J. E., and K. E. Vanover. 1993. "5-HT Receptors as Targets for the Development of Novel Anxiolytic Drugs: Models, Mechanisms and Future Directions." *Psychopharmacology* 112 (1): 1–12. 10.1007/BF02247357

Belzung, Catherine, and Maël Lemoine. 2011. "Criteria of Validity for Animal Models of Psychiatric Disorders: Focus on Anxiety Disorders and Depression." *Biology of Mood & Anxiety Disorders* 1 (1): 9. https://doi.org/10.1186/2045-5380-1-9. 10.1186/2045-5380-1-9.

Borsini, F., A. Lecci, G. Volterra, and A. Meli. 1989. "A Model to Measure Anticipatory Anxiety in Mice?" *Psychopharmacology* 98 (2): 207–11. https://doi.org/10.1007/BF00444693.

Bourin, Michel, and Martine Hascoët. 2003. "The Mouse Light/Dark Box Test." *European Journal of Pharmacology* 463 (1–3): 55–65. https://doi.org/10.1016/S0014-2999(03)01274-3.

Bourin, Michel. 2015. "Animal Models for Screening Anxiolytic-like Drugs: A Perspective." *Dialogues in Clinical Neuroscience* 17 (3): 295–303.

Britton, K. T., J. Morgan, J. Rivier, W. Vale, and G. F. Koob. 1985. "Chlordiazepoxide Attenuates Response Suppression Induced by Corticotropin-Releasing Factor in the Conflict Test." *Psychopharmacology* 86 (1–2): 170–74. https://doi.org/10.1007/BF00431704.

Burghardt, Nesha S., Gregory M. Sullivan, Bruce S. McEwen, Jack M. Gorman, and Joseph E. LeDoux. 2004. "The Selective Serotonin Reuptake Inhibitor Citalopram Increases Fear after Acute Treatment but Reduces Fear with Chronic Treatment: A Comparison with Tianeptine." *Biological Psychiatry* 55 (12): 1171–78. https://doi.org/10.1016/j.biopsych.2004.02.029.

Campos, Alline C., Manoela V. Fogaca, Daniele C. Aguiar, and Francisco S. Guimaraes. 2013. "Animal Models of Anxiety Disorders and Stress." *Revista Brasileira de Psiquiatria* 35 (suppl 2): S101–11. https://doi.org/10.1590/1516-4446-2013-1139.

Carobrez, A. P., and L. J. Bertoglio. 2005. "Ethological and Temporal Analyses of Anxiety-like Behavior: The Elevated plus-Maze Model 20 Years On." *Neuroscience & Biobehavioral Reviews* 29 (8): 1193–1205. https://doi.org/10.1016/j.neubiorev.2005.04.017.

Castanheira, Lígia, Miguel F. Ferreira, Ana M. Sebastião, and Diogo Telles-Correia. 2018. "Anxiety Assessment in Pre-Clinical Tests and in Clinical Trials: A Critical Review." *Current Topics in Medicinal Chemistry* 18 (19): 1656–76. https://doi.org/10.2174/1568026618666181115102518.

Celada, Pau, Analía Bortolozzi, and Francesc Artigas. 2013. "Serotonin 5-HT1A Receptors as Targets for Agents to Treat Psychiatric Disorders: Rationale and Current Status of Research." *CNS Drugs* 27 (9): 703–16. https://doi.org/10.1007/s40263-013-0071-0.

Corda, Maria G., Maria A. Piludu, Francesco Sanna, Giovanna Piras, Marianna Boi, Fabrizio Sanna, Alberto Fernández Teruel, and Osvaldo Giorgi. 2018. "The Roman High- and Low-Avoidance Rats Differ in the Sensitivity to Shock-Induced Suppression of Drinking and to the Anxiogenic Effect of Pentylenetetrazole." *Pharmacology Biochemistry and Behavior* 167 (April): 29–35. https://doi.org/10.1016/j.pbb.2018.02.004.

Cueto-Escobedo, Jonathan, Carlos M. Contreras, Blandina Bernal-Morales, Gabriel Guillén-Ruiz, and Juan F. Rodríguez-Landa. 2013. "Defensive Burying Test in Postweaning Rats: Use of a Small Round Chamber." *Behavioural Pharmacology* 24 (8): 693–98. https://doi.org/10.1097/FBP.0000000000000008.

Davis, M. 1986. "Pharmacological and Anatomical Analysis of Fear Conditioning Using the Fear-Potentiated Startle Paradigm." *Behavioral Neuroscience* 100 (6): 814–24. http://dx.doi.org/10.1037/0735-7044.100.6.814.

Davis, M. 1990. "Animal Models of Anxiety Based on Classical Conditioning: The Conditioned Emotional Response (CER) and the Fear-Potentiated Startle Effect." *Pharmacology & Therapeutics* 47 (2): 147–65. https://doi.org/10.1016/0163-7258(90)90084-F.

Davis, M., W. A. Falls, S. Campeau, and M. Kim. 1993. "Fear-Potentiated Startle: A Neural and Pharmacological Analysis." *Behavioural Brain Research* 58 (1–2): 175–98.

Davis, M, David L Walker, Leigh Miles, and Christian Grillon. 2010. "Phasic vs Sustained Fear in Rats and Humans: Role of the Extended Amygdala in Fear vs Anxiety." *Neuropsychopharmacology* 35 (1): 105–35. https://doi.org/10.1038/npp.2009.109.

De Boer, Sietse F., and Jaap M. Koolhaas. 2003. "Defensive Burying in Rodents: Ethology, Neurobiology and Psychopharmacology." *European Journal of Pharmacology* 463 (1–3): 145–61. https://doi.org/10.1016/S0014-2999(03)01278-0.

de Brouwer, Geoffrey de, and De Wet Wolmarans. 2018. "Back to Basics: A Methodological Perspective on Marble-Burying Behavior as a Screening Test for Psychiatric Illness." *Behavioural Processes* 157 (December): 590–600. https://doi.org/10.1016/j.beproc.2018.04.011.

De Jesús-Burgos, María I., Stephanie González-García, Yanira Cruz-Santa, and Nivia L. Pérez-Acevedo. 2016. "Amygdalar Activation of Group I Metabotropic Glutamate Receptors Produces Anti- and pro-Conflict Effects Depending upon Animal Sex in a Sexually Dimorphic

Conditioned Conflict-Based Anxiety Model." *Behavioural Brain Research* 302 (April): 200–212. https://doi.org/10.1016/j.bbr.2016.01.009.

Demyttenaere, Koen, Ronny Bruffaerts, Jose Posada-Villa, Isabelle Gasquet, Viviane Kovess, Jean Pierre Lepine, Matthias C. Angermeyer, et al. 2004. "Prevalence, Severity, and Unmet Need for Treatment of Mental Disorders in the World Health Organization World Mental Health Surveys." *JAMA* 291 (21): 2581–90. https://doi.org/10.1001/jama.291.21.2581.

Ennaceur, Abdelkader, and Paul L. Chazot. 2016. "Preclinical Animal Anxiety Research - Flaws and Prejudices." *Pharmacology Research & Perspectives* 4 (2): e00223. https://doi.org/10.1002/prp2.223.

Farach, Frank J., Larry D. Pruitt, Janie J. Jun, Alissa B. Jerud, Lori A. Zoellner, and Peter P. Roy-Byrne. 2012. "Pharmacological Treatment of Anxiety Disorders: Current Treatments and Future Directions." *Journal of Anxiety Disorders* 26 (8): 833–43. https://doi.org/10.1016/j.janxdis.2012.07.009.

Franco, Nuno Henrique. 2013. "Animal Experiments in Biomedical Research: A Historical Perspective." *Animals : An Open Access Journal from MDPI* 3 (1): 238–73. https://doi.org/10.3390/ani3010238

Fuchs, Eberhard, and Gabriele Flügge. 2006. "Experimental Animal Models for the Simulation of Depression and Anxiety." *Dialogues in Clinical Neuroscience* 8 (3): 323–33.

Fucich, Elizabeth, and David Morilak. 2018. "Shock-Probe Defensive Burying Test to Measure Active versus Passive Coping Style in Response to an Aversive Stimulus in Rats." *BIO-PROTOCOL* 8 (17). https://doi.org/10.21769/BioProtoc.2998.

Ganella, Despina E, and Jee Hyun Kim. 2014. "Developmental Rodent Models of Fear and Anxiety: From Neurobiology to Pharmacology: Pharmacological Studies in Developmental Anxiety." *British Journal of Pharmacology* 171 (20): 4556–74. https://doi.org/10.1111/bph.12643.

Geller, Irving, John T. Kulak, and Joseph Seifter. 1962. "The Effects of Chlordiazepoxide and Chlorpromazine on a Punishment

Discrimination." *Psychopharmacologia* 3 (5): 374–85. https://doi.org/10.1007/BF00408322.

Griebel, G. 1995. "5-Hydroxytryptamine-Interacting Drugs in Animal Models of Anxiety Disorders: More than 30 Years of Research." *Pharmacology & Therapeutics* 65 (3): 319–95. https://doi.org/10.1016/0163-7258(95)98597-J.

Gross, Cornelius, Luca Santarelli, Dani Brunner, Xiaoxi Zhuang, and René Hen. 2000. "Altered Fear Circuits in 5-HT1A Receptor KO Mice." *Biological Psychiatry* 48 (12): 1157–63. https://doi.org/10.1016/S0006-3223(00)01041-6.

Hamed, Adam, Tomasz Jaroszewski, Piotr Maciejak, Janusz Szyndler, Małgorzata Lehner, Ita Kamecka, Mieszko Olczak, Urszula Kuzinska, Ewa Taracha, and Adam Płaźnik. 2009. "The Effects of Buspirone and Diazepam on Aversive Context- and Social Isolation-Induced Ultrasonic Vocalisation." *Physiology & Behavior* 98 (4): 474–80. https://doi.org/10.1016/j.physbeh.2009.07.013.

Heisler, L. K., H. M. Chu, T. J. Brennan, J. A. Danao, P. Bajwa, L. H. Parsons, and L. H. Tecott. 1998. "Elevated Anxiety and Antidepressant-like Responses in Serotonin 5-HT1A Receptor Mutant Mice." *Proceedings of the National Academy of Sciences of the United States of America* 95 (25): 15049–54. https://doi.org/10.1073/pnas.95.25.15049.

Hogg, Sandy. 1996. "A Review of the Validity and Variability of the Elevated Plus-Maze as an Animal Model of Anxiety." *Pharmacology Biochemistry and Behavior* 54 (1): 21–30. https://doi.org/10.1016/0091-3057(95)02126-4.

Kash, S. F., L. H. Tecott, C. Hodge, and S. Baekkeskov. 1999. "Increased Anxiety and Altered Responses to Anxiolytics in Mice Deficient in the 65-KDa Isoform of Glutamic Acid Decarboxylase." *Proceedings of the National Academy of Sciences of the United States of America* 96 (4): 1698–1703. https://doi.org/10.1073/pnas.96.4.1698.

Kaufman, D. L., C. R. Houser, and A. J. Tobin. 1991. "Two Forms of the Gamma-Aminobutyric Acid Synthetic Enzyme Glutamate Decarboxylase Have Distinct Intraneuronal Distributions and Cofactor

Interactions." *Journal of Neurochemistry* 56 (2): 720–23. https://doi.org/10.1111/j.1471-4159.1991.tb08211.x.

Keenan, Ryan J., Jacky Chan, Paul S. Donnelly, Kevin J. Barnham, and Laura H. Jacobson. 2018. "The Social Defeat/Overcrowding Murine Psychosocial Stress Model Results in a Pharmacologically Reversible Body Weight Gain but Not Depression - Related Behaviours." *Neurobiology of Stress* 9 (November): 176–87. https://doi.org/10.1016/j.ynstr.2018.09.008.

Kessler, Ronald C., Ayelet Meron Ruscio, Katherine Shear, and Hans-Ulrich Wittchen. 2010. "Epidemiology of Anxiety Disorders." *Current Topics in Behavioral Neurosciences* 2: 21–35. 10.1007/7854_2009_9.

Koe, A S, A Ashokan, and R Mitra. 2016. "Short Environmental Enrichment in Adulthood Reverses Anxiety and Basolateral Amygdala Hypertrophy Induced by Maternal Separation." *Translational Psychiatry* 6 (2): e729–e729. https://doi.org/10.1038/tp.2015.217.

Korte, S. Mechiel, and Sietse F. De Boer. 2003. "A Robust Animal Model of State Anxiety: Fear-Potentiated Behaviour in the Elevated plus-Maze." *European Journal of Pharmacology* 463 (1–3): 163–75. https://doi.org/10.1016/s0014-2999(03)01279-2.

Kulesskaya, Natalia, and Vootele Voikar. 2014. "Assessment of Mouse Anxiety-like Behavior in the Light–Dark Box and Open-Field Arena: Role of Equipment and Procedure." *Physiology & Behavior* 133 (June): 30–38. https://doi.org/10.1016/j.physbeh.2014.05.006.

Kumar, Vijender, Zulfiqar Ali Bhat, and Dinesh Kumar. 2013. "Animal Models of Anxiety: A Comprehensive Review." *Journal of Pharmacological and Toxicological Methods* 68 (2): 175–83. https://doi.org/10.1016/j.vascn.2013.05.003.

Kuniishi, Hiroshi, Satoshi Ichisaka, Miki Yamamoto, Natsuko Ikubo, Sae Matsuda, Eri Futora, Riho Harada, Kohei Ishihara, and Yoshio Hata. 2017. "Early Deprivation Increases High-Leaning Behavior, a Novel Anxiety-like Behavior, in the Open Field Test in Rats." *Neuroscience Research* 123 (October): 27–35. https://doi.org/10.1016/j.neures.2017.04.012.

Lamontagne, Steven J., Mary C. Olmstead, and Janet L. Menard. 2016. "The Lateral Septum and Anterior Hypothalamus Act in Tandem to Regulate Burying in the Shock-Probe Test but Not Open-Arm Avoidance in the Elevated plus-Maze." *Behavioural Brain Research* 314 (November): 16–20. https://doi.org/10.1016/j.bbr.2016.07.034.

Lapiz-Bluhm, M. D. S., C. O. Bondi, J. Doyen, G. A. Rodriguez, T. Bédard-Arana, and D. A. Morilak. 2008. "Behavioural Assays to Model Cognitive and Affective Dimensions of Depression and Anxiety in Rats." *Journal of Neuroendocrinology* 20 (10): 1115–37. https://doi.org/10.1111/j.1365-2826.2008.01772.x.

LeDoux, Joseph E., and Daniel S. Pine. 2016. "Using Neuroscience to Help Understand Fear and Anxiety: A Two-System Framework." *American Journal of Psychiatry* 173 (11): 1083–93. https://doi.org/10.1176/appi.ajp.2016.16030353.

Lightowler, S., G. A. Kennett, I. J. R. Williamson, T. P. Blackburn, and I. F. Tulloch. 1994. "Anxiolytic-like Effect of Paroxetine in a Rat Social Interaction Test." *Pharmacology Biochemistry and Behavior* 49 (2): 281–85. https://doi.org/10.1016/0091-3057(94)90422-7.

Mathiasen, L., and N. R. Mirza. 2005. "A Comparison of Chlordiazepoxide, Bretazenil, L838,417 and Zolpidem in a Validated Mouse Vogel Conflict Test." *Psychopharmacology* 182 (4): 475–84. https://doi.org/10.1007/s00213-005-0119-z.

McGregor, N. W., J. J. Dimatelis, P. J. Van Zyl, S. M. J. Hemmings, C. Kinnear, V. A. Russell, D. J. Stein, and C. Lochner. 2018. "A Translational Approach to the Genetics of Anxiety Disorders." *Behavioural Brain Research* 341 (April): 91–97. https://doi.org/10.1016/j.bbr.2017.12.030.

McKinney, W. T., and W. E. Bunney. 1969. "Animal Model of Depression. I. Review of Evidence: Implications for Research." *Archives of General Psychiatry* 21 (2): 240–48. 10.1001/archpsyc.1969.01740200112015

Müller, Iris, Gürsel Çalışkan, and Oliver Stork. 2015. "The GAD65 Knock out Mouse - a Model for GABAergic Processes in Fear- and Stress-Induced Psychopathology." *Genes, Brain, and Behavior* 14 (1): 37–45. https://doi.org/10.1111/gbb.12188.

Nakamura, Kazuhiro. 2015. "Neural Circuit for Psychological Stress-Induced Hyperthermia." *Temperature (Austin, Tex.)* 2 (3): 352–61. https://doi.org/10.1080/23328940.2015.1070944.

Olivier, B., T. Pattij, S. J. Wood, R. Oosting, Z. Sarnyai, and M. Toth. 2001. "The 5-HT(1A) Receptor Knockout Mouse and Anxiety." *Behavioural Pharmacology* 12 (6–7): 439–50.

Olivier, Berend, Theo Zethof, Tommy Pattij, Meg van Boogaert, Ruud van Oorschot, Christina Leahy, Ronald Oosting, et al. 2003. "Stress-Induced Hyperthermia and Anxiety: Pharmacological Validation." *European Journal of Pharmacology* 463 (1–3): 117–32. https://doi.org/10.1016/s0014-2999(03)01326-8.

Orso, Rodrigo, Luis Eduardo Wearick-Silva, Kerstin Camile Creutzberg, Anderson Centeno-Silva, Laura Glusman Roithmann, Rafaelly Pazzin, Saulo Gantes Tractenberg, Fernando Benetti, and Rodrigo Grassi-Oliveira. 2018. "Maternal Behavior of the Mouse Dam toward Pups: Implications for Maternal Separation Model of Early Life Stress." *Stress* 21 (1): 19–27. https://doi.org/10.1080/10253890.2017.1389883.

Otto, Michael W., R. Kathryn McHugh, Naomi M. Simon, Frank J. Farach, John J. Worthington, and Mark H. Pollack. 2010. "Efficacy of CBT for Benzodiazepine Discontinuation in Patients with Panic Disorder: Further Evaluation." *Behaviour Research and Therapy* 48 (8): 720–27. https://doi.org/10.1016/j.brat.2010.04.002.

Padurariu, Manuela, Iulia Antioch, Ioana Balmus, Alin Ciobica, Heba S. El-Lethey, and Mervat M. Kamel. 2017. "Describing Some Behavioural Animal Models of Anxiety and Their Mechanistics with Special Reference to Oxidative Stress and Oxytocin Relevance." *International Journal of Veterinary Science and Medicine* 5 (2): 98–104. https://doi.org/10.1016/j.ijvsm.2017.08.003.

Picazo, O., and A. Fernández-Guasti. 1998. "Antianxiety Effects of Diazepam and Buspirone in Rats under Different Hormonal Status." *Proceedings of the Western Pharmacology Society* 41: 205–6.

Prut, Laetitia, and Catherine Belzung. 2003. "The Open Field as a Paradigm to Measure the Effects of Drugs on Anxiety-like Behaviors: A Review."

*European Journal of Pharmacology* 463 (1–3): 3–33. https://doi.org/10.1016/s0014-2999(03)01272-x.

Ramboz, S., R. Oosting, D. A. Amara, H. F. Kung, P. Blier, M. Mendelsohn, J. J. Mann, D. Brunner, and R. Hen. 1998. "Serotonin Receptor 1A Knockout: An Animal Model of Anxiety-Related Disorder." *Proceedings of the National Academy of Sciences of the United States of America* 95 (24): 14476–81. https://doi.org/10.1073/pnas.95.24.14476.

Ravindran, Lakshmi N., and Murray B. Stein. 2010. "The Pharmacologic Treatment of Anxiety Disorders: A Review of Progress." *The Journal of Clinical Psychiatry* 71 (7): 839–54. https://doi.org/10.4088/JCP.10r06218blu.

Resstel, L. B. M., R. F. Souza, and F. S. Guimarães. 2008. "Anxiolytic-like Effects Induced by Medial Prefrontal Cortex Inhibition in Rats Submitted to the Vogel Conflict Test." *Physiology & Behavior* 93 (1–2): 200–205. https://doi.org/10.1016/j.physbeh.2007.08.009.

Rodgers, R. J. 1997. "Animal Models of 'Anxiety': Where Next?" *Behavioural Pharmacology* 8 (6–7): 477–96; discussion 497-504. http://dx.doi.org/10.1097/00008877-199711000-00003.

Rodríguez-Landa, Juan Francisco, Fabiola Hernández-López, Jonathan Cueto-Escobedo, Emma Virginia Herrera-Huerta, Eduardo Rivadeneyra-Domínguez, Blandina Bernal-Morales, and Elizabeth Romero-Avendaño. 2019. "Chrysin (5,7-Dihydroxyflavone) Exerts Anxiolytic-like Effects through GABAA Receptors in a Surgical Menopause Model in Rats." *Biomedicine & Pharmacotherapy* 109 (January): 2387–95. https://doi.org/10.1016/j.biopha.2018.11.111.

Rodríguez-Landa, Juan Francisco, Rosa Isela García-Ríos, Jonathan Cueto-Escobedo, Blandina Bernal-Morales, and Carlos M. Contreras. 2013. "Participation of GABA A Chloride Channels in the Anxiolytic-Like Effects of a Fatty Acid Mixture." *BioMed Research International* 2013: 1–7. https://doi.org/10.1155/2013/121794.

Rudy, J. W., N. C. Huff, and P. Matus-Amat. 2004. "Understanding Contextual Fear Conditioning: Insights from a Two-Process Model."

*Neuroscience and Biobehavioral Reviews* 28 (7): 675–85. https://doi.org/10.1016/j.neubiorev.2004.09.004.

Sampedro-Piquero, P., E. Castilla-Ortega, C. Zancada-Menendez, L. J. Santín, and A. Begega. 2016. "Environmental Enrichment as a Therapeutic Avenue for Anxiety in Aged Wistar Rats: Effect on Cat Odor Exposition and GABAergic Interneurons." *Neuroscience* 330 (August): 17–25. https://doi.org/10.1016/j.neuroscience.2016.05.032.

Seetharaman, Shyam, Monika Fleshner, Collin R. Park, and David M. Diamond. 2016. "Influence of Daily Social Stimulation on Behavioral and Physiological Outcomes in an Animal Model of PTSD." *Brain and Behavior* 6 (5). https://doi.org/10.1002/brb3.458.

Shekhar, A., U. D. McCann, M. J. Meaney, D. C. Blanchard, M. Davis, K. A. Frey, I. Liberzon, et al. 2001. "Summary of a National Institute of Mental Health Workshop: Developing Animal Models of Anxiety Disorders." *Psychopharmacology* 157 (4): 327–39. https://doi.org/10.1007/s002130100859.

Shin, Sang Yep, Nam Jun Baek, Seung Ho Han, and Sun Seek Min. 2019. "Chronic Administration of Ketamine Ameliorates the Anxiety- and Aggressive-like Behavior in Adolescent Mice Induced by Neonatal Maternal Separation." *The Korean Journal of Physiology & Pharmacology* 23 (1): 81. https://doi.org/10.4196/kjpp.2019.23.1.81.

Shimada, T., K. Matsumoto, M. Osanai, H. Matsuda, K. Terasawa, and H. Watanabe. 1995. "The Modified Light/Dark Transition Test in Mice: Evaluation of Classic and Putative Anxiolytic and Anxiogenic Drugs." *General Pharmacology* 26 (1): 205–10. https://doi.org/10.1016/0306-3623(94)00148-G.

Shimizu, H., Y. Kumasaka, H. Tanaka, A. Hirose, and M. Nakamura. 1992. "Anticonflict Action of Tandospirone in a Modified Geller-Seifter Conflict Test in Rats." *Japanese Journal of Pharmacology* 58 (3): 283–89. 10.1254/jjp.58.283.

Silverstone, Peter H., and Eliseo Salinas. 2001. "Efficacy of Venlafaxine Extended Release in Patients With Major Depressive Disorder and Comorbid Generalized Anxiety Disorder." *The Journal of Clinical Psychiatry* 62 (7): 523–29. http://dx.doi.org/10.4088/JCP.v62n07a04.

Steele, Floyd F., Shannon C. Whitehouse, Jacob S. Aday, and Adam J. Prus. 2017. "Neurotensin NTS 1 and NTS 2 Receptor Agonists Produce Anxiolytic-like Effects in the 22-KHz Ultrasonic Vocalization Model in Rats." *Brain Research* 1658 (March): 31–35. https://doi.org/10.1016/j.brainres.2017.01.012.

Steimer, Thierry. 2011. "Animal Models of Anxiety Disorders in Rats and Mice: Some Conceptual Issues." *Dialogues in Clinical Neuroscience* 13 (4): 495–506.

Stork, O., H. Yamanaka, S. Stork, N. Kume, and K. Obata. 2003. "Altered Conditioned Fear Behavior in Glutamate Decarboxylase 65 Null Mutant Mice." *Genes, Brain, and Behavior* 2 (2): 65–70. https://doi.org/10.1034/j.1601-183X.2003.00008.x.

Sturman, Oliver, Pierre-Luc Germain, and Johannes Bohacek. 2018. "Exploratory Rearing: A Context- and Stress-Sensitive Behavior Recorded in the Open-Field Test." *Stress* 21 (5): 443–52. https://doi.org/10.1080/10253890.2018.1438405.

Tan, Shawn, Hin San Ho, Anna Yoonsu Song, Joey Low, and Hyunsoo Shawn Je. 2017. "Maternal Separation Does Not Produce a Significant Behavioral Change in Mice." *Experimental Neurobiology* 26 (6): 390. https://doi.org/10.5607/en.2017.26.6.390.

Toth, Iulia, and Inga D. Neumann. 2013. "Animal Models of Social Avoidance and Social Fear." *Cell and Tissue Research* 354 (1): 107–18. https://doi.org/10.1007/s00441-013-1636-4.

Trujillo, Verónica, Patricia E. Durando, and Marta M. Suárez. 2016. "Maternal Separation in Early Life Modifies Anxious Behavior and Fos and Glucocorticoid Receptor Expression in Limbic Neurons after Chronic Stress in Rats: Effects of Tianeptine." *Stress* 19 (1): 91–103. https://doi.org/10.3109/10253890.2015.1105958.

Valvassori, Samira S., Josiane Budni, Roger B. Varela, and João Quevedo. 2013. "Contributions of Animal Models to the Study of Mood Disorders." *Revista Brasileira De Psiquiatria (Sao Paulo, Brazil: 1999)* 35 Suppl 2: S121-131. https://doi.org/10.1590/1516-4446-2013-1168. 10.1590/1516-4446-2013-1168.

Van der Heyden, J. A., T. J. Zethof, and B. Olivier. 1997. "Stress-Induced Hyperthermia in Singly Housed Mice." *Physiology & Behavior* 62 (3): 463–70. https://doi.org/10.1016/S0031-9384(97)00157-1.

Vinkers, Christiaan H., Meg J. V. van Bogaert, Marianne Klanker, S. Mechiel Korte, Ronald Oosting, Taleen Hanania, Seth C. Hopkins, Berend Olivier, and Lucianne Groenink. 2008. "Translational Aspects of Pharmacological Research into Anxiety Disorders: The Stress-Induced Hyperthermia (SIH) Paradigm." *European Journal of Pharmacology* 585 (2–3): 407–25. https://doi.org/10.1016/j.ejphar.2008.02.097.

Varga, Zoltán K., Áron Zsigmond, Diána Pejtsik, Máté Varga, Kornél Demeter, Éva Mikics, József Haller, and Manó Aliczki. 2018. "The Swimming Plus-Maze Test: A Novel High-Throughput Model for Assessment of Anxiety-Related Behaviour in Larval and Juvenile Zebrafish (Danio Rerio)." *Scientific Reports* 8 (1). https://doi.org/10.1038/s41598-018-34989-1.

Willner, P. 1984. "The Validity of Animal Models of Depression." *Psychopharmacology* 83 (1): 1–16. https://doi.org/10.1007/BF00427414.

Wilson, Tyler K., and Jayson Tripp. 2019. "Buspirone." In *StatPearls*. Treasure Island (FL): StatPearls Publishing. http://www.ncbi.nlm.nih.gov/books/NBK531477/.

World Health Organization (WHO). 2017. *Depression and Other Common Mental Disorders: Global Health Estimate*. Switzerland.

Zewde, Ashenafi Mebratu, Frances Yu, Sunil Nayak, Christopher Tallarida, Allen B. Reitz, Lynn G. Kirby, and Scott M. Rawls. 2018. "PLDT (Planarian Light/Dark Test): An Invertebrate Assay to Quantify Defensive Responding and Study Anxiety-like Effects." *Journal of Neuroscience Methods* 293 (January): 284–88. https://doi.org/10.1016/j.jneumeth.2017.10.010.

In: Laboratory Animals and Neurosciences ISBN: 978-1-53618-462-4
Editors: B. Hernandez Godinez et al.© 2020 Nova Science Publishers, Inc.

*Chapter 3*

# EFFECTS ON MEMORY, LEARNING AND HISTOLOGICAL ANALYSIS OF MYELIN SHEATHS OF RATS LONG EVANS BLACK INTOXICATED WITH ARSENIC

***Javier Morán Martínez[1,7,*], Omar Zambrano Ortiz[1,7], Alfonso Zambrano Martínez[1,7], Esperanza Calleros Rincón[2], María Del Pilar Carranza Rosales[3], Ruben García Garza[4], Marisela Del Rocio González Martínez[1], Hector Delgado Aguirre[5], Natalia Ortega Morales[6] and Nadia Denys Betancourt Martínez[1,7]***

[1]Departamento de Biología Celular y Ultraestrucutura,
Centro de Investigación Biomédica, Facultad de Medicina,
Universidad Autónoma de Coahuila Unidad Torreón,
Torreón, Coahuila, México

[*] Corresponding Author's E-mail:javmoran@yahoo.com.

[2]Facultad de Ciencias Químicas,
Universidad Juárez del Estado de Durango, Campus Gómez Palacio,
Gómez Palacio, Durango, México
[3]Departamento de Biología Celular y Molecular,
Centro de Investigación Biomédica del Noreste,
Instituto Mexicano del Seguro Social. Monterrey, Nuevo León, México
[4]Departamento de Histología, Facultad de Medicina,
Universidad Autónoma de Coahuila Unidad Torreón,
Torreón, Coahuila, México
[5]Departamento de Investigación,
Unidad Médica de Alta Especialidad,
Instituto Mexicano del Seguro Social. Torreón, Coahuila, México
[6]Universidad Autónoma Agraria Antonio Narro Unidad Laguna
[7]CICUAL, Bioterio Facultad de Medicina,
Universidad Autónoma de Coahuila Campus Torreón, Mexico

## Abstract

At present, several investigations have been carried out to discover the harmful effects of heavy metal exposure, due to the diverse work activities of each region. In the Lagunera Region, located in the north of Mexico, arsenic in the water of all uses is an endemic problem that triggers diverse health problems. Problems that have caught the attention of local, national and international health professionals comparing this situation with other parts of the world. The brain is especially susceptible to arsenic toxicity (As), because it crosses the blood-brain barrier. Exposure to this metal is associated with some neurological complications. It is believed that arsenic neurotoxicity involves oxidative stress, increased reactive oxygen species among others. The objective of this study was to demonstrate the affectations that this metalloid has in the basic cognitive functions such as memory and learning through a model of exposure to arsenic in rats. On the other hand, assessing the effects of As in myelin sheaths in rat brains was another of the priorities of this work. 24 Long Evans rats were used: 8 groups of 3 rats each administering $AsO3$ (sub groups Adults and youth). The classification of the groups and their dosage of As was: G 1: Control; G2: at 0.025mg/L, G3: at 0.050mg/L, G4: at 0.070mg/L. Obtaining brain:

The rats were sacrificed and the brain was immediately removed and 10% neutral formalin was placed. It was processed with the conventional histological technique. The Klüver Barrera technique was used for the study of myelin sheaths. The Morris Water Labyrinth was used to evaluate learning and memory. In the adult and young rats in the G1 no visible alterations were found, in the rest of the groups an apparent decrease in myelin areas could be observed, areas of demyelination were observed in axonal trajectories and vacuolization in the white matter of the cerebellum. On the other hand, in the aquatic labyrinth test no significant differences were found that point to a damage caused by the exposure. Discussion. There are some studies that associate variants of the concentration of As and its effects at the level of the central nervous system. In our study, the concentrations to which the animals were exposed would correspond to the chronic exposure of hydroarsenicism in the Comarca Lagunera (Northern Mexico), in our country, which represents a risk of environmental exposure and public health. Conclusion. Rats exposed to As showed dose-dependent alterations in the cerebellar and cerebellar myelin sheaths.

**Keywords**: arsenic, memory, learning, myelin sheaths, long Evans rats

## INTRODUCTION

Arsenic is an element that is naturally found in the earth's crust, its exposure by various air, earth and mainly water pathways is considered a serious current health problem since it presents acute effects such as abdominal pain, vomiting, diarrhea, numbness of limbs, muscle cramps In the long term, hyperkeratosis occurs in the skin, in addition to being a carcinogen. Currently, its effects on other aspects of human health are still being investigated, such is the case of the ability to learn and remember that they are some of the most important characteristics of the human being. Man can recognize stimuli he has seen before, make associations between them and even orient himself according to the relationships he establishes between stimuli. Most of the animals are also oriented in the space to organize their behaviors in relation to the environment in which they are in each moment. Spatial navigation is important for many of the behavioral repertoires of animals: search for food, parental and reproductive behavior, return to the nest or escape to a safe place. Learning and spatial memory are related to the ability to acquire and retain associations of the characteristics of the environment, which allows the organism to function in space. Spatial memory consists of multiple specialized mechanisms to encode, store and retrieve information about routes, configurations and spatial locations. There are several tests and psychometric tests that have the function and purpose of evaluating intelligence and memory to cite some characteristics. An example of this is Wechsler's scales. However, these have some disadvantages such as socio-cultural deprivation that may have an impact on their results, on the other hand in the case of experimental animals it is not possible to evaluate aspects such as memory with conventional methods, there are tests designed specifically for it, as the aquatic labyrinth of Morris directed to rats and mice, which has the characteristic of isolating the rodent from the olfactory stimulus, so it will only use visual stimuli to locate the platform, translating it into memory.

## Effect of Arsenic on Health

For some years now it has been known that arsenic exposure from water intake is linked to harmful effects on health, it is counted as one of the records studies conducted by Hutchington in 1888 in which they related arsenic in water and some skin lesions such as hyper pigmentation, hyperkeratosis (in the palms of the hands, soles of the foot, thorax as well as in any part of the skin) and skin cancer (Carabantes et al., 2003; Fumal et al., 2005; Watson et al., 2004). Chronic exposure to water and food (Chiou et al., 2001) contaminated with arsenic are causes of liver, lung and bladder skin cancer, in addition to causing toxicity in the intestine and brain (Bashir et al., 2006). As noted (Berbel., et al., 2004) pain in the abdominal area, cardiac arrhythmias, dermatological abnormalities and haematological disorders are some signs of acute poisoning by this metal, in addition they are also attributed alterations in the Central Nervous System (CNS) that include affectations in recent memory, learning and concentration (Chatterjee et al., 2010).

## Arsenite-Induced Neurotoxicity

The brain is especially susceptible to arsenic toxicity, because it easily crosses the blood-brain barrier (Yadav et al., 2010; Brinkel et al., 200). Exposure to this metal is associated with some neurological complications such as problems of memory, lack of concentration, Parkinson's disease, Guillain-Barre syndrome, neuropathy, verbal comprehension, encephalopathy, and peripheral neuropathy (Piao et al., 2005).

It is believed that arsenic neurotoxicity involves oxidative stress with increased reactive oxygen species, lipid peroxides along with decreased superoxide dismutase, and reduced glutathione levels. Arsenic exposure has been reported to alter the metabolism of various neurotransmitters, such as monoamines, acetylcholine, gamma amino butyric acid, and glutamate (Dwivedi et al., 2011). The reduction of monoamines (adrenaline, norepinephrine, dopamine and serotonin) in the striatum, frontal cortex and some areas of the hippocampus. On the other hand, its exposure causes destabilization and disruption of the cytoskeleton framework that leads to axonal degeneration. Arsenic-induced oxidative stress in the brain causes oxidative DNA damage and the death of subsequent brain cells and induces the degeneration of dopaminergic neurons resulting in n symptoms such as Parkinson's (Namgung et al., 2001).

On the other hand, arsenic affects the peripheral nervous system by disrupting the neuroeskeleton and therefore markedly decreases the nerve conduction velocity (NMVC) in the peripheral nerves to cause peripheral neuropathy (Pohl et al., 2011; Vahidnia et al., 2008). Exposure to arsenic and its metabolites of monomethyl arsenic acid and monomethyl arsenic acid suppresses NMDA receptors in the hippocampus, which play a fundamental role in synaptic plasticity, learning and memory, leading to neurobehavioral disorders and cognitive dysfunction (Dwivedi & Flora., 2011).

## Memory and Learning

One of the most important characteristics of the human being is his ability to learn and remember. Man can recognize stimuli he has seen before, make associations between them and even orient himself according to the relationships he establishes between stimuli. There is relatively little research on the effects of As in the intellect of children, one from Mexico (Calderón et al., 2001) and the other in Taiwan (Tsai et al., 2001). However, it is worth mentioning that in both of them a small number of people were evaluated, in addition that when talking about intelligence it should be remembered that there are factors that have a direct impact on their development such as inheritance, access to education, food and of course their social environment (Wang et al., 2007). This can be divided into implicit (non-declarative) which is the result of habits and unconscious abilities given by stimulation or sensitization, and explicit (declarative) in which the information is consciously retained, consists in safeguarding places and facts (Navarrete et al., 2008). Spatial memory consists of multiple factors mainly responsible for encoding the storage and retrieval of vital information regarding space locations. Rodents are capable of carrying out four main forms of navigation related to space tasks (Santín, 2000). Despite the tremendous advance of knowledge in neurosciences, research in human beings is limited, which makes experimental studies with animals essential to understand the different types of cognitive dysfunction (Navarrete et al., 2008).

## Intelligence

Despite current advances in techniques and knowledge in different branches related to neurology, early implementation in human patients is still limited, so experimental studies in animals become important, evaluating in these various types of cognitive functions (Navarrete et al., 2008). Cognition includes the processes of learning and memory and of functionality, in the first it includes spatial or non-spatial learning, associative learning and short and long-term memory, in the second it includes pre-attention processes, in which they discriminate certain external stimuli to concentrate on the most important ones, the alteration of this could favor the appearance of different psychological disorders, on the other hand a process of attention refers to the visual orientation, learned, reflexive attention, habituation and maintained, selective attention or divided (Navarrete et al., 2008). There is evidence that arsenic exposure can affect both growth and intelligence (Rosado et al., 2007; Wang et al., 2007). There are specific studies where the effect highlighted by the research indicates a decrease in the IQ and the long-term memorandum (Parvez et al., 2008; Rocha et al., 2007; Wasserman et al., 2007).

## Morris Water Maze

Mostly animals, like humans, organize their behaviors based on the stimuli that surround them, space navigation plays an important role in them since it is used in the search for breath and behaviors as basic as reproductive until Threat refuge is why memory and learning play such an important role in processing data from our environment and then develop properly in it (Vicens et al., 2003). The MWM (water maze test) by its acronym in English, It was first described in the year 1981, is an open field test in which the rats when submitted to a swim learn to find a platform placed below the Water level (Adelson et al., 2013) It is also one of the major models used for the study of memory in rats and mice, it also has the advantage that it is not required to deprive him of food, drinking water much less some type of electric shock to model behavior (Vicens et al., 2003). Its purpose is to evaluate the learning of the rat/mouse that depends on the brain area known as the hippocampus, as well as short-term and spatial memory (Bromley et al., 2011; Bromley et al., 2011) and among its advantages is the shape of the pool minimizes that the sense of smell can act as a bias in the acquisition of the location of the platform (Block, 1999), it is even used to assess the neuronal effects of Alzheimers (Qing et al., 2008).

# Materials and Methods

The present study was carried out in the facilities of the Laboratory of Cellular Biology and Ultra Structure and the Bioterium of the Faculty of Medicine of the Autonomous University of Coahuila, Campus Torreón, where the evaluation of 24 Long Evans Black male rats was performed, which were submitted at different arsenic poisoning treatments live reagents were provided by the Bioterio of the Faculty of Medicine, of the Autonomous University of Coahuila (Figure 1).

Type of Study: Experimental.

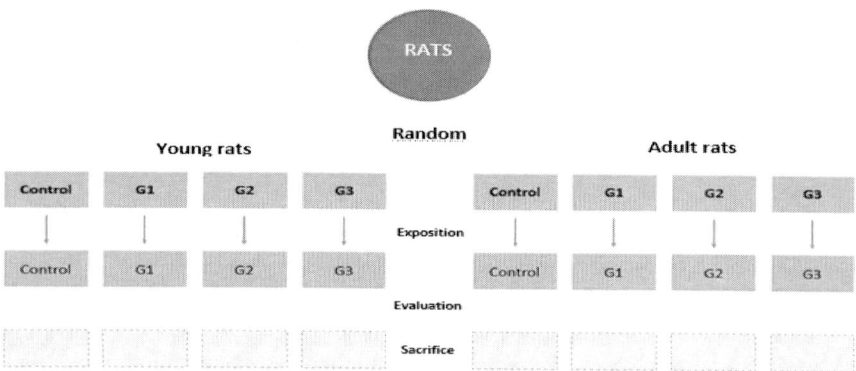


Figure 1. Experimental Model. Shows the experimental strategy in the treated rats.

## Animal in Experimentation

The study included 24 males long evans black rats divided into (8) groups of 3 rats each. The classification of the groups and their dosage of As was as described below.

- Group 1: Healthy adult control
- Group 2: Exposed to 0.025mg/L of $As_2O_3$

- Group 3: Exposed to 0.050 mg/L of $As_2O_3$
- Group 4: Exposed to 0.070 mg/L of $As_2O_3$
- Group 1: Healthy control Weaning
- Group 2: Exposed to 0.025mg/L of $As_2O_3$
- Group 3: Exposed to 0.050 mg/L of $As_2O_3$
- Group 4: Exposed to 0.070 mg/L of $As_2O_3$

## Driving Conditions

Rats in the exposed groups were treated with arsenic trioxide in the drinking water at a rate of 50 mL daily. For one month in adult rats and two months in young rats.

The rats were obtained from the Bioterio of the Faculty of Medicine of the Autonomous University of Coahuila, the rats will adapt in the Bioterio with a stay during a week of cycles of light and dark from 12-12 h at a temperature of 25°C. The rats were fed with rodent food from Purina® with 18% protein and purified water at a rate of 50 mL daily, as marked by Mexican Official Standard NOM-062-ZOO-1999, of technical specifications for production, care and use of laboratory animals (NOM-062-ZOO).

## Ethical Considerations

The present study was presented to the Internal Committee for the Care and Use of Laboratory Animals (CICUAL) of the Torreón unit School of Medicine for proper review and/or approval, in order to proceed to the experimental phase of the same.

## Behavior Tests (Morris Water Maze)

**Table 1. Order of the Morris Labyrinth, North, (N) South, (S), East (E), West (O), Northwest (NO) Northeast (NE), Southwest (SO), Southeast (SE), Center (C)**

| | **Day 1** | | **Day 2** | **Day 3** | **Day 4** | **Day 5** | **Day 6** |
|---|---|---|---|---|---|---|---|
| | Platform location | Starting direction | Platform Location: SW Starting Location as No Platform follows: | | | | |
| Trial 1 | SW | S | W | N | N | E | N |
| Trial 2 | NW | N | S | W | E | S | |
| Trial 3 | NE | S | N | E | W | W | |
| Trial 4 | Center | E | E | W | S | E | |
| Trial 5 | SE | W | S | S | N | N | |

Bromley-Brits (2011).

The Morris Water Maze consists of a pool with water 150cm in diameter and 50cm deep that is divided into four quadrants NW, NE, SW and SE, corresponding to the north, south east and west wind rose, within it is placed a platform that was installed in the different quadrants depending on the day and in a pre-established order. Thus the test consists of three phases, the first with the visible platform of transparent acrylic of 10 cm in diameter above the water level, is taken to the rat and placed at the established starting point trying to submerge the body first, if the tail rat will be taken, it will be stressed, once inside the rat is allowed to swim to find the platform of salvation, it will be given a minute of time, if it fails to find the platform, it will go towards it leaving it 1 minute in the same to identify you. In the second phase where the platform is below the water level, being this time fixed in a specific quadrant, you will also be given a minute to find it and twenty seconds in it before removing it. The third phase removes the platform and will also be granted a minute of swimming, but this time special attention will be given to the record of swimming that you perform in a certain sector. It will be carried out at the rate of four weeks, thus being five consecutive days of the exhibition for two days of rest, the three groups will be submitted before and after (test-retest) of the exposure to the MWM metalloid being this the preferred form of evaluate memory and rodent learning, as shown in Table 1.

## Obtaining Brain

Once exposed to the contaminant and the aquatic labyrinth, the animal was taken to a procedure room, the rats were sacrificed by cervical dislocation, a blood sample was taken by cardiac puncture and immediately the brain was removed, it was placed in containers with formalin 10% neutral, representative samples were collected for further analysis. After fixing, a wash was carried out with the aid of a dehydration train ranging from 60% alcohol to absolute alcohol, then a rinse process with Xilol was carried out according to the conventional method. Once dehydrated and rinsed, it was included with 60°C paraffin that penetrates and surrounds the tissue for hardening. Blocks were formed to be cut to a thickness of 10 micrometers in the Leitz Model 1512 microtome (Austria), and then passed to a flotation bath where the cut extends to be "fish" with a slide previously prepared with a solution of albumin. After the corresponding staining the sections were mounted with synthetic resin and coverslips, leaving them to dry for later analysis by light microscopy.

## Histological Technique

### *Klüver Barrera (Luxol Blue) Technique for the Study of Myelin Sheaths*

The 10-micron cuts were stained with the Kluver-Barrier technique, this is intended to identify myelin sheaths and neuronal bodies in the central nervous system. Staining occurs in the lipoproteins and basic proteins that make up myelin, the proposed mechanism is an acid-base reaction with the formation of a salt; the anionic dye (luxol blue) is attracted to the cationic sites of the tissue so all components are stained while the cationic dye (cresyl violet) remains in solution. After staining, the sections were mounted with synthetic resin and coverslips, and analyzed by light microscopy using a Leitz Model 1512 microtome (Austria).

## Statistical Analysis

A database with Microsoft Excel V2013 of the times obtained in the Morris Aquatic Labyrinth test was created. Descriptive statistics of the variables included in the study were carried out. The KS test was performed to test the normality in the distribution of the data. Nonparametric statistics were used with the Wilcoxon rank test for group comparison. The statistical software SPSS Statistics Base V22.00 was used for the corresponding analysis. Those $p < 0.05$ values with 95% confidence intervals (95% ic, if you are going to put them) were considered significant. For histological cuts, the participation of a Morphologist will be required to observe the differences in the cuts taken compared to the control groups.

# RESULTS

The Kolmogórov-Smirnov test (also K-S test) was found that the data has a non-normal distribution (Figure 2 and Figure 3). Statistical analyzes of the times obtained with respect to the control group before exposure to Arsenic, a median of 2.69 and an IQR of 2.35 were found. In the group 1 corresponding to the 0.025 mg/L dose of $As_2O_3$, it yielded a median of 4.56 and an IQR of 4.34, group 2 obtained a median of 4.40 and an IQR of 4.69 and group three a median of 7.31 and an IQR of 2.19, after the exposure, he again underwent the Morris labyrinth test, finding that the control group had a median of 2.24 and an IQR of 1.05, of group 1 of 2.90 and an IQR of 1.04, of group 2 of 2.66 an IQR 1.50 and group 3 of 2.75 with an IQR of 0.91 (Table 2).

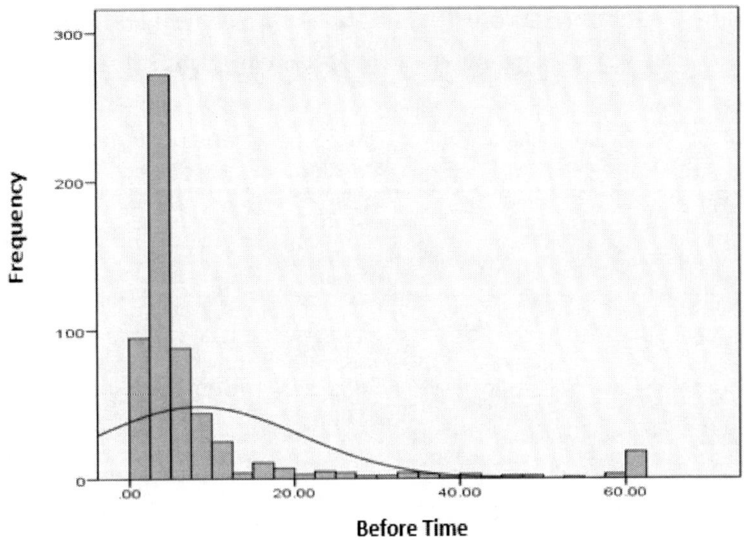


Figure 2. KS test of the time variable before poisoning with As.

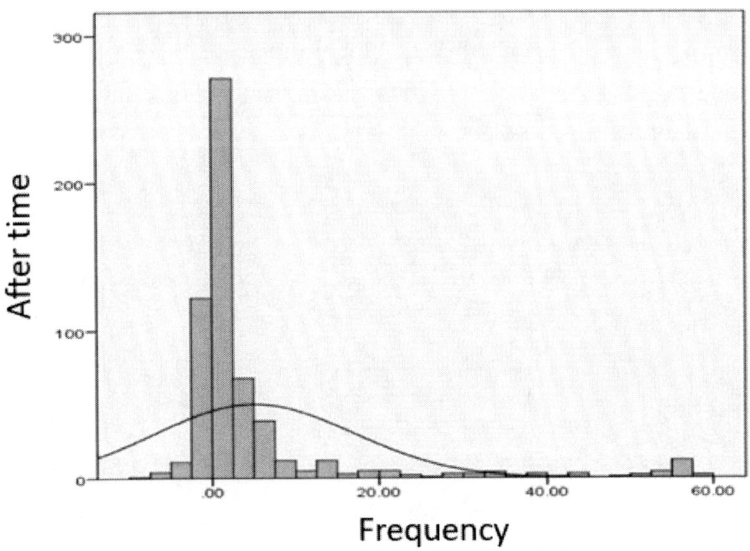


Figure 3. KS test of the variable time after poisoning with As.

**Table 2. Comparison of the times in seconds obtained in the Morris water maze in the adult rat groups**

| ADULT RATS | TIME 1 Before (IQR) | TIME 2 After (IQR) | DIFERENCE (IQR) | p < 0.05 |
|---|---|---|---|---|
| CONTROL | 2.69 (2.35) | 2.34 (1.05) | 0.09 (1.63) | p < 0.05 |
| GROUP 1 | 4.56 (4.34) | 2.90 (1.04) | 0.94 (3.41) | p < 0.05 |
| GROUP 2 | 4.40 (4.69) | 2.66 (1.50) | 1.43 (3.99) | p < 0.05 |
| GROUP 3 | 7.31 (2.19) | 2.75 (0.91) | 0.63 (2.04) | p < 0.05 |

In the Wilcoxon range test it was applied to all groups, obtaining the following results in the group (control) of adult rats (Figure 4) significant differences were found between the measurements before and after the swim time with a p value < 0.005, group 1 of Adult rats (Figure 5) significant differences were found between the measurements before and after the swim time with a p value < 0.005, Group 2 of Adult rats (Figure 6) found significant differences between Measures before and after the swim time with a p value < 0.005, group 3 of Adult rats (Figure 7) significant differences were found between the measurements before and after the swim time with a p value < 0.005.

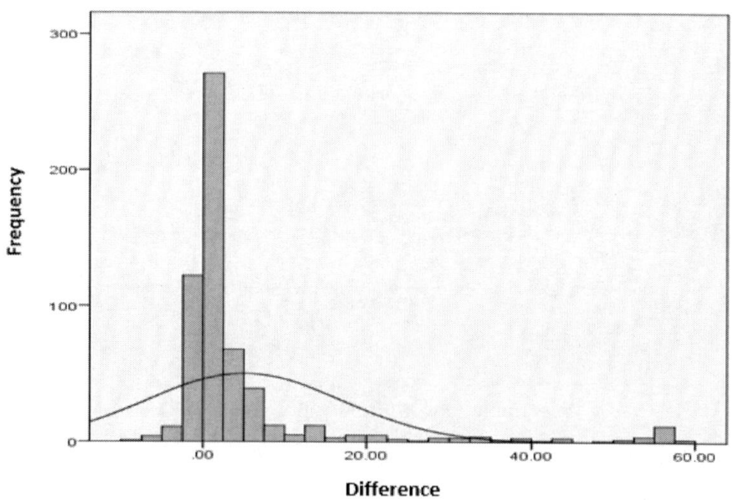

Figure 4. KS test of the time difference variable before As poisoning *vs* time after As poisoning.

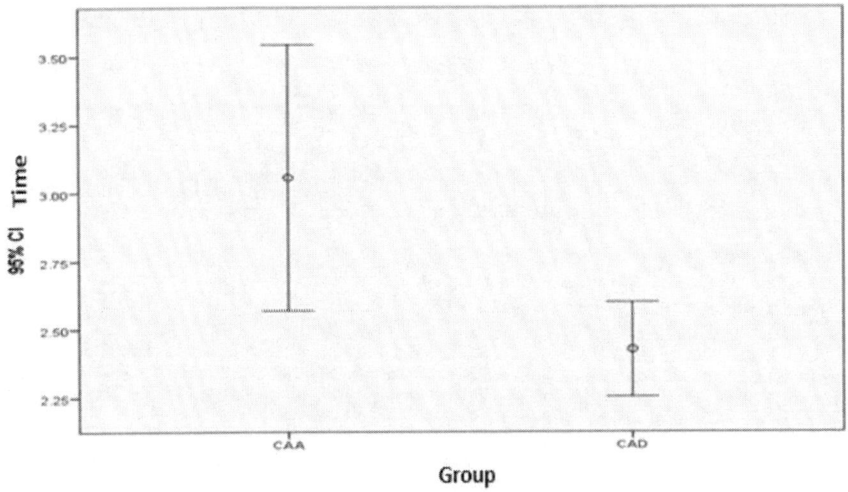


Figure. 5 Adult Control Group Measurement Test - Retest ** $p < 0.01$.

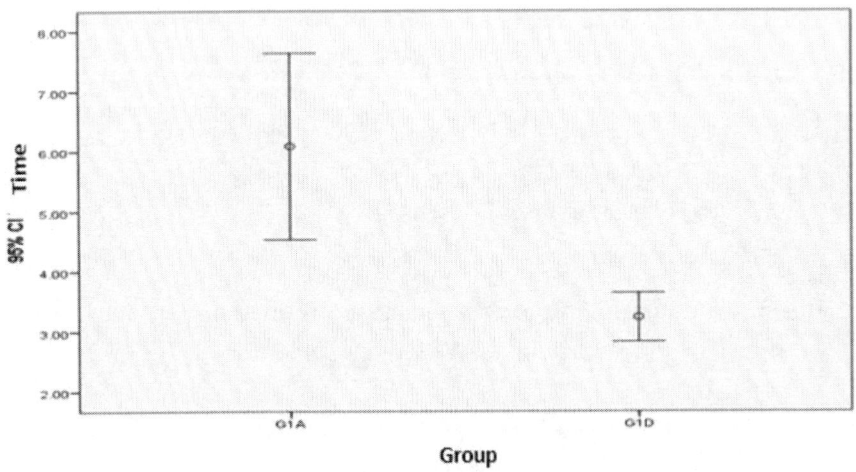


Figure 6. Group 1. Adult rats treated with 0.025mg/L of $As_2O_3$ memory measurement before and after poisoning (4 weeks) ** $p < 0.01$.

Statistical analyzes with respect to the adult control group before exposure to Arsenic, a median of 5.22 and an IQR of 12.03 were found. In the group 1 corresponding to the 0.025 mg/L dose of $As_2O_3$, it showed a median of 4.2 and an IQR of 4.12, group 2 obtained a median of 4.82 and an IQR of 5.28 and group three a median of 4.87 and an IQR of 5.15, after exposure, the Morris labyrinth test was re-tested and the control group found a median of 3.1 and an IQR of 1.32, of group 1 of 3.2 and an IQR of 1.53, of group 2 of 3.2 an IQR 1.59 and group 3 of 3.22 with an IQR of 1.40 (Table 3).

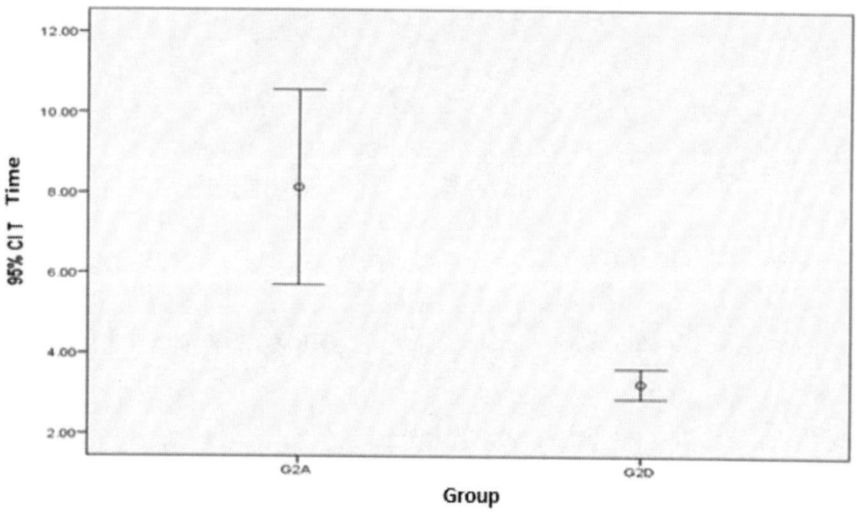


Figure 7. Group 2. Adult Rats Treated with 0.050 mg/l of $As_2O_3$ memory measurement before and after poisoning (4 weeks). ** $p < 0.01$.

**Table 3. Comparison of times in seconds, obtained in the Morris water maze in the Young Rats groups**

| YOUNG RATS | TIME 1 Before (IQR) | TIME 2 After (IQR) | DIFERENCE (IQR) | p < 0.05 |
|---|---|---|---|---|
| CONTROL | 5.22 (12.03) | 3.1 (1.32) | 1.67 (8.82) | p < 0.05 |
| GROUP 1 | 4.2 (4.12) | 3.2 (1.53) | 0.79 (3.96) | p < 0.05 |
| GROUP 2 | 4.82 (5.28) | 3.2 (1.59) | 1.90 (4.75) | p<0.05 |
| GROUP 3 | 4.87 (5.15) | 3.22 (1.40) | 1.27 (5.62) | p<0.05 |

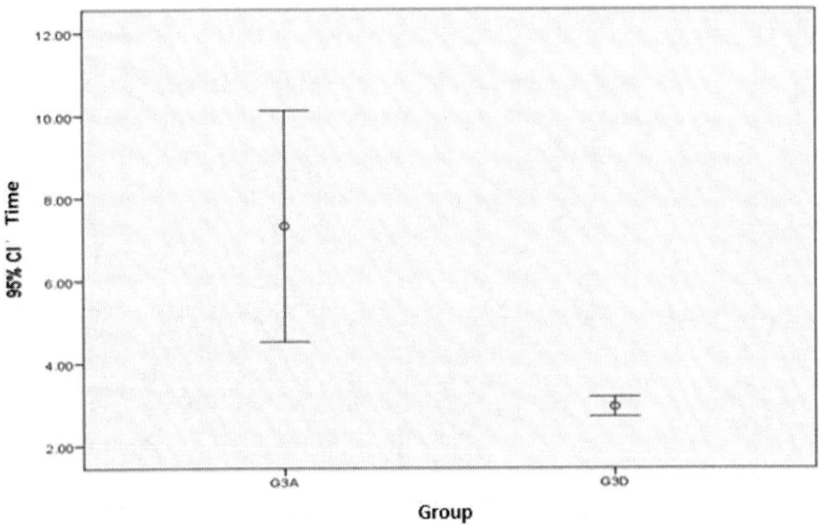


Figure 8. Group 3. Adult Rats Treated with 0.075 mg/L of $As_2O_3$ memory measurement before and after poisoning (4 weeks). ** $p < 0.01$.

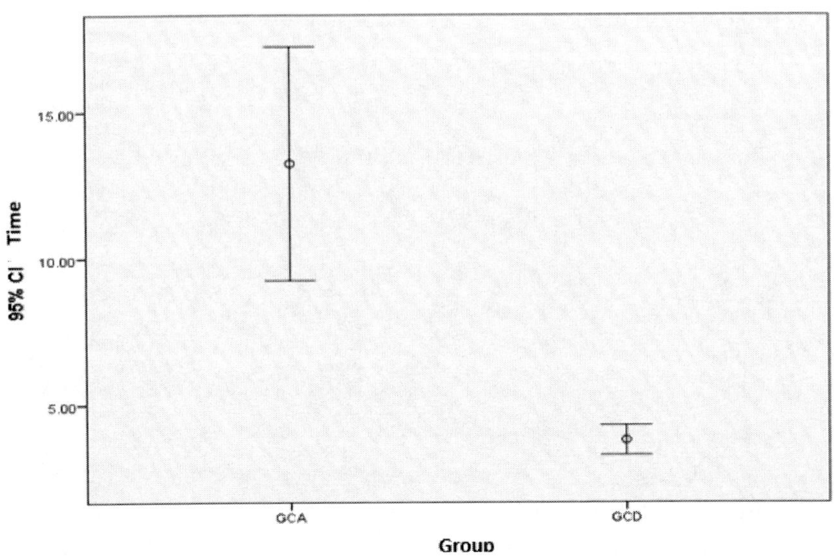


Figure 9. Young Control Group test - retest measurement. ** $p < 0.01$ ks). ** $p < 0.01$.

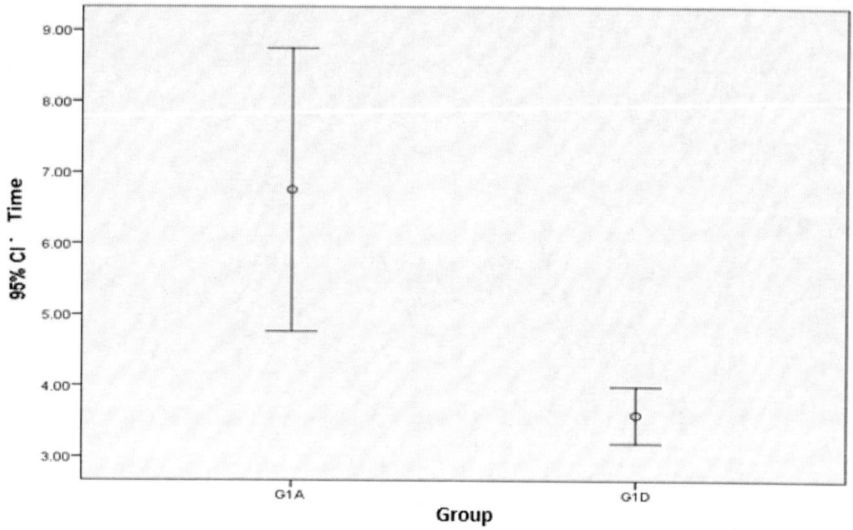


Figure 10. Group 1. Young Rats Treated with 0.025 mg/L of $As_2O_3$ memory measurement before and after poisoning (8 weeks). ** $p < 0.01$.

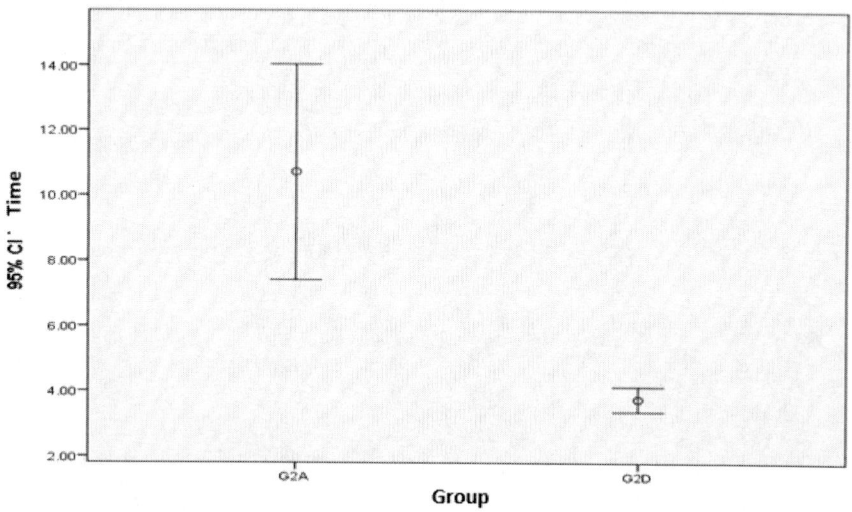


Figure 11. Group 2. Young Rats Treated with 0.050 mg/L of $As_2O_3$ memory measurement before and after poisoning (8 weeks). ** $p < 0.01$.

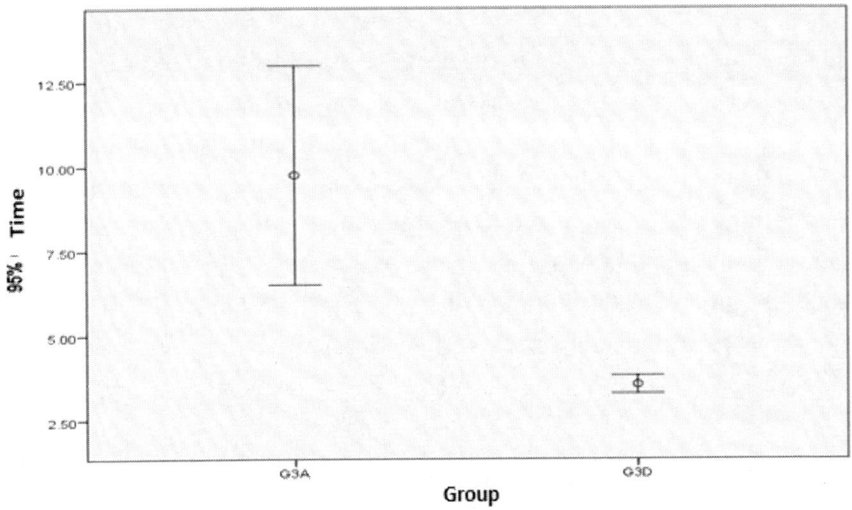


Figure 12. Group 3. Young Rats Treated with 0.075 mg/L of $As_2O_3$ memory measurement before and after poisoning (8 weeks). ** $p < 0.01$.

In the Wilcoxon range test with respect to the groups of young rats, it is found that in the Control group of Young rats (Figure 8) significant differences were found between the measurements before and after the swim time with a p value < 0.005 in group 1 of young rats (Figure 9) found significant differences between the measurements before and after the swim time with a p value < 0.005 in group 2 of young rats (Figure 10) significant differences were found between the measures before and after the swim time with a p value < 0.005 in group 3 of Young rats (Figure 11, 12) significant differences were found between the measurements before and after the swim time with a p value < 0.005.

## Histological Results

The lamellae were examined with 10 micron cuts, stained with Kluver Barrier technique, finding areas of myelin of normal distribution in the white matter of the brain and cerebellum; in group 1 (concentration of 0.025 mg/L) no visible alterations were found, in group 2 (concentration of 0.05 mg/L) an apparent decrease in myelin areas was observed, in group 3 (concentration of 0.075 mg/L) areas of demyelination in axonal paths and vacuolization were observed in the white matter of the cerebellum; in the case of young rats, in groups 1 (concentration of 0.025 mg/L) areas of demyelination and vacuolization were found in the white matter of the cerebellum, in group 2 (concentration of 0.050 mg/L) areas of Mild demyelination and vacuolization areas, large areas of demyelination were found in group 3 (concentration of 0.075 mg/L). Additionally, in the latter group, more erratic movements were observed during rat manipulation (Figure 13).

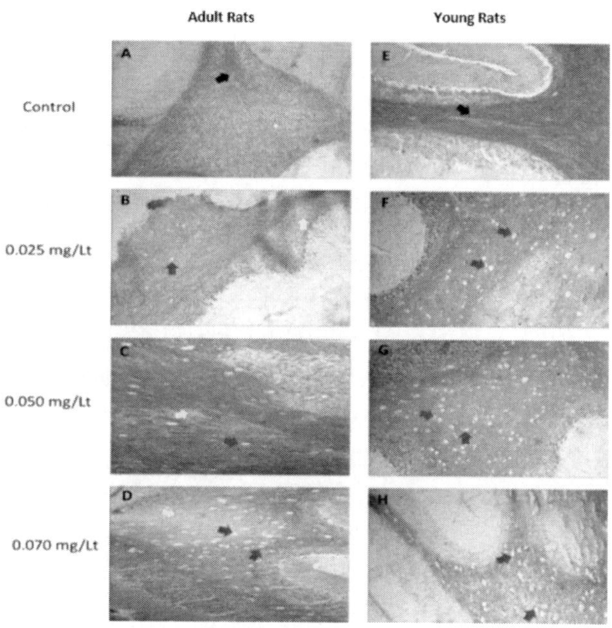


Figure 13. Cerebral microphotographs of adult rats; in the control group (A) the white substance with the presence of myelin (black arrow) is observed; In the groups treated with 0.025mg of mg/L of $As_2O_3$ (B), 0.050mg/L of $A_s2O_3$ (C), 0.070mg/L of $As_2O_3$ (D), variable areas of vacuolization were observed in the white matter (red arrows), in addition to myelin-free areas (yellow arrow), which increased in relation to the dose. In the Group of young rats the rats of the control group (E) presented areas of myelination similar to those of the control of adult rats; In the experimental groups 0.025mg of mg/L of $As_2O_3$.025 (F), 0.050mg/L of $As_2O_3$ (G) and 0.070mg/L of $As_2O_3$ (H) the presence of abundant vacuoles in the white matter (red arrows) was observed, as well as accentuated areas of demyelination (yellow arrows).

## Discussion

With the results obtained in the present study of damage caused by As in the area of the cerebellum we can contrast it with other works since as it is well known not only the arsenic is believed to be involved in memory and learning effects also lead It is as indicated (Quadros et al., 2016) in whose study a significant reduction in the number and size of neurons was also found at the histopathological level, in addition to being densely stained and highly shrunk, following a treatment of thirty days with lead acetate. Its arsenic exposure is also associated with other pathologies, it is documented the carcinogenic effects that it has, as is the case that a study of the ecological type was recently carried out in the United States in which arsenic levels and the incidence of cancer were measured, being able to obtain positive associations in bladder cancer in women and men as well as lung cancer in women, however this result should be taken with caution due to the limitations of the type of study (Mendez et al., 2016). However, we can also observe reproductive effects in which the oxidative damage was accompanied by a significant decrease in both the quantity and quality of sperm in the rats exposed to the metalloid compared to the control group (Adedaraetal, 2017) and the doses of 25, 50 and 100 ppm of sodium arsenite in the drinking water were exposed for 90 days, the results show that this exposure increased the levels of triglycerides and cholesterol of low-density lipoproteins (LDL-C), and electrolytes (Waghe et al., 2016). In this work the Morris aquatic labyrinth was also used, which has been widely used in the environment to assess the memory of rats and mice, we can observe that in a 2008 study in which mice were exposed to a treatment of one month with valproic acid (VPA) from 7 months of age, so the aquatic labyrinth of morris was used to assess spatial memory, having as one of its results that motility and vision were not significantly affected mouse, also in another group but of young mice they were also evaluated cognitive function which showed that despite the reduction of plaque there were no significant differences in the morris water maze between the groups undergoing treatment and the control group ($p > 0.05$,) (Qing et al., 2008). These results coincide at a certain point since, as stated in the results section, there were no affectations in memory due to the exposure, although it is different substance the employee can start making inferences. In another study, the combined effects of lead and arsenic were sought in different areas such as anxiety, learning and deterioration in spatial memory, mice were exposed to 10 mg/kg of body weight and 10 mg/kg of body weight, it was found that the group exposed to the combination of metals was significantly less time in the desired square of the psychine compared to the unexposed group, it was also found that in both metals combined the individual accumulation of As was inhibited (arsenic) and Pb (lead), so taken together it can be suggested that there are toxic effects on changes at the neurobehavioral level (Aktar et al., 2016). In another study the aquatic labyrinth of morris was supplied to measure learning capacity and memory recovery, to thirty-two male wistar strain rats, divided into four groups, Control, sham (saline solution injection, Aβ and (β - amyloid) AβCr (β-amyloid creatine) and during 10 weeks that the study in which the neuroprotective effect of creatine was investigated, resulting in a retention deficit in AβCr and Aβ and in terms of escape latency was significantly higher in AβCr than in Aβ. (Alimohammadi et al., 2016) in telling you it would be advisable to expand the study and measure escape latencies to try to cover all situations in which the metalloid could affect in this case the reaction. that is, where he exposed both rats and humans to scopolamine in order to emulate the cognitive dysfunction observed in Alzheimer's disease (AD) and donepezil, the navigation tests consist On 4 sessions of HGT hidden platform at a rate of 2.4 and 8 hours after dosing them in humans and 1, 2.5 and 5 hours for rats, finding that scopolamine negatively altered the performance in both species deteriorating the navigation place (Laczo et al., 2016). Another example of this was that in human patients with hippocampal lesions they had difficulty finding the platform in a virtual water maze test (Astur et al., 2002). In a 2007 article, neurotoxicity and its influence on oxidative stress in chickens were investigated, with one seventy-two male chickens from one day of age at different doses 7.5, 15 and 30 mg/kg, of Arsenic Trioxide being these corresponding to four groups L, M, H, and Group C (control) (N = 18 chickens each group) respectively, in group H (30mg/kg) a slight swelling can be observed in the thalamus and in the brainstem, brainstem vaculoization, focal and cerebrospinal nerve cells. In general, the antioxidant activities of the GSH-Px and CAT enzymes were diminished while the MDA concentrations saw a dose-dependent increase, after 90 days of treatment with the metalloid. (Zhao et al., 2017) also found the case of the presence of vacuums in the tissue in a clinical case of a 40-year-old woman, whose autopsy results revealed the presence of vacuoles in the white matter and within some of these macrophages, it should be clarified that the patient had previously been diagnosed with AIDS de novo and associated interstical pneumonia, which led to a ventilatory failure, which triggered a multiple organ failure (Serna et al., 2013), on the other hand (Du et to 2010) vacuoles were found in mice lacking neuropeptide Y (NPY) but they did not find these in wild mice, so according to the researchers their presence is associated with areas of high virus infection in the inner capsule, which suggests that There is a possible variation between the rat strains. In a study with nur7 mice (mutant mouse) it was found by means of histological analysis vacuoles in the brain and spinal cord specifically in animals where the activity of Aspartoacilase (Aspa) was increased, also deduce that the degeneration of myelin leads to axonal loss in the cerebellum, in addition to the axonal pathology due to the effects of myelin on the central nervous system may be the basis of neurological diseases of people suffering from Canavan disease (CD) which is characterized by progressive degeneration of white matter in the brain (Traka et al., 2008).

## CONCLUSION

Learning basically responds to external stimuli, whether experience or practice causes a permanent change in our behavior. Several studies have talked about its importance and how external agents can have a positive and negative impact.

In this study a comparison was made between male rats exposed and not exposed to the metalloid in various concentrations, it was not demonstrated that the swim time was extended since it is one of the factors evaluated to determine a learning impairment, however studies Histopathological determined morphological abnormalities in the cerebellum which is believed to have a fundamental role in memory and learning processes.

Demyelination refers to the pathological process in which the myelin layer of nerve fibers is damaged, which could be detected in each exposed group except for the control groups, this can be related to diseases such as Multiple Sclerosis, encephalomyelitis, leukodystrophies and some encephalopathies, however the list of demyelinating diseases is almost unknown for now. For future studies it is recommended to evaluate the effects of chronic exposure, using specific stains to determine the nature of the histological findings found.

## References

Abernathy, C. O., Thomas, D. J., and Calderon, R. L. 2003. "Health effects and risk assessment of arsenic." *Journal of Nutrition* 133 (1): 1536-1538. http://doi:10.1093/jn/133.5.1536S.

Adedara, I. A., Abolaji, A. O., Awogbindin, I. O., and Farombi, E. O. 2017. "Suppression of the brain-pituitary-testicular axis function following acute arsenic and manganese co-exposure and withdrawal in rats." *Journal of Trace Elements in Medicine and Biology* 39: 21-29. http://doi:10.1016/j.jtemb.2016.07.001.

Adelson, P. D., Fellows-Mayle, W., Kochanek, P. M., and Dixon, C. E. 2013. "Morris water maze function and histologic characterization of two age-at-injury experimental models of controlled cortical impact in the immature rat." *Child's Nervous System*, 29(1): 43-53. http://doi:10. 1007/s00381-012-1932-4.

Aktar, S., Jahan, M., Alam, S., Mohanto, N. C., Arefin, A., Rahman, A., and Saud, Z. A. 2016. "Individual and Combined Effects of Arsenic and Lead on Behavioral and Biochemical Changes in Mice." *Biological Trace Element Researh* 177(2): 288-296. http://doi:10. 1007/s12011-016-0883-0.

Alimohammadi-Kamalabadi, M., Eshraghian, M., Zarindast, M. R., Aliaghaei, A., and Pishva, H. 2016. "Effect of creatine supplementation on cognitive performance and apoptosis in a rat model of amyloid-beta-induced Alzheimer's disease." *Iranian Journal of Basic Medical Sciences* 19(11): 1159-1165. http://doi:10. 22038/ijbms.2016.7814.

Astur, R. S., Taylor, L. B., Mamelak, A. N., Philpott, L., and Sutherland, R. J. 2002. "Humans with hippocampus damage display severe spatial memory impairments in a virtual Morris water task." *Behavioural Brain Research* 132(1): 77-84. http://doi:10.1016/s0166-4328(01) 00399-0.

Bashir, S., Sharma, Y., Irshad, M., Gupta, S. D., and Dogra, T. D. 2006. "Arsenic induced cell death in liver and brain of experimental rats." *Basic and Clinical Pharmacoly and Toxicology* 98(1): 38-43. http://doi:10.1111/j.1742-7843.2006.pto_170.x.

Berbel-Garcia, A., Gonzalez-Aguirre, J. M., Botia-Paniagua, E., Orts-Castro, E., Lopez-Zuazo, I., Rodriguez-Garcia, J. L., and Gil-Madre, J. 2004. "Acute polyneuropathy and encephalopathy caused by arsenic poisoning." *Revista de Neurología* 38(10): 928-930. https://doi.org/ 10.33588/rn.3810.2004011.

Block, F. 1999. "Global ischemia and behavioural deficits." *Progress in Neurobiology* 58(3): 279-295. 41. https://doi.org/10.1016/S0301-0082(98)00085-9.

Brinkel, J., Khan, M. H., and Kraemer, A. 2009. "A systematic review of arsenic exposure and its social and mental health effects with special reference to Bangladesh." *International Journal of Environmental Research and Public Health* 6(5): 1609-1619. http://doi:10.3390/ijerph 6051609.

Bromley-Brits, K., Deng, Y., and Song, W. 2011. "Morris water maze test for learning and memory deficits in Alzheimer's disease model mice." *Journal of Visualized Experiments* (53)e2920. http://doi:10.3791/2920.

Calderon, J., Navarro, M. E., Jimenez-Capdeville, M. E., Santos-Diaz, M. A., Golden, A., Rodriguez-Leyva, I., and Diaz-Barriga, F. 2001. "Exposure to arsenic and lead and neuropsychological development in Mexican children." *Environmental Research* 85(2): 69-76. http://doi: 10.1006/enrs.2000.4106.

Carabantes, A. G., and de Fernicola, N. A. G. G. 2003. "Arsénico en el agua de bebida:un problema de salud pública." *Revista Brasileira de Ciências*

*Farmacêuticas* 39(4): 365-372. ["Arsenic in drinking water: a public health problem." *Brazilian Journal of Pharmaceutical Sciences*]

Centeno, J. A., Mullick, F. G., Martinez, L., Page, N. P., Gibb, H., Longfellow, D., and Ladich, E. R. 2002. "Pathology related to chronic arsenic exposure." *Environmental Health Perspectives* 110(5): 883-886. http://doi:10.1289/ehp.02110s5883.

Chatterjee, A., and Chatterji, U. 2010. "Arsenic abrogates the estrogen-signaling pathway in the rat uterus." *Reproductive Biology and Endocrinology* 8: 80- 80. http://doi:10.1186/1477-7827-8-80.

Chiou, H. Y., Chiou, S. T., Hsu, Y. H., Chou, Y. L., Tseng, C. H., Wei, M. L. and Chen, C. J. 2001. "Incidence of Transitional Cell Carcinoma and Arsenic in Drinking Water: A Follow-up Study of 8,102 Residents in an Arseniasis-endemic Area in Northeastern Taiwan." *American Journal of Epidemiology* 153(5): 411-418. http://doi:10.1093/aje/ 153.5.411.

Coronado-Gonzalez, J. A., Del Razo, L. M., Garcia-Vargas, G., Sanmiguel-Salazar, F., and Escobedo-de la Pena, J. 2007. Inorganic arsenic exposure and type 2 diabetes mellitus in Mexico. *Environmental Research* 104(3): 383-389. http://doi:10.1016/j.envres. 2007.03.004.

Du, M., Butchi, N. B., Woods, T., Morgan, T. W. and Peterson, K. E. 2010. "Neuropeptide Y has a protective role during murine retrovirus-induced neurological disease." *Journal of virology* 84(21): 11076-11088. http://doi:10.1128/JVI.01022-10.

Dwivedi, N. and Flora, S. J. 2011. "Concomitant exposure to arsenic and organophosphates on tissue oxidative stress in rats." *Food and chemical toxicology* 49(5): 1152-1159. http://doi:10.1016/j.fct.2011. 02.007.

Fumal, I., Pierard-Franchimont, C. and Pierard, G. E. 2005. "Arsenical keratoses and carcinomas." *Revue médicale de Liège* 60(4): 217-221. 42. [*Liège medical journal*]

Garcia Salcedo, J. J., Hernández Serrano, M.C., Rodriguez Arredondo, P., Valdés Anaya, B., Valdés Anaya, B., García Rodriguez, D. and Albores Medina, A. 2010. "Carga Corporal de arsénico." *Revista Medicina de Torreon* 3: 25-28. ["Body Burden of Arsenic." *Torreon Medicine Magazine*]

Guyton, A., C., and Hall J., E. 2001. "Fisiologia de la membrana, del nervio y del musculo" in M.H. I. Editores (Ed.), *Tratado de Fisiologia Medica* (10 ed., pp. 47-112). ["Physiology of the membrane, the nerve and the muscle" in *Treatise on Medical Physiology*]

Laczo, J., Markova, H., Lobellova, V., Gazova, I., Parizkova, M., Cerman, J. and Stuchlik, A. 2016. "Scopolamine disrupts place navigation in rats and humans: a translational validation of the Hidden Goal Task in the Morris water maze and a real maze for humans." *Psychopharmacology* (Berl) 234(4): 535-547. http://doi:10.1007/ s00213-016-4488-2.

Leslie P. Gartner, J. L. H. 2015. "Sistema Nervioso." In W. K. Health (Ed.), *Biología Celular e Histología* 7: 143-161. Philadelphia. (Reprinted from: 7). ["Nervous system." In *Cell Biology and Histology*]

Marin, O., Smeets, W. J., and Gonzalez, A. 1998. "Evolution of the basal ganglia in tetrapods: a new perspective based on recent studies in amphibians." *Trends in neurosciences* 21(11), 487-494. http://doi:10. 1016/s0166-2236(98)01297-1.

Mendez, W. M., Jr., Eftim, S., Cohen, J., Warren, I., Cowden, J., Lee, J. S. and Sams, R. 2016. "Relationships between arsenic concentrations in drinking water and lung and bladder cancer incidence in U.S. counties." *Journal of exposure science & environmental* 27(3): 235-243. http://doi:10.1038/jes.2016.58.

Morris, C. G. and Maisto, A. A. 2005. "Bases Biologicas de la Conducta." In P. H. INC (Ed.), *Psicología* (12 ed., pp. 712). ["Biological bases of behavior." In *Psychology*]

Mukherjee, A., Sengupta, M. K., Hossain, M. A., Ahamed, S., Das, B., Nayak, B. and Chakraborti, D. 2006. "Arsenic contamination in groundwater: a global perspective with emphasis on the Asian scenario." *Journal of health, population, and nutrition* 24(2): 142- 163.

Namgung, U. and Xia, Z. 2001). Arsenic induces apoptosis in rat cerebellar neurons via activation of JNK3 and p38 MAP kinases. *Toxicology and applied pharmacology* 174(2): 130-138. http://doi:10.1006/taap.2001. 9200.

Navarrete, F., Perez-Ortiz, J. M., Femenia, T., Garcia-Gutierrez, M. S., Garcia-Paya, M. E., Leiva-Santana, C. and Manzanares, J. 2008.

"Methods to evaluate cognitive disorders in animal models." *Revista de neurologia* 47(3): 137-145.

Parvez, F., Chen, Y., Brandt-Rauf, P. W., Bernard, A., Dumont, X., Slavkovich, V. and Ahsan, H. 2008. "Nonmalignant respiratory effects of chronic arsenic exposure from drinking water among never-smokers in Bangladesh." *Environmental health perspectives* 116(2): 190-195. http://doi:10.1289/ehp.9507.

Piao, F., Ma, N., Hiraku, Y., Murata, M., Oikawa, S., Cheng, F., and Yokoyama, K. 2005. "Oxidative DNA damage in relation to neurotoxicity in the brain of mice exposed to arsenic at environmentally relevant levels." *Journal of Occupational Health* 47(5): 445-449. http://doi:10.1539/joh.47.445.

Pohl, H. R., Roney, N., and Abadin, H. G. 2011. "Metal ions affecting the neurological system." *Metal Ions in Life Sciences* 8: 247-262.

Qing, H., He, G., Ly, P. T., Fox, C. J., Staufenbiel, M., Cai, F., and Song, W. 2008. "Valproic acid inhibits Abeta production, neuritic plaque formation, and behavioral deficits in Alzheimer's disease mouse models." *Journal of Experimental Medicine* 205(12): 2781-2789. http://doi:10.1084/jem.20081588.

Quadros, L. S., Bangera, H., Kotian, S. R., and Bhat, K. M. R. 2016. "Effects of lead in various preparatory stages of Nagabhasma on function and histopathology of *Cornu Ammonis* of Hippocampus." *Journal of Clinical and Diagnostic Research* 10(10): AF01-AF04. http://doi:10.7860/JCDR/2016/20424.8748.

Rocha-Amador, D., Navarro, M. E., Carrizales, L., Morales, R., and Calderon, J. 2007. "Decreased intelligence in children and exposure to fluoride and arsenic in drinking water." *Cuadernos de Salud Publica* 23(4): S579-587. http://doi:10.1590/S0102-311X2007001600018.

Rosado, J. L., Ronquillo, D., Kordas, K., Rojas, O., Alatorre, J., Lopez, P., and Stoltzfus, R. J. 2007. "Arsenic Exposure and Cognitive Performance in Mexican Schoolchildren." *Environmental Health Perspectives* 115(9): 1371-1375. http://doi:10.1289/ehp.9961.

Santín, L. R. S., Begega, A., Miranda, R., and Arias, JL. 2000. "Aprendizaje espacial e hipocampo." *Revista de Neurología* 31: 455-462.

http://doi:https://doi.org/10.33588/rn.3105.2000103. ["Spatial learning and hippocampus." *Journal of Neurology*]

Serna Ortiz, C. A., Muñoz Ortiz, É., Arias Restrepo, L. F., and Cataño Correa, J. C. 2013. "Conferencia Clínico Patológica (CPC): paciente previamente sana con insuficiencia respiratoria debida a neumonía intersticial." *Iatreia* 26(1): 83-94. ["Clinical Pathological Conference (CPC): previously healthy patient with respiratory failure due to interstitial pneumonia." *Iatreia*]

Singh, A. P., Goel, R. K., and Kaur, T. 2011. "Mechanisms pertaining to arsenic toxicity." *Toxicology International* 18(2): 87-93. http://doi:10.4103/0971-6580.84258.

Squire, L. R., and Knowlton, B. J. 1995. "Learning about categories in the absence of memory." *Proceedings of the National Academy of Sciences of the United States of America* 92(26): 12470-12474. http://doi:10.1073/pnas.92.26.12470.

Traka, M., Wollmann, R. L., Cerda, S. R., Dugas, J., Barres, B. A., and Popko, B. 2008. "Nur7 is a nonsense mutation in the mouse aspartoacylase gene that causes spongy degeneration of the central nervous system." *Journal of Neuroscience* 28(45): 11537- 11549. http://doi:10.1523/JNEUROSCI.1490-08.2008.

Tsai, S. Y., Chou, H. Y., The, H. W., Chen, C. M., and Chen, C. J. 2003. The effects of chronic arsenic exposure from drinking water on the neurobehavioral development in adolescence. *Neurotoxicology* 24(4-5): 747-753. http://doi:10.1016/S0161-813X(03)00029-9.

Vahidnia, A., Romijn, F., van der Voet, G. B., and de Wolff, F. A. 2008. "Arsenicinduced neurotoxicity in relation to toxicokinetics: effects on sciatic nerve proteins." *Chemico-Biological Interactions* 176(2-3): 188-195. 44. http://doi:10.1016/j.cbi.2008.07.001.

Vicens, P., Redolat, R., and Carrasco, M. d. C. 2003. "Aprendizaje espacial y Laberinto de agua: metodología y apliaciones." *Psicothema* 15 (4): 539-544. ["Spatial learning and the Water Labyrinth: methodology and applications." *Psychothema*]

Waghe, P., Sarkar, S. N., Sarath, T. S., Kandasamy, K., Choudhury, S., Gupta, P., and Mishra, S. K. 2016. "Subchronic Arsenic Exposure

Through Drinking Water Alters Lipid Profile and Electrolyte Status in Rats." *Biological Trace Element Research* 176(2): 350-354. http://doi:10.1007/s12011-016-0851-8.

Wang, S. X., Wang, Z. H., Cheng, X. T., Li, J., Sang, Z. P., Zhang, X. D., and Wang, Z. Q. 2007. "Arsenic and Fluoride Exposure in Drinking Water: Children's IQ and Growth in Shanyin County, Shanxi Province, China." *Environmental Health Perspectives* 115(4): 643-647. http://doi:10.1289/ehp.9270.

Wasserman, G. A., Liu, X., Parvez, F., Ahsan, H., Factor-Litvak, P., Kline, J., and Graziano, J. H. 2007. "Water arsenic exposure and intellectual function in 6-yearold children in Araihazar, Bangladesh." *Environmental Health Perspectives* 115(2): 285-289. http://doi:10. 1289/ehp.9501.

Watson, K., and Creamer, D. 2004. "Arsenic-induced keratoses and Bowen's disease." *Clinical and Experimental Dermatology* 29(1): 46-48. http://doi:10.1111/j.1365-2230.2004.01447.x.

Yadav, R. S., Shukla, R. K., Sankhwar, M. L., Patel, D. K., Ansari, R. W., Pant, A. B., Islam, F., and Khanna, V. K. 2010. "Neuroprotective effect of curcumin in arsenic-induced neurotoxicity in rats." *Neurotoxicology* 31(5): 533-539. http://doi:10.1016/j.neuro.2010. 05.001.

Zhao, P., Guo, Y., Zhang, W., Chai, H., Xing, H., and Xing, M. 2017. "Neurotoxicity induced by arsenic in Gallus Gallus: Regulation of oxidative stress and heat shock protein response." *Chemosphere* 166: 238-245. http://doi:10.1016/j.chemosphere.2016.09.060.

In: Laboratory Animals and Neurosciences ISBN: 978-1-53618-462-4
Editors: B. Hernandez Godinez et al.


*Chapter 4*

# EFFECT OF CARBAMAZEPINE ON ELECTROLYTE LEVELS IN AN ANIMAL MODEL OF EPILEPSY

***Alfonso Alfaro Rodríguez***[1]***, Samuel Reyes Long***[1,3]***, Angelica Gonzalez Maciel***[3]***, Herlinda Bonilla Jaime***[4]***, Cindy Bandala***[1, 3] ***and Jose Luis Cortes-Altamirano***[1,2,*]

[1]División de Neurociencias, Instituto Nacional de Rehabilitación "Luis Guillermo Ibarra Ibarra", Ciudad de México, México

[2]Universidad Estatal del Valle de Ecatepec (UNEVE), Ecatepec de Morelos, Estado de México, México

[3]Escuela Superior de Medicina., Instituto Politécnico Nacional, Ciudad de México, México

[4]Laboratorio de Morfología Celular y Tisular, Instituto Nacional de Pediatría, Ciudad de México, México

Departamento de Biología de la Reproducción, Universidad Autónoma Metropolitana-Iztapalapa, Ciudad de México

[*] Corresponding Author's E-mail: jose_luiscortesalta@hotmail.com.

## ABSTRACT

### Introduction

Epilepsy affects approximately 1% of the world population and it involves changes at various physiological levels. Carbamazepine (CBZ) is a well-known and commonly prescribed anticonvulsant with the ability to decrease the epileptic effects of Pentylenetetrazole (PTZ).

### Objective

Evaluate the regulator effect of CBZ on blood electrolyte levels in an animal model of epilepsy induced by PTZ, and the histological changes present in the brain.

### Method

Ten male Wistar rats were divided into two groups: G1 (n = 5) was administered PTZ (70 mg/kg i.p.) and G2 a dose of CBZ (50 mg/kg i.p.) prior to the dose of PTZ. The parameters evaluated were pH, serum electrolytes (Na+, K+, Ca++), glucose, lactate, hematocrit, and total hemoglobin.

### Results

The administration of PTZ produced electrolyte imbalance and caused dilatation of vascular capillaries and vessels, and in some cases, a break in the endothelium. A darkening and condensation of neuronal perikarya was observed. Frontal cortex, hippocampus, and cerebellum were deeply affected.

### Conclusion

The treatment with CBZ contributes to the equilibrium of electrolyte and avoids the neuronal death.


**Keywords:** epilepsy, serum electrolytes, Pentylenetetrazole, Carbamazepine

# INTRODUCTION

Epilepsy is one of the most common neurological disorders (Zhao et al., 2007; Filocamo et al., 2019) and is characterized by recurrent and spontaneous seizures (Kurt, Bosnak, Inan, Celik, & Uremis, 2016). Approximately 60 million people worldwide suffer from this neurological disorder and about one third of them present drug-resistant seizures (Thurman et al., 2011). Epileptogenesis involves histological, biochemical, and physiological alterations that, over time, alter the excitatory-inhibitory neurotransmission balance in multiple brain structures (Sasa, 2006). The orderly function of the nervous system depends on its electrical excitability, which is maintained through a voltage gradient across neuronal and glial membranes by means of metabolically driven ion channels. It is known that the body's electrolytes are involved in epilepsy, as several reports stated that they (sodium, potassium, calcium, and magnesium) are altered in epileptic patients (Hamed, Abdellah, & El-Melegy, 2004). These effects are usually occasioned by a failure of the Blood-Brain Barrier (BBB) which contributes to ictogenesis, epileptogenesis, and sustainment of seizures (Friedman, 2011; Marchi, Granata, Ghosh, & Janigro, 2012). The BBB is a dynamic barrier with regulation of cerebral blood flow, transport, metabolic, and immunological aspects and was initially considered a static barrier to the passage of blood components or drugs into the brain; however, today it is recognized as a factor participating in the pathophysiology of several Central Nervous System (CNS) disorders (Abbott, Patabendige, Dolman, Yusof, & Begley, 2010; Neuwelt et al., 2011).

The systemic administration of high doses of Pentylenetetrazole (PTZ) in rats produces a typical seizure pattern (Ramos-Morales et al., 2012). Plus, Carbamazepine (CBZ) is widely administered for the treatment of partial seizures and generalized tonic-clonic seizures due to their extensive and complex metabolism, which involves several metabolic pathways and multiple enzymes (Djordjevic et al., 2016). Therefore, the aim of the study was to analyze the values obtained of blood electrolytes levels in an animal model of epilepsy induced by PTZ for 4 days and compared against a PTZ-

and CBZ-treated group, as well as to evaluate histological changes in the frontal cortex, hippocampus, and cerebellum.

# Methods

## Subjects

Ten male Wistar rats (350-420g) were used. The animals were maintained under controlled laboratory conditions at a cycle of 12-h light/12-h dark at 22 °C; with food and water ad libitum. The Research Ethics Committee of the National Rehabilitation Institute (INR) "Luis Guillermo Ibarra Ibarra" approved all procedures.

Because of blood sampling and experimental procedures of the present study, the *n* was employed in accordance with the Guide for the Care and Use of Experimental Animals (Olfert, Cross, & McWilliam, 1993), the number of subjects is considered statistically significant for this study.

To evaluate the effect of CBZ on pH, serum electrolytes (Na+, K+, Ca++), glucose, lactate, hematocrit, and total hemoglobin in a PTZ-induced model of epilepsy, the rats were divided into two groups: Group 1, PTZ group (n = 5), was anesthetized with sodium Pentobarbital (PB) at a dose of 50 mg/kg intraperitoneally (i.p.), and 1 h later a basal sample of blood was obtained; later the animals were given a dose of PTZ (70 mg/kg i.p.) (Sigma, USA) and 30 min after, blood samples were obtained for analysis and processing by a gas analyzer. Group 2, CBZ+PTZ group (n = 5) was given a single dose of CBZ (50 mg/kg i.p.) 30 min prior to being anesthetized and the same procedure of G1 was followed. The basal measurements of both groups were considered as Control conditions. All samples were obtained at the same hour and under the same procedure and it was carried out for 4 consecutive days

Blood samples of 100 µl of arterial blood were obtained by cardiac puncture, and the blood was transferred into a heparinized capillary microtube and further processed by a third-generation gas and blood electrolyte analyzer (GEM Premier 3000; Instrumentation Laboratory

Diagnostics, USA and Italy). The parameters evaluated were pH, serum electrolytes: $Na^+$, $K^+$, and $Ca^{++}$ (mmol/L); substrates: glucose (mg/dL) and lactate (mg/dL), Hematocrit (Hct) (%), and Total Hemoglobin (THbc).

## Histology

Five animals from each group were euthanized with an overdose of PB (1 ml/kg body weight). They were then transcardially perfused with a cold solution of phosphate buffer saline (PBS) 0.1 M, pH 7.4, followed by 10% formaldehyde in PBS. Brains were removed from the skull and blocked in a coronal stereotaxic plane and kept in the same fixing solution during 24 h. To verify neuropathological changes the tissues were embedded in paraffin. Ten sections of 7 μm thick with a separation of 40 μm between cuts were obtained per animal/region. The orientation of the tissues was: cortex in coronal plane, dorsal hippocampus throughout the rostro-caudal axis and cerebellum in midsagittal plane. Slices were stained with Cresyl Violet. The researcher in charge of evaluating the tissues was blind to the identification of the groups. A microscope Carl Zeiss Axioskop 2 Plus equipped with a Zen 2.3 imaging system and camera Axiocam 503 color (Zeiss) was used, under 20x magnification.

## Statistical Analysis

Normality tests were performed for all variables examined. The values obtained were expressed as Mean ± Standard Errors of the Mean (*SEM*). For the results of the blood electrolytes, Analysis of Variance (ANOVA) and the post hoc Tukey test were conducted. Origin 7 for Windows (U.S.A.) was employed and a value of $p < .05$ was considered statistically significant.

## RESULTS

Table 1, depicts the results of the different indicators evaluated and the significant differences observed in the values of Na+, K+, Ca++, Glu, Lac, Hct, and THbc of G1 PTZ rats for 4 days presented consecutively. In Na+, there were significant differences between basal and day 2 ($p = .02$); similarly, values between basal and day 4 ($p = .05$) are present. For K+, significant differences were found between basal and day 4 ($p = .02$) and between day 1 and 4 ($p = .01$). In Ca++ there were significant differences between basal compared with days 1 ($p = .04$) and 2 ($p = .01$). Glucose values demonstrated a highly significant difference between basal and day 1 ($p = .0005$) and 4 ($p = .03$). Lactate only exhibited a significant difference between basal and day 1 ($p = .03$). Regarding Hct, significant differences were recorded between basal and day 1 ($p = .02$), 2 ($p = .01$), and 4 ($p = .05$). In THbc significant differences were found between basal and day 1 ($p = .02$), 2 ($p = .01$), and 4 ($p = .05$) were observed.

On the other hand, when comparing each group significant differences were found in different blood electrolytes, Na+ presented an increase in G1 in comparison with Control and G2 ($p < .05$), however no differences were found between G2 and Control, in K+ a significant decrease was found in G2 in comparison with Control ($p < .05$), glucose was decreased in G1 when comparing it with G2 and Control, ($p < .05$) and finally THbc was reduced significantly in G1 in comparison with G2 and Control ($p < .05$), but no difference was found between G2 and Control.

**Table 1. Blood electrolyte and metabolites levels in an animal model of PTZ-induced epilepsy**

| | | Day 1 | | Day 2 | | Day 3 | |
|---|---|---|---|---|---|---|---|
| Variable | Basal | G1 | G2 | G1 | G2 | G1 | G2 |
| pH | 7.426 ± 0.02 | 7.406 ± 0.02 | 7.398 ± 0.01 | 7.372 ± 0.02 | 7.328 ± 0.04 | 7.413 ± 0.02 | 7.400 ± 0.01 |
| Na+ | 147.2 ± 3.13 | 154.2 ± 2.70 | 151.8 ± 1.71 | 158.8 ± 2.63* | 153 ± 1.14 | 153.6 ± 1.76 | 156.8 ± 0.58 |
| K+ | 3.80 ± 0.31 | 3.46 ± 0.20** | 3.28 ± 0.13 | 3.12 ± 0.28 | 3.18 ± 0.13 | 3.10 ± 0.17 | 3.18 ± 0.34 |
| Ca++ | 0.898 ± 0.12 | 0.648 ± 0.06* | 0.792 ± 0.06 | 0.602 ± 0.11** | 0.784 ± 0.07 | 0.713 ± 0.12 | 0.596 ± 0.05 |
| Glu | 147.2 ± 9.15 | 78 ± 8.61*** | 105.4 ± 5.50 | 102.8 ± 24.51 | 152 ± 21.68 | 97 ± 17.08 | 88.6 ± 18.51 |
| Lac | 2.75 ± 0.31 | 0.92 ± 0.25* | 0.66 ± 0.06* | 1.58 ± 0.42 | 2.02 ± 0.26* | 1.33 ± 0.26 | 1.06 ± 0.34** |
| Hct | 43.6 ± 2.33 | 28.2 ± 4.45* | 36 ± 4.08 | 29 ± 3.86* | 39.2 ± 1.98 | 34 ± 4.16 | 30 ± 4.13 |
| THbc | 13.54 ± 0.72 | 10.06 ± 0.97* | 11.16 ± 1.26 | 9 ± 1.18* | 12.18 ± 0.61 | 10.53 ± 1.28 | 10.04 ± 0.24 |

Note. Data are expressed as M ± SEM. Compared with Basal/Control. G1=Group PTZ, G2=Group CBZ+PTZ. *$p < .05$, **$p < .01$, ***$p < 0.001$.

## Histology

Single injection of PTZ (70mg/kg, i.p.) provoked dilatation of vascular capillaries and blood vessels, with clearly break of the endothelium in frontal cortex, hippocampus and cerebellum (Figure 1. 4 A, B, C); in addition, conspicuous cytopathologic changes are present in neurons of the dentate gyrus and cerebellum; the granular cells, hilar interneurons and Purkinje neurons are picnotic and shrunken. The average thickness of eight granular cells in the dorsal layer of dentate gyrus is significantly lower ($p < .01$) in both PTZ and PTZ-CBZ groups. In control (Figure 1. D, E, F) or CBZ-PTZ (Figure 1. G, H, I) groups no more detectable cytopathologic changes were evident.

# DISCUSSION

The main purpose of this study was to analyze the regulator effect of CBZ on blood electrolyte levels in an animal model of PTZ-induced epilepsy. In both groups, pH values exhibited no abnormalities, this may be due to the effect of PB because this anesthetic performs a fundamental role in various cell processes, including pH control, volume homeostasis, and cell growth (Eloqayli, Dahl, Götestam, Unsgård, & Sonnewald, 2004), and can significantly lessen the seizure-severity rate.

The increase that Na+ underwent in G1 in contrast with the CBZ-treated group, and the decrease of K+ that was recorded on day 1 are directly related with the Na+, K+-Adenine TriPhosphatase (ATP) enzyme, these membrane protein aims at the export of Na+ and K+ import plus they are the main ones responsible for regulating brain excitability. Funk et al., (2015) concluded that inhibition of Na+, K+-ATPase system leads to neuronal excitability, which in turn creates the appearance of seizures. The above is consistent with our results, as it allows us to infer that the increase of Na+ and the decrease of K+ in blood of the PTZ-induced group is due to the inhibition of the Na+, K+ system-ATPase, which generates an electrolyte imbalance and increases extracellular Na+ and K+ intracellular loss, resulting at the end in the appearance of seizures. The effect of CBZ might comprise the same output level modulating Na+ and K+ entry into the cell, thus maintaining homeostasis at the neuronal level. In our results, Ca++ showed a significant decrease in blood level during days 1 and 2 in the PTZ-induced group. This agrees with De Bock et al., (2012) who proposed that decreased amounts of extracellular Ca++ are closely linked with a deficiency in the BBB, which generates the excessive passage of various electrolytes, in turn generating an osmotic imbalance, depolarizing the membrane, and giving rise to neuronal hyperexcitation.

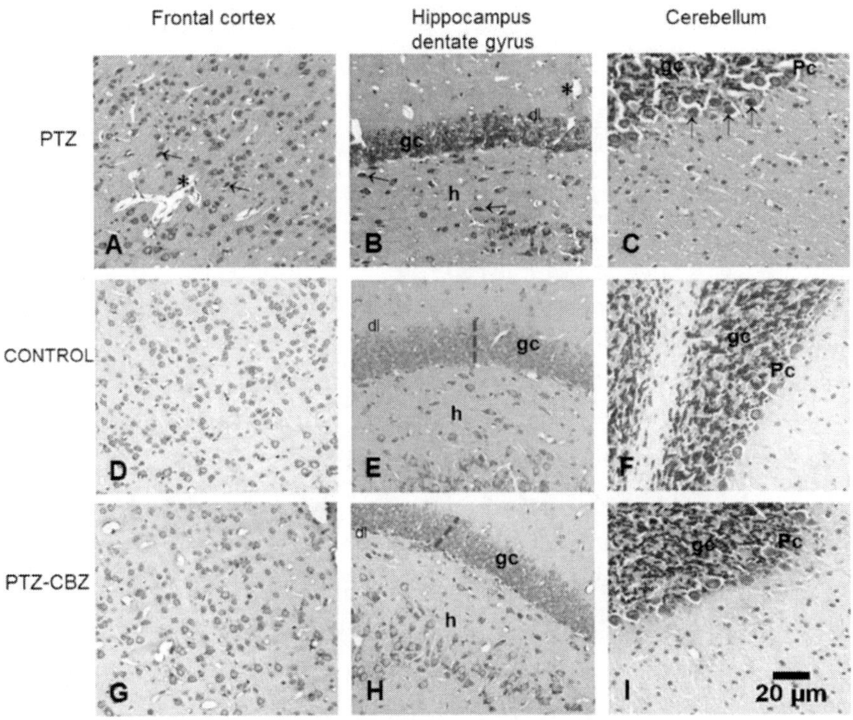


Figure 1. Representative photomicrographs of frontal cortex, dentate gyrus (hippocampus) and cerebellum.

We observed large amounts of Na+, but decreased amounts of Ca++, in the blood level of the PTZ group; however, no significant differences were found in the PTZ + CBZ group. These findings allow us to infer that CBZ is closely linked with the depolarization of neuron signaling, modulating the Na+, K+, and Ca++ T-type channel, avoiding an osmotic imbalance.

Changes in Glucose levels due to the administration of PTZ were expressed mainly in a decrease at day 1 of G1, leading us to think that the fact of membrane depolarization comprises an active transport; therefore, the consumption of energy is necessary for the reorganization of intracellular glucose. It is noteworthy that the group treated with CBZ exhibited no significant difference.

Van Hall et al., (2009) point out that glycolysis in the presence of oxygen (aerobic glycolysis) is an interesting feature of brain metabolism and that, under resting conditions, there is a net efflux of lactate from the CNS, i.e., lactate concentration in venous blood is higher than in the arterial blood supplying the brain. In our baseline measurements, lactate is increased in both groups, probably due to the effect of PB.

Hct and THbc, exhibited a significant decrease in the PTZ-induced group, possibly deriving from the processes that cause PZT apnea during Cmax. The most relevant of these results is the effect of CBZ, in that the group treated with the drug did not exhibit statistically significant differences and maintained its values in baseline levels: Shariff et al., (2006) on the other hand, indicate that, for an indefinite period of time, CBF is inadequate for meeting the metabolic demands of the epileptic neurons, leading to a decrease in both tissue and hemoglobin oxygenation. However, significant controversy remains because cortical oxygenation may vary depending on systemic oxygenation, blood pressure, and seizure duration. There are reports that the systemic injection of PTZ induces apoptotic-type neurodegeneration in hippocampal neurons and amygdalae (Park, Cho, Kim, & Kim, 2006). A feature of the PTZ model is the appearance of hyperchromic neurons and alterations, such as dark degeneration of neurons, and the nearly total chromatolysis of some cells or substantial pathologies of cytoplasmic organelles might be considered irreversible (Zhvania, Ksovreli, Japaridze, & Lordkipanidze, 2015). Among these features, we also find capillary dilation and endothelium disruption throughout the brain, but there are greater in hippocampus. However, the dose of CBZ 30 min prior to being anesthetized and administering a 70mg/kg dose of PTZ i.p.

prevented cellular alterations; again, these results allow us to infer that CBZ regulates PTZ-induced imbalances and prevents neuronal damage. The results of this study suggest that treatment with CBZ in rats with PTZ-induced seizures contributes to the restoration of the balance of Na+, K+, and Ca++, and that this treatment allows the products of metabolism, such as glucose and hemodynamic parameters (Hct and THbc), to return to baseline levels and prevents neurodegeneration and the death of neurons.

## References

Abbott, N. J., Patabendige, A. A., Dolman, D. E., Yusof, S. R., & Begley, D. J. (2010). Structure and function of the blood–brain barrier. *Neurobiology of disease, 37*(1), 13-25. Doi: 10.1016/j.nbd.2009.07.030.

De Bock, M., Culot, M., Wang, N., da Costa, A., Decrock, E., Bol, M., . . . Leybaert, L. (2012). Low extracellular Ca2+ conditions induce an increase in brain endothelial permeability that involves intercellular Ca2+ waves. Brain researc*h, 1487*, 78-87. Doi: 10.1016/j.brainres.2012.06.046.

Djordjevic, N., Milovanovic, D. D., Radovanovic, M., Radosavljevic, I., Obradovic, S., Jakovljevic, M., . . . Jankovic, S. (2016). CYP1A2 genotype affects carbamazepine pharmacokinetics in children with epilepsy. *European journal of clinical pharmacology, 72*(4), 439-445. Doi: 10.1007/s00228-015-2006-9.

Eloqayli, H., Dahl, C. B., Götestam, K. G., Unsgård, G., & Sonnewald, U. (2004). Changes of glial–neuronal interaction and metabolism after a subconvulsive dose of pentylenetetrazole. *Neurochemistry international, 45*(5), 739-745. 10.1016/j.neuint.2004.02.002.

Filocamo, M., Procopio, E., & Morrone, A. (2019). Lysosomal Disorders and Epilepsy. *The Causes of Epilepsy: Diagnosis and Investigation*, 234. ISBN: 1108420753, 9781108420754.

Friedman, A. (2011). Blood–brain barrier dysfunction, status epilepticus, seizures, and epilepsy: a puzzle of a chicken and egg? *Epilepsia, 52*(s8), 19-20. Doi: 10.1111/j.1528-1167.2011.03227.x.

Funck, V., Ribeiro, L., Pereira, L., De Oliveira, C., Grigoletto, J., Della-Pace, I., . . . Larrick, J. (2015). Contrasting effects of Na+, K+-ATPase activation on seizure activity in acute versus chronic models. *Neuroscience, 298*, 171-179. Doi: 10.1016/j.neuroscience.2015.04.031.

Hamed, S. A., Abdellah, M. M., & El-Melegy, N. (2004). Blood levels of trace elements, electrolytes, and oxidative stress/antioxidant systems in epileptic patients. *Journal of pharmacological sciences, 96*(4), 465-473. Doi: 10.1254/jphs.FPJ04032X.

Kurt, A. H., Bosnak, M., Inan, S. Y., Celik, A., & Uremis, M. M. (2016). Epileptogenic effects of G protein-coupled estrogen receptor 1 in the rat pentylenetetrazole kindling model of epilepsy. *Pharmacological Reports, 68*(1), 66-70. Doi: 10.1016/j.pharep.2015.07.001.

Marchi, N., Granata, T., Ghosh, C., & Janigro, D. (2012). Blood–brain barrier dysfunction and epilepsy: pathophysiologic role and therapeutic approaches. *Epilepsia, 53*(11), 1877-1886. Doi: 10.1111/j.1528-1167.2012.03637.x.

Neuwelt, E. A., Bauer, B., Fahlke, C., Fricker, G., Iadecola, C., Janigro, D., . . . Povlishock, J. T. (2011). Engaging neuroscience to advance translational research in brain barrier biology. *Nature Reviews Neuroscience, 12*(3), 169. Doi: 10.1038/nrn2995.

Olfert, E. D., Cross, B. M., & McWilliam, A. A. (1993). *Guide to the care and use of experimental animals* (Vol. 1): Canadian Council on Animal Care Ottawa.

Park, J.-H., Cho, H., Kim, H., & Kim, K. (2006). Repeated brief epileptic seizures by pentylenetetrazole cause neurodegeneration and promote neurogenesis in discrete brain regions of freely moving adult rats. *Neuroscience, 140*(2), 673-684. Doi: 10.1016/j.neuroscience.2006.02.076.

Ramos-Morales, F., Correa-Basurto, J., Saavedra-Vélez, M., Acosta-Hernández, M., Gasca-Pérez, E., Pérez-Palacios, A., & Trujillo-Ferrara, J. (2012). Modelo PTZ: un screening primario para el desarrollo de nuevas moléculas con actividad anticonvulsivante. *Archivos de Neurociencias, 17*(1), 45-48. [PTZ model: a primary screening for the development of new molecules with anticonvulsant activity. *Neuroscience Archives*]

Sasa, M. (2006). A new frontier in epilepsy: novel antiepileptogenic drugs. *Journal of pharmacological sciences, 100*(5), 487-494. Doi: 10.1254/jphs.CPJ06010X.

Shariff, S., Suh, M., Zhao, M., Ma, H., & Schwartz, T. H. (2006). Recent developments in oximetry and perfusion-based mapping techniques and their role in the surgical treatment of neocortical epilepsy. *Epilepsy & Behavior, 8*(2), 363-375. Doi: 10.1016/j.yebeh.2005.11.006.

Thurman, D. J., Beghi, E., Begley, C. E., Berg, A. T., Buchhalter, J. R., Ding, D., . . . Kobau, R. (2011). Standards for epidemiologic studies and surveillance of epilepsy. *Epilepsia, 52*, 2-26. Doi: 10.1111/j.1528-1167.2011.03121.x.

Van Hall, G., Stømstad, M., Rasmussen, P., Jans, Ø., Zaar, M., Gam, C., . . Nielsen, H. B. (2009). Blood lactate is an important energy source for the human brain. *Journal of Cerebral Blood Flow & Metabolism, 29*(6), 1121-1129. Doi: 10.1038/jcbfm.2009.35.

Zhao, M., Suh, M., Ma, H., Perry, C., Geneslaw, A., & Schwartz, T. H. (2007). Focal increases in perfusion and decreases in hemoglobin oxygenation precede seizure onset in spontaneous human epilepsy. *Epilepsia, 48*(11), 2059-2067. Doi: 10.1111/j.1528-1167.2007.01229.x.

Zhvania, M. G., Ksovreli, M., Japaridze, N. J., & Lordkipanidze, T. G. (2015). Ultrastructural changes to rat hippocampus in pentylenetetrazol- and kainic acid-induced status epilepticus: A study using electron microscopy. *Micron, 74*, 22-29. Doi: 10.1016/ j.micron.2015.03.015.

In: Laboratory Animals and Neurosciences ISBN: 978-1-53618-462-4
Editors: B. Hernandez Godinez et al.© 2020 Nova Science Publishers, Inc.

*Chapter 5*

# SURGICAL BIOMODELS IN NEUROLOGY: CEREBRAL ISCHEMIA

***Jessica Vanessa Gálvez-Susano[1], Eduardo Vega-Sánchez[2], Stella Viviana Arias-Santiago[1] and Yolanda Cruz[1,*]***

[1]Centro de Investigación en Ciencias de la Salud (CICSA); Universidad Anáhuac México, Huixquilucan, Estado de Mexico
[2]Anestesiología, Hospital regional de Tlalnepantla ISSEMYM, Tlalnepantla, Estado de Mexico

## ABSTRACT

The surgical biomodels currently being used to emulate pathologies in neurology research have evolved to be less invasive, for it has been shown that less invasive procedures lead to less unwanted effects; it has to be considered that the biomodels are structured with enormous similarity to the condition that is being studied thus adapting to our experimental needs.

* Corresponding Author's E-mail: yolanda.cruz@anahuac.mx.

Through this chapter, we will discuss key points of the main focal cerebral ischemia biomodels in laboratory animals: intraluminal occlusion, electrocoagulation occlusion and intracranial suture occlusion. These models have revolutionized the way of inducing focal cerebral ischemia in animal models since they are closer to the pathophysiology of the real disorder and have allowed the development of new pharmacological and physical rehabilitation therapies, which we will review throughout this chapter.

**Keywords:** cerebral ischemia, stroke, surgical biomodels, occlusion artery

## INTRODUCTION

An aging population and the rise of risk factors such as diabetes, hypertension and dyslipidemia as well as sedentary lifestyles contribute to the development of chronic-degenerative illness such as cerebrovascular diseases (CVD), among which, cerebral ischemia (Boehme, Esenwa, and Elkind 2017)

According to the World Health Organization (WHO), CVDs are the second cause of death worldwide (WHO 2018b) and it is considered the third cause of any kind disability, whether temporary or permanent (WHO 2018b); this implies a high economic impact for families and governments, as well as an enormous social impact for the communities.

Given these conditions there is a great need to develop primary, secondary and tertiary prevention alternatives aimed to reduce the incidence and mortality of this disease, which is why further research of its pathophysiology, the development of pharmacological agents and physiotherapy techniques that allow to solve such a big problem is an urgent need. For this, the creation of experimental models that represent the in vivo characteristics of the CVD is utmost priority.

According to the international classification of diseases (ICD-11), CVDs are classified by their etiology, being it hemorrhagic, ischemic or of unknown origin (WHO 2018a); Ischemic CVD is the one with the highest incidence (85-87% of cases) due mainly to thromboembolic occlusions in large arteries (Banerjee and Chimowitz 2017).

Considering that a percentage as high as 85% of the cases of CVD have ischemic origin and that a great amount of them presents later reperfusion, meaning that the blood flow is reestablished either spontaneously (from 50 to 70%) or induced by medical interventions either pharmacological or surgical (L, X, and Z 2016), and that large arteries such as the middle cerebral artery (MCA) is the most commonly occluded (Tsivgoulis et al. 2018); biomodels of transient ischemia (where reperfusion is allowed) or permanent (constant occlusion) biomodels have been developed, mainly for MCA occlusion, in order to trigger the biochemical and molecular processes as close as possible to real events.

## Physiopathological Characteristics of Cerebral Ischemia

Ischemia pathophysiology is characterized by the following biochemical and molecular events. It begins when there is a transient or permanent decrease in cerebral blood flow sufficient enough to cause metabolic and functional impairment (X.M. Hu et al. 2017). Neural tissue is not affected homogeneously as cerebral ischemia causes areas with different damage degrees. The area directly exposed to the blood flow obstruction mechanism becomes an infarct zone (Uzdensky 2019) which is surrounded by a penumbra zone, penumbra presents itself with disorders ranging from ionic alterations to electrical silencing, it is nevertheless viable and potentially salvageable (Yao et al. 2017)

Oxygen and glucose supply interruption during ischemia causes the failure of the Na+ and K+ pumps then causing a rapid intracellular of K+ and Na+ increase resulting in membrane depolarization and Ca2 + entry through voltage-dependent channels and vesicular release (H.-J. Hu and Song 2017) These mechanisms cause the release of excitatory neurotransmitters, glutamate, and aspartate (Alvarez-Sabin et al. 2003)

Released glutamate stimulates membrane ionotropic receptors N-methyl-D-aspartate (NMDA) and α-amino-3-hydroxy-5-methyl-4-

isoxazolepropionic acid (AMPA). AMPA receptor stimulation achieves greater depolarization inducing the release of more glutamate causing cellular edema and the opening of new voltage-dependent channels permeable to Ca2 + (Rama and García 2016).

Ca2 +, in turn, activates the constitutive nitric oxide synthase (NOSc), causing an increase in NO synthesis; In addition to the arrival of different inflammatory cells, the expression of inducible NOS (iNOS) is also increased, which is independent of Ca2 + and produces large amounts of NO. On the other hand, free radicals and Ca2 + rise activate a whole series of enzymes that intervene in catabolic processes that lead to neuronal death such as calpains, phospholipases, endonucleases, etc. (Won, Kim, and Gwag 2002; Lai, Zhang, and Wang 2014).

Both the initial lesions of the endothelium and in the brain parenchyma during blood flow obstruction, induce the release of inflammatory molecules such as interleukins (IL) IL-6, IL-1ß and tumor necrosis factor-alpha (TNF-α), molecular patterns associated with damage, free radicals and chemokines, which together allow the activation of the immune system and the subsequent infiltration of leukocytes (Vidale et al. 2017).

When reperfusion is carried out, that is to say, the restoration of blood flow, oxygen and glucose molecules arrive so substrate (ATP) becomes available and cell death pathway such as apoptosis can be concluded, oxygen molecules participate in reactions that produce free radicals as in the activity of xanthine oxidase, NADPH oxidase and/or cyclooxygenase (Rama and García 2016); these events produce a greater injury since they facilitate the rupture of the blood-brain barrier and the formation of edema (Sun et al. 2018).

In the regions in the heart of the infarction, microglia (innate immune cells of the central nervous system) is activated acquiring phagocytic characteristics and pro-inflammatory phenotype although it also has been demonstrated that it is capable of releasing neuroprotective molecules such as brain-derived neurotrophic factor (BDNF), insulin-like growth factor-1 (IGF-1), IL-4, and IL-10 that drive neural tissue repair (Khoshnam et al. 2017).

The activation of microglia and the infiltration of neutrophils, macrophages, and lymphocytes create a mainly pro-inflammatory environment that contributes to the increase of the neural death area transforming the penumbra zone in an infarcted region.

Several animal models have tried to reproduce these biochemical events, they can be classified into two groups; models that induce permanent ischemia and those that induce transient ischemia; the first seek to reproduce mainly the physiopathological characteristics that occur after a myocardial infarction or events that produce a strong cerebral hypoperfusion (Plesnila 2013) meanwhile models of transient ischemia try to emulate a thrombo-embolic event (Sommer 2017).

Choosing the model type basically depends on what is intended to be studied, whether it is knowing more about the pathophysiology of the event or trying out pharmacological therapies such as thrombolytics, antioxidants, anti-inflammatories, immunomodulators, etc.

## Surgical Biomodels in Cerebral Ischemia

Among the main models that cause permanent ischemia are electrocoagulation, photothrombosis, and middle cerebral artery occlusion (MCAO) either by intracranial ligation or by the insertion of a monofilament that remains permanently in place. Transient ischemia models use a suture filament placed intraluminal in the MCA for a certain time causing ischemia, it is then removed. Another model consists of thrombin microinjection, this forms a thrombus that is maintained for a defined time and is then removed when a thrombolytic agent is applied.

Of the aforementioned models, in the last year (2019), the intraluminal MCAO model has been used more frequently when attempting to cause transient ischemia (Figure 1) while electrocoagulation has been used when trying to cause permanent ischemia followed by phototrombosis; we consider that this is due to the advantages presented by these models which we will discuss later.

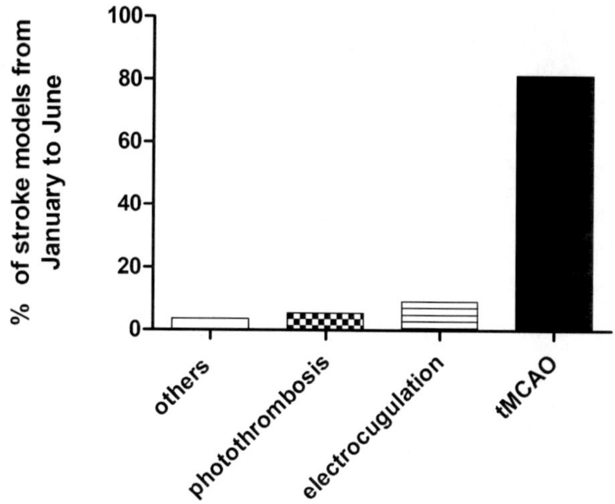


Figure 1. Most used animal models from January-July 2019 (articles found in Pub Med, search words used "cerebral ischemia").

## OCCLUSION BY ELECTROCOAGULATION/ ELECTROCAUTERY

The electrocoagulation model used to cause permanent cerebral blood flow occlusion in rats was published by Akira Tamura in 1981. The surgery is performed under a microscope, the rodent, which is previously anesthetized, is placed in a lateral position. It begins with an incision to the skin between the ear and the orbit on the left side, the division of the temporal muscle is identified, a craniotomy is performed until an orifice is obtained at the junction of the zygomatic arch and the squamous bone, afterward the middle cerebral artery is occluded by electrocoagulation (A. Tamura et al. 1981), in some cases the artery is cut to ensure that there is no reperfusion.

This model has presented modifications through its use with the intention of improving the original technique(M. Tamura et al. 2001); In the conventional model, the left middle cerebral artery (MCA) is occluded between its cortical branches and lateral striate arteries. In the modified technique, the left MCA is occluded by performing electrocoagulation distal to the lateral striatal arteries (Ma et al. 2012) to provoke a defined and greater infarct. Different temperatures with which electrocoagulation is performed have also been evaluated, for example, Da Silva H. and cols. in 2018 determined that the ideal temperature of the probe to produce the vascular lesion should be between 300-400 °C, this allows us to specify an infarction that possesses all the histological and functional characteristics of focal ischemia.

When compared with other models, this one has the advantage of a very short operating time, approximately 10 minutes when performed by a trained scientist. Therefore, short anesthesia times can be achieved, thus clearing the neuroprotective variable of anesthetics (Nunes et al. 2013) . The general mortality of this technique is regularly around 5%. Among the limitations of this model is that a craniotomy is required as access to coagulate the artery, which facilitates the development of infections; In addition, mechanical damage to the cortex during preparation and coagulation cannot be excluded although it can be limited by careful perforation and removal of the skull, constant humidification of the surgical site and minimal necessary electrocoagulation. But the most important disadvantage of this technique is that due to the permanent coagulation of the MCA, reperfusion cannot be obtained, which is a characteristic observed in a substantial percentage of patients with stroke due to the lysis of clots (Llovera et al. 2014). That is why today the use of other techniques is preferred because its high invasiveness and secondary complications limit the emulation of the stroke (Fluri, Schuhmann, and Kleinschnitz 2015)

Despite the limitations of the model, it has allowed defining the core terms of ischemic infarction and penumbra, as well as being able to evaluate some neuroprotective agents (Colak, Filiano, and Johnson 2011) of importance such as D-Deprenyl, also known as selegiline, which has been shown to possess neuroprotective qualities since it reduced the size of the infarction by 50%, the number of apoptotic cells and the ability to induce neuroplasticity (Simon et al. 2001); in 2015, it was tested in 47 patients who met the inclusion criteria in an Italian clinic where they evaluated that selegiline is capable of stimulating cognitive and motor recovery (Bartolo et al. 2015), this drug is still undergoing evaluation.

## OCCLUSION BY PHOTOTHROMBOSIS

The photothrombosis model was proposed by Rosenblum WI and EL-Sabban F. in the '70s, in this model 2% sodium fluorescein was added intravenously (IV), then the animals were anesthetized and subjected to craniotomy where the dura mater was perforated in order to expose the tissue that would later receive the mercury light, which allowed the formation of platelet aggregates due to the endothelial denudation just in the area where the light affected (Rosenblum and El-Sabban 1977).

Subsequently, the use of sodium fluorescein was replaced by pink bengal dye, the latter also belongs to the family of fluorescein dyes, but the advantage of its use is that a craniotomy is not necessary to allow the effect of light on the dye, so this variant of the technique is less invasive; In addition, it causes a greater volume of thrombosis because the extent of the infarction can increase for several hours, another advantage is that it allows to specifically choose the location of the ischemic lesion (Watson et al. 1985) although it has the limitation of not allowing reperfusion

This model allowed the evaluation of several neuroprotective drugs which were then evaluated in the clinic context as chlormethiazole, which showed promising neuroprotective effects in basic research, as Snape MF and cols showed in 1993 when it was able to reduce the size of the infarct by up to 50%; unfortunately in clinical trials when it was administered to patients who had suffered ischemia and showed cortical dysfunction they did not show any improvement (Lyden et al. 2002); In the same way, lubeluzole showed neuroprotective effects in murine patients, reducing the infarct area by up to 24% (De Ryck et al. 1996); in 2002 Gandolfo C. and cols. concluded by analyzing several articles of clinical evaluations that lubeluzole does not present real benefits in the clinic, on the contrary, they found that it exacerbates cardiac disorders.

Years later in 1988 Nakayama H and cols. proposed modifications to the technique with the intention of specifically occluding the middle cerebral artery (MCA) and allowing reperfusion after photothrombosis caused by rose bengal; for this, the artery region has to be exposed, so it is necessary to remove part of the jaw and retract the masseter muscle after injecting the rose bengal in an I.V. access; subsequently, the animals were placed in the stereotaxic in a position in which the laser first touches the region of the proximal MCA, then in the distal region of the olfactory tract and proximal to the rinal branch. To allow recanalization, one hour after thrombosis the dura mater were perforated along the MCA then topical nimodipine was applied, this is a calcium channel blocker that allows vasodilation. The results showed that although the possibility of reperfusion was allowed, the ischemic lesions presented severe edema and hemorrhage, so the model was not widely used.

Currently, although this model is scarcely used (Figure 1) some researchers use it because the mortality rate of experimental animals is low, platelet aggregation and the consequent formation of thrombi (as the original cause of ischemia) is allowed, the area where the infarction is needed can be specifically selected and enables preservation of the cellular changes that develop during ischemia such as edema and infiltration of inflammatory cells; however, the main limitation is that the rapid and massive coagulation within the area of illumination during the development of the model differs from the way in which ischemia actually occurs (Liu et al. 2017).

## Thrombus/Embolic Occlusion

With the intention of creating an injury as similar as possible to the events taking place in the human brain during ischemia, in 1982 Kudo and cols adapted a model that had been used previously in dogs by Hill NC and cols. in 1955 (Braeuninger and Kleinschnitz 2009). Kudo injected thrombi created in situ with autologous whole blood in the carotid artery of each rat, achieving heterogeneous cerebral infarctions because the thrombi were fragile due to the high amount of red blood cells; this easily allowed spontaneous recanalization and with it a huge variability in the size and location of the infarcts, so the technique was difficult to reproduce (Overgaard et al. 1992)

Kudo's model underwent several modifications, for example in 1958 Chandler AB. created *in vitro* a more resistant clot with citrated whole blood that maintained characteristics very similar to a thrombus (Ardlie, Raelene, and Kinlough 1966), this model also did not allow homogeneous infarctions, so later, in 1992 Overgaard K and cols injected through the internal carotid artery (ACI) clots created with a mixture of thrombin and whole blood in a 4: 1 ratio; In 1997, Zhang Z and cols.et directly injected thrombin into the ICA, creating highly reproducible infarctions. Subsequently, the thrombin injection also began to be applied directly to the middle cerebral artery (MCA).

In this technique, rodents are anesthetized then placed in a stereotaxic, a skin incision is made between the right eye and the right ear so the temporal muscle is exposed, the masseter muscle is dissociated from the edge of the skull and is cut vertically exposing the skull to perform a craniotomy. A Doppler probe is placed in the distal part of the MCA to record the speed of blood flow, the pipette containing the thrombin is mounted in the micromanipulator and connected to a syringe filled with air, the tip of the pipette is inserted into the lumen of the MCA and thrombin is injected by applying a positive air pressure with the syringe, the pipette is removed 10 minutes after thrombin injection to allow clot stabilization (Ansar et al. 2014).

This surgical model is of vital importance because it was used to test the only pharmacological treatment authorized by the Food and Drugs Administration (FDA) for acute ischemic stroke, which is the activator of intravenous recombinant tissue-type plasminogen (r-tPA), which can be administered within 4.5 hours after the onset of stroke, however, it can only be administered to very few patients who met criteria for reperfusion, achieving early arterial recanalization in less than 50% of cases and it is known it could cause harmful effects such as intracranial hemorrhage; hence, the need to develop new acute strategies for the treatment of stroke (Orset et al. 2007).

That is the reason there has been a great development in research regarding Stroke, for example, it was stated recently at the International Stroke Conference that there are benefits to the administration of r-tPA in an extended therapeutic window of up to 9 hours in selected patients candidates for reperfusion (Mark 2019).

There are several techniques for achieving embolic occlusion, among the ones used frequently in recent protocols is ferric chloride-induced thrombosis in rats where the same procedure is performed but instead of inserting thrombin, a plastic tube is wrapped around the MCA, then a filter paper soaked with 35% ferric chloride is placed around the tube. 4 minutes after initiating the treatment, the filter paper is removed, the artery is washed with normal saline and the blood flow is monitored continuously for 30 minutes (Sawada et al. 2014).

Another of the modifications that this technique has are the models based on micro and macrospheres; the microsphere model includes spheres with a diameter of 20 to 50 μm of different materials, such as dextran, supraparamagnetic iron oxide, $TiO_2$, and ceramics. The procedure consists of inserting microspheres in the ACM or ICA through the ECA using a microcatheter, which is passively rinsed in the cerebral circulation by the blood flow, this model produces multifocal and heterogeneous infarctions. The macrosphere model uses spheres with a diameter of 100–400 μm, which are inserted into the ICA, providing a reproducible occlusion of the main stem of the MCA, resulting in focal ischemic lesions that are comparable to the MCAO suture model. In contrast to the MCAO model, this technique preserves the blood supply to the hypothalamus and, therefore, prevents hypothalamic infarctions and suffering from post-surgical hyperthermia (Fluri, Schuhmann, and Kleinschnitz 2015).

## Occlusion by Intracranial Suture

This biomodel was described by Shigeno T. in 1985, it was one of the first techniques to be used worldwide to emulate focal cerebral ischemia with reperfusion; although other less invasive methods are preferred today, it is still used by many authors.

In the Shigeno technique, the trunk of the middle cerebral artery is isolated between the rhinocortical branch and the lenticulostriated artery and the trunk is surrounded with a loose suture. The suture is externalized through a small polyethylene catheter, which is previously inserted into the craniectomy site through a hole drilled in the zygomatic bone. The occlusion of the middle cerebral artery is achieved by retracting the nylon filament, which is then fixed with biological glue and recirculation is achieved by cutting and removing the thread. Under the operating microscope, the complete cessation of blood flow and subsequent restoration of blood circulation are confirmed.

During occlusion of the ACM, blood flow is reduced by up to 75% in the cortex while in the caudate nucleus up to 65%, the decrease is even less pronounced at the periphery of the adjacent ischemic area (penumbra zone) to the cingulate cortex. When reperfusion is allowed it is possible to observe an increase in blood flow that exceeds the values of the contralateral hemisphere, the increased flow persists between 30 minutes and 2 hours after ischemia. As time progresses, post-occlusion flow tends to be subnormal and late hypoperfusion is limited to the central region, with good recovery of blood flow over the penumbra zone (Shigeno et al. 1985).

In 1986 Bederson JB. concluded that an important limitation of this model is that it caused various lesions in the frontal cortex and the striatum of the animal, causing an increase in the size of the lesion thus causing behavioral, learning and sensory abnormalities, which may be the result of altered levels of norepinephrine, this is why this model is not recommended for investigations of memory dysfunctions (Leker and Constantini 2002).

## Intraluminal Monofilament Model

The intraluminal suture or monofilament model in the MCAO is one of the most used techniques in the investigation of cerebrovascular accidents (Vital and Gavins 2016) since it is the least invasive method of the MCAO models because it does not require craniectomy and, therefore, prevents damage to cranial structures (Fluri, Schuhmann, and Kleinschnitz 2015).

In this surgical model, there are important variables such as survival rate, lesion volume, neurological scores, cerebral blood flow and body weight, including suture type and filament diameter (Morris et al. 2016).

This surgery is performed under a microscope, the rodent is placed in ventral position with the neck in extension to achieve maximum exposure of the surgical site, then an incision is made in the midline between the manubrium and the mandible (Fluri, Schuhmann, and Kleinschnitz 2015)

The underlying submandibular glands are exposed and dissection is continued until reaching the omohyoid muscle, the common carotid artery (CCA) is exposed, once its identification is complete the adjacent vagus nerve is separated from the bifurcation of the CCA in the external carotid artery (ECA) and the internal carotid artery (ICA). The superior thyroid artery (STA) and the occipital artery (OA) are isolated and cauterized (Morris et al. 2016)

Next, the ECA is permanently ligated as distally as possible to the CCA bifurcation and then cauterized. At this point, some operators suggest the removal of the pterygopalatine artery, which bifurcates from the ICA (Chen et al. 2008). The insertion of the intraluminal suture, which is ultimately the one that will cause the blood blockage of the MCA, can be incorporated either through the ECA (Longa method) or through the ICA (Koizumi method) (Vital and Gavins 2016). After the occlusion surgery, the incision sites in the neck are sutured and the animal is left to recover from anesthesia until reperfusion must be performed (Chiang, Messing, and Chou 2011).

This model has allowed us to evaluate a long list of neuroprotectors ranging from those that try to avoid initial ionic alterations in ischemia and those that capture free radicals to those that avoid or modulate the immune response. For example, metformin; this is an oral hypoglycemic agent that has demonstrated neuroprotective effects in basic research and in some clinical studies where at a dose of 200 mg/kg it exerts neuroprotection through the increase in AMPK activity (AMP-activated protein kinase); although on the contrary if different doses are applied, it presents a decrease, so the dose and duration of treatment have yet to be determined in order to have favorable results (Leech, Chattipakorn, and Chattipakorn 2019).

Another drug tested with this model is copolymer-1 (Cop-1) which is a peptide formed by L-alanine, L-lysine, L-glutamic acid and L-tyrosine (Ibarra, Avendano, and Cruz 2007), which has been shown to have neuroprotective effects and at the same time induce neurogenesis, which allows to preserve the neural tissue and promote a remarkable motor recovery (Cruz et al. 2015); this is because Cop-1 modulates the immune response by inducing a change in the Th-2 phenotype of activated lymphocytes during the development of the pathology, this change induces the secretion of anti-inflammatory cytokines and neurotrophic factors that in turn modulate the cerebral microenvironment (Cruz et al. 2018).

Fingolimod is another immunomodulator that has been shown to have neuroprotective effects since it is able to reduce the size of infarction in rodents, neurological deficit and edema using the OACM model (Wei et al. 2011); Such encouraging results led to it being tested in the clinical environment where it has had encouraging results since it has avoided secondary tissue injury, attenuating the neurological deficit and promoting recovery (Fu et al. 2014), but its safety and posterior adverse effects are yet to be established.

## CONCLUSION

Experimental models that cause cerebral ischemia have provided an enormous knowledge of pathology at the molecular level and have allowed the evaluation of a large number of drugs, unfortunately r-tPA is the only one approved by the FDA that is considered effective for treatment of the stroke so it is very important to continue experimenting to propose more and different alternatives until a range of safe and effective drugs that allow the extensive recovery of people with stroke is achieved and for this it is of utmost importance to refine and maintain animal models.

## REFERENCES

Alvarez-Sabin, J., A. Davalos, E. Martinez-Vila, J. Vivancos, J. J. Zarranz, J. Castillo-Dominguez, E. Diez-Tejedor, and I Lizasoain. 2003. "Revisión de consenso. Neuroprotección farmacológica en la isquemia cerebral: ¿es todavía una opción terapéutica?". *Neurologia* 18: 369-384. [Consensus Review Pharmacological neuroprotection in cerebral ischemia: is it still a therapeutic option?. *Neurology*. 18 (7): 369-384.].

Ansar, S., E. Chatzikonstantinou, A. Wistuba-Schier, S. Mirau-Weber, M. Fatar, M. G. Hennerici, and S. Meairs. 2014. "Characterization of a new model of thromboembolic stroke in C57 black/6J mice." *Transl Stroke Res* 5 (4): 526-33. Accessed September 23, 2019. doi.org/10.1007/s12975-013-0315-9.

Ardlie, N. G., L. Raelene, and R. L. Kinlough. 1966. "In vitro thrombosis and platelet aggregation in myocardial infarction." *Br Med J* 1 (5492): 888-91.

Banerjee, C., and M. I. Chimowitz. 2017. "Stroke Caused by Atherosclerosis of the Major Intracranial Arteries." *Circ Res* 120 (3): 502-513. Accessed September 23, 2019. doi.org/10.1161/circresaha.116.308441.

Bartolo, M., C. Zucchella, A. Capone, G. Sandrini, and F. Pierelli. 2015. "An explorative study regarding the effect of l-deprenyl on cognitive and functional recovery in patients after stroke." *J Neurol Sci* 349 (1-2): 117-23. Accessed September 23, 2019. doi.org/10.1016/j.jns.2014.12.039.

Boehme, A. K., C. Esenwa, and M. S. Elkind. 2017. "Stroke Risk Factors, Genetics, and Prevention." *Circ Res* 120 (3): 472-495. Accessed September 23, 2019. doi.org/10.1161/circresaha.116.308398.

Braeuninger, S., and C. Kleinschnitz. 2009. "Rodent models of focal cerebral ischemia: procedural pitfalls and translational problems." *Exp Transl Stroke Med* 1: 8. Accessed September 23, 2019. doi.org/10.1186/2040-7378-1-8.

Chen, Y., A. Ito, K. Takai, and N. Saito. 2008. "Blocking pterygopalatine arterial blood flow decreases infarct volume variability in a mouse model of intraluminal suture middle cerebral artery occlusion." *J*

*Neurosci Methods* 174 (1): 18-24. Accessed September 24, 2019. doi.org/10.1016/j.jneumeth.2008.06.021.

Chiang, Terrance, Robert O Messing, and Wen-Hai Chou. 2011. "Mouse model of middle cerebral artery occlusion." *JoVE (Journal of Visualized Experiments)* (48): e2761.

Colak, G., A. J. Filiano, and G. V. Johnson. 2011. "The application of permanent middle cerebral artery ligation in the mouse." *J Vis Exp* (53). Accessed September 24, 2019. doi.org/10.3791/3039.

Cruz, Y., E. E. Garcia, J. V. Galvez, S. V. Arias-Santiago, H. G. Carvajal, R. Silva-Garcia, H. Bonilla-Jaime, J. Rojas-Castaneda, and A. Ibarra. 2018. "Release of interleukin-10 and neurotrophic factors in the choroid plexus: possible inductors of neurogenesis following copolymer-1 immunization after cerebral ischemia." *Neural Regen Res* 13 (10): 1743-1752. Accessed September 24, 2019. doi.org/10.4103/1673-5374.238615.

Cruz, Y., J. Lorea, H. Mestre, J. H. Kim-Lee, J. Herrera, R. Mellado, V. Galvez, L. Cuellar, C. Musri, and A. Ibarra. 2015. "Copolymer-1 promotes neurogenesis and improves functional recovery after acute ischemic stroke in rats." *PLoS One* 10 (3): e0121854. Accessed September 24, 2019. doi.org/10.1371/journal.pone.0121854.

De Ryck, M., R. Keersmaekers, H. Duytschaever, C. Claes, G. Clincke, M. Janssen, and G. Van Reet. 1996. "Lubeluzole protects sensorimotor function and reduces infarct size in a photochemical stroke model in rats." *J Pharmacol Exp Ther* 279 (2): 748-58.

Fluri, F., M. K. Schuhmann, and C. Kleinschnitz. 2015. "Animal models of ischemic stroke and their application in clinical research." *Drug Des Devel Ther* 9: 3445-54. Accessed September 24, 2019. doi.org/10.2147/dddt.s56071.

Fu, Y., N. Zhang, L. Ren, Y. Yan, N. Sun, Y. J. Li, W. Han, R. Xue, Q. Liu, J. Hao, C. Yu, and F. D. Shi. 2014. "Impact of an immune modulator fingolimod on acute ischemic stroke." *Proc Natl Acad Sci U S A* 111 (51): 18315-20. Accessed September 25, 2019. doi.org/10.1073/pnas.1416166111.

Hu, Hui-Jie, and Mingke Song. 2017. "Disrupted Ionic Homeostasis in Ischemic Stroke and New Therapeutic Targets." *Journal of Stroke and Cerebrovascular Diseases* 26 (12): 2706-2719. Accessed September 25, 2019. doi.org/10.1016/j.jstrokecerebrovasdis.2017.09.011.

Hu, X. M., T. M. De Silva, J. Chen, and F. M. Faraci. 2017. "Cerebral Vascular Disease and Neurovascular Injury in Ischemic Stroke." *Circulation Research* 120 (3): 449-471. Accessed September 25, 2019 doi.org/10.1161/circresaha.116.308427.

Ibarra, A., H. Avendano, and Y. Cruz. 2007. "Copolymer-1 (Cop-1) improves neurological recovery after middle cerebral artery occlusion in rats." *Neurosci Lett* 425 (2): 110-3. Accessed September 26, 2019 doi.org/10.1016/j.neulet.2007.08.038.

Khoshnam, Seyed Esmaeil, William Winlow, Maryam Farzaneh, Yaghoob Farbood, and Hadi Fathi Moghaddam. 2017. "Pathogenic mechanisms following ischemic stroke." *Neurological Sciences* 38 (7): 1167-1186. Accessed September 26, 2019. doi.org/10.1007/s10072-017-2938-1. https://doi.org/10.1007/s10072-017-2938-1.

L, L., W. X, and Y. Z. 2016. "Ischemia-reperfusion Injury in the Brain: Mechanisms and Potential Therapeutic Strategies." *Biochem Pharmacol (Los Angel)* 5 (4). Accessed September 26, 2019. doi.org/10.4172/2167-0501.1000213.

Lai, T. W., S. Zhang, and Y. T. Wang. 2014. "Excitotoxicity and stroke: identifying novel targets for neuroprotection." *Prog Neurobiol* 115: 157-88. Accessed September 26, 2019. doi.org/10.1016/j.pneurobio.2013.11.006.

Leech, T., N. Chattipakorn, and S. C. Chattipakorn. 2019. "The beneficial roles of metformin on the brain with cerebral ischaemia/reperfusion injury." *Pharmacol Res* 146: 104261. Accessed September 26, 2019. doi.org/10.1016/j.phrs.2019.104261.

Leker, R. R., and S. Constantini. 2002. "Experimental models in focal cerebral ischemia: are we there yet?" *Acta Neurochir Suppl* 83: 55-9. Accessed September 26, 2019. doi.org/10.1007/978-3-7091-6743-4_10.

Liu, N. W., C. C. Ke, Y. Zhao, Y. A. Chen, K. C. Chan, D. T. Tan, J. S. Lee, Y. Y. Chen, T. W. Hsu, Y. J. Hsieh, C. W. Chang, B. H. Yang, W. S.

Huang, and R. S. Liu. 2017. "Evolutional Characterization of Photochemically Induced Stroke in Rats: a Multimodality Imaging and Molecular Biological Study." *Transl Stroke Res* 8 (3): 244-256. Accessed September 26, 2019. doi.org/10.1007/s12975-016-0512-4.

Llovera, G., S. Roth, N. Plesnila, R. Veltkamp, and A. Liesz. 2014. "Modeling stroke in mice: permanent coagulation of the distal middle cerebral artery." *J Vis Exp* (89): e51729. Accessed September 27, 2019. doi.org/10.3791/51729.

Lyden, P., A. Shuaib, K. Ng, K. Levin, R. P. Atkinson, A. Rajput, L. Wechsler, T. Ashwood, L. Claesson, T. Odergren, and E. Salazar-Grueso. 2002. "Clomethiazole Acute Stroke Study in ischemic stroke (CLASS-I): final results." *Stroke* 33 (1): 122-8. Accessed September 27, 2019 doi.org/10.1161/hs0102.101478.

Ma, J., C. Peng, W. Guo, Y. F. Dong, X. H. Dong, X. Sun, and H. H. Xie. 2012. "A modified model of middle cerebral artery electrocoagulation in mice." *CNS Neurosci Ther* 18 (9): 796-8. Accessed September 27, 2019 doi.org/10.1111/j.1755-5949.2012.00370.x.

Mark, Parson. 2019. "Safety Window for tPA Extended Up to 9 Hours for Ischemic Stroke". *International Stroke Conference*, Honolulu.

Morris, G. P., A. L. Wright, R. P. Tan, A. Gladbach, L. M. Ittner, and B. Vissel. 2016. "A Comparative Study of Variables Influencing Ischemic Injury in the Longa and Koizumi Methods of Intraluminal Filament Middle Cerebral Artery Occlusion in Mice." *PLoS One* 11 (2): e0148503. Accessed September 27, 2019. doi.org/10.1371/journal.pone.0148503.

Nunes, Rogean Rodrigues, Gastão Fernandes Duval Neto, Júlio César Garcia de Alencar, Suyane Benevides Franco, Nayanna Quezado de Andrade, Danielle Maia Holanda Dumaresq, and Sara Lúcia Cavalcante. 2013. "Anestésicos, Pre-condicionamiento y Protección Cerebral." *Brazilian Journal of Anesthesiology (Edicion en Espanol)* 63 (1): 119-129. Accessed September 27, 2019. doi.org/10/10.16/j.bjanes.2013.07.002. [Anesthetics, cerebral protection and preconditioning. *Brazilian Journal of Anesthesiology*]

Orset, C., R. Macrez, A. R. Young, D. Panthou, E. Angles-Cano, E. Maubert, V. Agin, and D. Vivien. 2007. "Mouse model of in situ thromboembolic stroke and reperfusion." *Stroke* 38 (10): 2771-8. Accessed September 27, 2019. doi.org/10.1161/strokeaha.107.487520.

Overgaard, K., T. Sereghy, G. Boysen, H. Pedersen, S. Hoyer, and N. H. Diemer. 1992. "A rat model of reproducible cerebral infarction using thrombotic blood clot emboli." *J Cereb Blood Flow Metab* 12 (3): 484-90. Accessed September 27, 2019. doi.org/10.1038/jcbfm.1992.66.

Plesnila, N. 2013. "Pathophysiological Role of Global Cerebral Ischemia following Subarachnoid Hemorrhage: The Current Experimental Evidence." *Stroke Res Treat* 2013: 651958. Accessed September 27, 2019. doi.org/10.1155/2013/651958.

Rama, Ramon, and Julio César García. 2016. "Excitotoxicity and oxidative stress in acute stroke." *Ischemic Stroke-Updates*.

Rosenblum, W. I., and F. El-Sabban. 1977. "Platelet aggregation in the cerebral microcirculation: effect of aspirin and other agents." *Circ Res* 40 (3): 320-8. Accessed September 27, 2019. doi.org/10.1161/01.res.40.3.320.

Sawada, H., N. Nishimura, E. Suzuki, J. Zhuang, K. Hasegawa, H. Takamatsu, K. Honda, and K. Hasumi. 2014. "SMTP-7, a novel small-molecule thrombolytic for ischemic stroke: a study in rodents and primates." *J Cereb Blood Flow Metab* 34 (2): 235-41. Accessed September 27, 2019. doi.org/10.1038/jcbfm.2013.191.

Shigeno, T., G. M. Teasdale, J. McCulloch, and D. I. Graham. 1985. "Recirculation model following MCA occlusion in rats. Cerebral blood flow, cerebrovascular permeability, and brain edema." *J Neurosurg* 63 (2): 272-7. Accessed September 27, 2019. doi.org/10.3171/jns.1985.63.2.0272.

Simon, L., G. Szilagyi, Z. Bori, P. Orbay, and Z. Nagy. 2001. "(-)-D-Deprenyl attenuates apoptosis in experimental brain ischaemia." *Eur J Pharmacol* 430 (2-3): 235-41. Accessed September 27, 2019. doi.org/10.1016/s0014-2999(01)01375-9.

Sommer, C. J. 2017. “Ischemic stroke: experimental models and reality.” *Acta Neuropathol* 133 (2): 245-261. Accessed September 27, 2019. doi.org/10.1007/s00401-017-1667-0.

Sun, M. S., H. Jin, X. Sun, S. Huang, F. L. Zhang, Z. N. Guo, and Y. Yang. 2018. “Free Radical Damage in Ischemia-Reperfusion Injury: An Obstacle in Acute Ischemic Stroke after Revascularization Therapy.” *Oxid Med Cell Longev* 2018: 3804979. Accessed September 24, 2019. doi.org/10.1155/2018/3804979.

Tamura, A., D. I. Graham, J. McCulloch, and G. M. Teasdale. 1981. “Focal Cerebral Ischaemia in the Rat: 1. Description of Technique and Early Neuropathological Consequences following Middle Cerebral Artery Occlusion.” *Journal of Cerebral Blood Flow & Metabolism* 1 (1): 53-60. Accessed September 27, 2019. doi.org/10.1038/jcbfm.1981.6.

Tamura, Masaru, Yasuaki Aoki, Toshie Seto, Yoshinori Itoh, and Yojiro Ukai. 2001. “Cerebroprotective action of a Na+/Ca2+ channel blocker NS-7: II. Effect on the cerebral infarction, behavioral and cognitive impairments at the chronic stage of permanent middle cerebral artery occlusion in rats.” *Brain Research* 890 (1): 170-176. Accessed September 27, 2019 doi.org/https://doi.org/10.1016/S0006-8993(00)03168-1.

Tsivgoulis, G., A. Safouris, D. E. Kim, and A. V. Alexandrov. 2018. “Recent Advances in Primary and Secondary Prevention of Atherosclerotic Stroke.” *J Stroke* 20 (2): 145-166. Accessed September 27, 2019. doi.org/10.5853/jos.2018.00773.

Uzdensky, A. B. 2019. “Apoptosis regulation in the penumbra after ischemic stroke: expression of pro- and antiapoptotic proteins.” *Apoptosis* 24 (9-10): 687-702. Accessed September 27, 2019. doi.org/10.1007/s10495-019-01556-6.

Vidale, S., A. Consoli, M. Arnaboldi, and D. Consoli. 2017. “Postischemic Inflammation in Acute Stroke.” *J Clin Neurol* 13 (1): 1-9. Accessed September 27, 2019. doi.org/10.3988/jcn.2017.13.1.1.

Vital, S. A., and F. N. Gavins. 2016. “Surgical Approach for Middle Cerebral Artery Occlusion and Reperfusion Induced Stroke in Mice.” *J Vis Exp* (116). Accessed September 24, 2019. doi.org/10.3791/54302.

Watson, B. D., W. D. Dietrich, R. Busto, M. S. Wachtel, and M. D. Ginsberg. 1985. "Induction of reproducible brain infarction by photochemically initiated thrombosis." *Ann Neurol* 17 (5): 497-504. Accessed September 27, 2019. doi.org/10.1002/ana.410170513.

Wei, Y., M. Yemisci, H. H. Kim, L. M. Yung, H. K. Shin, S. K. Hwang, S. Guo, T. Qin, N. Alsharif, V. Brinkmann, J. K. Liao, E. H. Lo, and C. Waeber. 2011. "Fingolimod provides long-term protection in rodent models of cerebral ischemia." *Ann Neurol* 69 (1): 119-29. Accessed September 27, 2019 doi.org/10.1002/ana.22186.

WHO. 2018a. *The 11th Revision of the International Classification of Diseases (ICD- 11) is due by 2018.* Accessed September 27, 2019 http://www.who.int/classifications/icd/revision/en/.

WHO. 2018b. *The top 10 causes of death.* Accessed September 27, 2019. https://www.who.int/news-room/fact-sheets/detail/the-top-10-causes-of-death.

Won, Seok-Joon, Doo-Yeon Kim, and Byoung-Joo Gwag. 2002. "Cellular and molecular pathways of ischemic neuronal death." *BMB Reports* 35 (1): 67-86.

Yao, H., T. Ago, T. Kitazono, and T. Nabika. 2017. "NADPH Oxidase-Related Pathophysiology in Experimental Models of Stroke." *Int J Mol Sci.* 18 (10). Accessed September 27, 2019. doi.org/10.3390/ijms18102123.

In: Laboratory Animals and Neurosciences ISBN: 978-1-53618-462-4
Editors: B. Hernandez Godinez et al.© 2020 Nova Science Publishers, Inc.

*Chapter 6*

# STUDY OF ADDICTION IN GENETICALLY MODIFIED MICE

***Andrea Herrera Solís*[1,*], *Wendy Verónica Herrera Morales*[2], *Luis Núñez Jaramillo*[2], *Mónica Méndez Díaz*[3] *and Oscar Prospéro García*[3]**

[1]Efectos Terapéuticos de los Canabinoides, Subdirección de Investigación Biomédica, Hospital General Dr. Manuel Gea González, Ciudad de México, México

[2] División de Ciencias de la Salud, Universidad de Quintana Roo, Chetumal, Quintana Roo, México

[3]Laboratorio de Canabinoides, Departamento de Fisiología, Facultad de Medicina, Universidad Nacional de México, Ciudad de México, México

[*] Corresponding Author's E-mail:draandreahs@gmail.com.

## Abstract

Addiction to drugs is a complex health problem that involves genetic and environmental factors. In humans, studies of twins have shown that genetics is an important component of drug addiction. Genetic engineering has recently led to great advances in this field, and the use of knockout or transgenic mice to study addiction to several abused drugs has shown that various genes are involved in addiction, as a general psychiatric disorder or addiction to a specific abused substance. Some examples of these include genes that encode dopamine receptors (such as D4L), monoamine transporters (such as DAT and SERT), different nicotine receptor subunits (such as β2 and α7), and enzymes (such as ALDH2), among many others. Furthermore, it has been found that genes not only contribute to vulnerability, but some also protect against addiction. This chapter describes some of the genes that have been found to be involved in addiction to substances such as psychostimulants, nicotine, and alcohol, in terms of both risk and protection, based on the study of genetically modified mice.


**Keywords**: addiction, drug abuse, psychostimulants, alcohol, nicotine, genetically modified mice, knockout mice, transgenic mice

## Introduction

Addiction to legal and illegal drugs such as nicotine, alcohol, cocaine, amphetamines, heroin, and marijuana comes with high economic and social costs and is one of the most important health problems worldwide. Addiction to drugs is a neuropsychiatric disorder characterized by 1) loss of control over drug seeking and drug taking (compulsion), 2) the presentation of negative emotional states such as dysphoria, anxiety, and intense craving, and 3) a high propensity for relapse and withdrawal (Koob and Volkow 2016, American Psychiatric Association 2013).

Both environmental and genetic factors influence the risk of developing addiction to drugs. Estimates indicate that genetics accounts for 40 to 60% of the vulnerability to drug addiction (Uhl 2004). This is primarily based on the study of monozygotic and dizygotic twins from the same nuclear family or from different adoptive families.

Potentially addictive drugs produce reinforcing effects in both humans and other mammals. In laboratories, monkeys, rats, and mice have been found to voluntarily consume addictive substances such as heroin, cocaine, and alcohol e.g., and the characteristics of their oral and intravenous consumption are very similar to those of humans, validating the use of animals as experimental models of addiction (Spanagel 2017). The neurophysiologic mechanisms of addiction have primarily been studied using animal models and behavioral paradigms that allow us to evaluate the self-administration of drugs, their reinforcing effect, and withdrawal and relapse, among others factors.

While animal models cannot completely reproduce the complexity of addiction in humans, they do enable us to study mechanisms that underlie addiction and to identify the genes that are involved in vulnerability to addiction to certain drugs of abuse, as well as those involved in protection from addiction. In this way, the use of genetically modified animals as models of addiction has led to the discovery of the involvement of genes and the ability to better substantiate the findings reported by genome-wide association studies (GWAS).

In animals and humans, drugs of abuse activate the brain's reward system, increasing the likelihood of consuming drugs again. The meso-cortico-striatal dopamine system is composed of the ventral tegmental area (VTA), nucleus accumbens (NAcc), and prefrontal cortex, and is the principal circuitry for reward, responsible for mediating binging and intoxication stages (Uhl, Koob, and Cable 2019). However, there are other systems that participate in addiction, including those that are involved in negative emotional states such as withdrawal and craving. The extended amygdala hypothalamus and brainstem are implicated in withdrawal and the basolateral amygdala, hippocampus, prefrontal, orbital and anterior cingulate cortices are involved in craving (Uhl, Koob, and Cable 2019, Koob and Volkow 2010). While dopamine is the principal neurotransmitter associated with addiction, many other neurotransmitters or neuromodulators are also associated with it, including GABA, glutamate, serotonin, acetylcholine, endocanabinoids, opioid peptides, and corticotropin-releasing factor, among others (Koob and Volkow 2016).

## GENETICALLY MODIFIED MICE

Advances in genetic engineering have led to the ability to make specific genome modifications in animals and to develop techniques to produce genetically modified animals. While the use of these animals is recent in neuroscience, and more specifically in the study of addiction, it has had a large impact.

Since mice have been used in the majority of genetic modifications, throughout this chapter we will focus on this animal model. In the study of addictions, the use of genetically modified mice has contributed greatly to clarifying the importance of a particular gene or its product, such as a receptor, a subunit, or neurotransmitter, or even an inserted and overexpressed human gene cluster in a mouse, to name some examples. In this chapter, the effects produced by deletion, overexpression, re-expression, and the insertion of a cluster in mice are compared to wild-type (WT) littermate controls, which we will refer to as WT.

The most commonly used genetically modified mouse model is conventional or global knockout (KO) (Figure 1), which completely lacks the expression of one or several target genes. Gene trapping and gene targeting methods are most often used to introduce site-specific genetic mutations into the genome of mouse embryonic stem (ES) cells (Fowler and Kenny 2012). In these knockout mice, since gene deletion is performed during embryogenesis, it is important to take into account that developmental problems as well as compensatory mechanisms can occur, such as compensation by other genes of the same family or by unrelated genes (Pich and Epping-Jordan 1998).

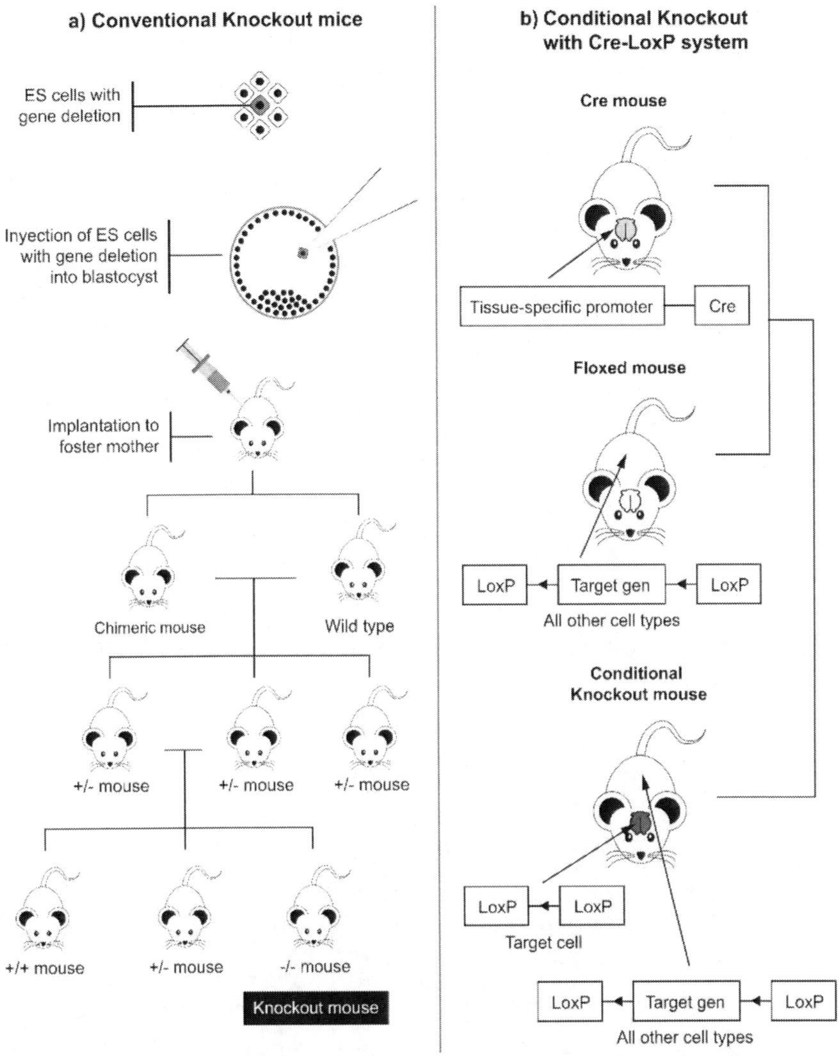


Figure 1. Genetically modified mice. a) Conventional knockout mice: embryonic stem cells with gene deletion are injected into a blastocyst that is implanted in a foster mother, resulting in a chimeric mouse. The cross between the chimeric mouse and a wild-type parent mouse produces heterozygote (+/-) mice. Lastly, the knock-out mice (-/-) are the product of a cross between heterozygote mice. b) Conditional knockout mice with Cre-LoxP system: a mouse expressing Cre recombinase with tissue-specific promoter is mated with a floxed mouse (LoxP sequences are flanked by a gene of interest in this mouse) and the offspring are tissue-specific mice.

After obtaining conventional knockout mice, the Cre recombinase system is used to remove or invert loxP-flanked DNA segments, or to create an intermolecular recombination between different DNA molecules. Conditional transgenics or conditional knockouts (Figure 1.) can be obtained by using recombinase activity as a genetic activation/deactivation switch (Nagy 2000). The advantage of this type of knockout is the ability to make more specific genetic modifications, such as disrupting the receptor gene in a cell-type specific or region-specific manner. And by combining several techniques, a mutation or homologous human receptor cDNAs can even be introduced through the homologous recombination of embryonic stem cells, in order to produce receptor knockins (Matsuda and Aiba 2004).

## Animal Models of Drug Addiction

The behavioral paradigms that are most used in animal models are conditioned place preference (CPP) and operant self-administration, including intravenous or oral self-administration, and oral non-operant self-administration (Figure 2).

These two types of operant self-administration make it possible to identify the amount of work that an animal exerts in order to obtain a dose of a drug, the process for acquiring drug consumption behavior based on the acquisition rate (between 70-80% stability in the response for three consecutive days, with a minimum of drug doses consumed), and the way in which the animal passes from initial consumption to drug seeking (behaviors aimed at obtaining a drug) and regular consumption (maintenance). Dose-response properties, withdrawal (period of time without drugs), and relapse (reinstatement of self-administration of drug after withdrawal) can also be observed. With intravenous self-administration, the animals are surgically implanted with a chronic jugular catheter, and an operant self-administration paradigm is conducted after a recovery period. In general terms, the animals are placed in operant conditioning chambers where they learn to perform a response (insert their nose in a hole or press a lever) in conjunction with an unconditioned stimulus and an intravenous dose of a drug (reinforcement).

There are various types of reinforcement schedules, such as varying the number of responses required from the animal to obtain a drug dose (ratio) or varying the waiting time between executing a response and obtaining the drug dose (interval). Another self-administration model is oral operant self-administration, which is the same as intravenous self-administration except that the animals do not undergo surgery and they are given drops of a liquid drug, usually alcohol, in the operant conditioning chamber.

The oral non-operant self-administration method known as two-bottle free-choice is a procedure in which the animal is offered the option of freely choosing to drink from two bottles, one containing a liquid drug and another containing water. While this oral self-administration model is used primarily for alcohol consumption research, it has also been used for opioids, nicotine, cocaine, and cannabinoids, among other substances (Spanagel 2017, Meisch 2001).

CPP is a procedure that demonstrates an animal's preference for a drug, that is, whether or not the drug reinforces drug-seeking behavior. This test uses a cage that contains two chambers having two different environments that are clearly distinguishable to the animal (for example, different textures and/or colors). These chambers are connected to each other through a small area that permits the animals to freely move between them. During the acquisition phase the animals are injected for each of the substances received. These are administered over the course of several days so that the drug is paired with a particular chamber. To prevent any type of bias, all CPP experiments introduce a counterbalance for the drug-chamber pairing, such that half of the animals receive the drug in one chamber and the other half receive it in the other chamber. During the test phase the animals are housed in the area that connects the two chambers, with free access to both. The amount of time that the animals spend in each chamber indicates the animal's preference for the drug of abuse, or its avoidance of the drug. In order to evaluate drug-seeking behavior, an extinction phase followed by drug priming is sometimes performed so as to quickly identify the animal's craving for the drug tested.

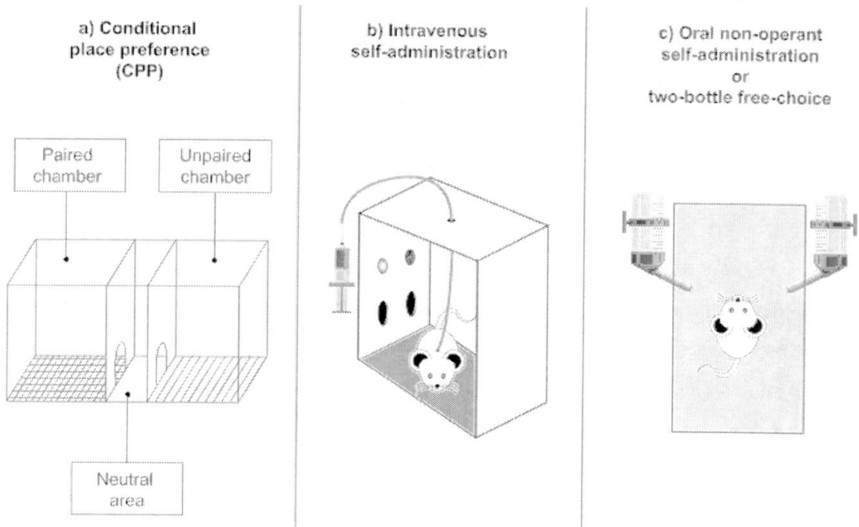


Figure 2. Behavioral paradigms used in animal models of drug addiction. a) Conditional place preference (CPP), b) Intravenous self-administration, c) Oral non-operant self-administration or two-bottle free-choice.

## PSYCHOSTIMULANTS

Psychostimulants are drugs that have a high heritability index for abuse or dependency. A heritability range of 0.42 to 0.73 has been estimated for the genetic influence of cocaine and other psychostimulants in male and female twins (van den Bree et al. 1998).

Cocaine, amphetamine, and methamphetamine are highly addictive psychostimulant drugs. Their consumption increases locomotion and reward effects. These psychostimulants bind to the plasma membrane transporters of dopamine (DA), norepinephrine (NE), and serotonin (5HT), inhibiting re-uptake of these monoamines (Seiden, Sabol, and Ricaurte 1993, dela Pena, Gevorkiana, and Shi 2015). Amphetamine can release monoamines from its vesicle into the cytoplasm, from where it leaves the cell through what is known as reverse transport (Seiden, Sabol, and Ricaurte 1993, Kahlig et al. 2005).

Increased locomotion is one of the most notable effects of consuming psychostimulants such as cocaine, amphetamine, and methamphetamine. It has been proposed that this locomotor activation is largely produced by the effects that these drugs have on the dopamine transporter (DAT). Nevertheless, it was not until the use of DAT KO mice (mice without the DA transporter) that a good deal of evidence was found to substantiate that locomotor activation is largely caused by DAT blocking, given that DAT KO mice do not exhibit increased locomotion as a result of the administration of cocaine, amphetamine, and methamphetamine (Giros et al. 1996, Zhuang et al. 2001, Spielewoy et al. 2001).

It is important to keep in mind that under baseline conditions, DAT KO mice have 5 to 6 times more diurnal and nocturnal locomotor activity than WT mice. In addition, since there is no reuptake of DA, its release into the extracellular space lasts at least 100 times longer than for WT mice, which is why they are also called hyperdopaminergic mice (Giros et al. 1996). These genetically modified mice also have a lower density of dopamine D1 and D2 receptors (between 45 and 55%) (Giros et al. 1996).

With regard to the effects produced by DAT deletion in models of CPP and the self-administration of cocaine, it has been shown that conditioned place preference in DAT KO mice substantially decreases or is not affected (Morice et al. 2004, Medvedev et al. 2005, Zhuang et al. 2001), except for one study that reported that DAT KO mice acquired conditioned place preference only with high doses of cocaine (Sora et al. 1998). And while DAT deletion generally decreases or does not affect place preference for cocaine with the CPP model, with intravenous self-administration DAT KO mice are able to self-administer cocaine, even with their low extracellular DA baseline levels (Rocha, Fumagalli, et al. 1998). Those authors attribute this to the ability of cocaine to maintain its reinforcing effect by acting on the serotonin transporter. They also found that the systemic administration of this drug increases extracellular DA in the nucleus accumbens (NAcc) of DAT KO mice (Carboni et al. 2001). Nonetheless, with a different line of DAT KO, in which an increase in DA in the NAcc was not produced after the administration of cocaine, the DAT KO did not acquire reliable self-administration of cocaine (Shen et al. 2004, Thomsen, Hall, et al. 2009), indicating the direct involvement of DAT in the reinforcing effect of cocaine.

Meanwhile, mutant mice expressing a knockin of a cocaine-insensitive but functional DAT (89-fold lower affinity for cocaine than WT) exhibit normal intravenous self-administration of amphetamine and do not self-administer cocaine intravenously, showing that DAT plays a key role in mediating the reinforcing effect of cocaine (Thomsen, Han, et al. 2009). Even in these mutant mice, cocaine does not produce more locomotion or extracellular DA in the NAcc, as compared to WT mice (Chen et al. 2006).

DAT KO mice have been found to exhibit quicker and longer conditioned place preference for amphetamine than WT, lasting weeks after the extinction of conditioned place preference behavior in WT mice. Furthermore, the systemic administration of amphetamine can increase extracellular DA in the NAcc, but not when it is directly administered into the NAcc. Since pre-treatment with a 5-HT1A serotonin receptor antagonist prevents conditioned place preference in DAT KO mice, the serotonergic system may be responsible for the reinforcing effects of amphetamine in the absence of DAT, and for the increase in extracellular DA in the NAcc during systemic administration of amphetamine (Budygin et al. 2004). In humans, nine- or fewer repeat alleles of the DAT polymorphism has been shown to be a significant risk factor for the consumption of methamphetamine and psychosis (Ujike et al. 2003).

In heterozygous vesicular monoamine transporter 2 (VMAT2) knockout mice with VMAT2 levels that are half those of WT, the knockout mice administer more amphetamine than WT, but they have less conditioned place preference than WT mice. This suggests that VMAT2 is more important for amphetamine-conditioned reward than for amphetamine-induced locomotion (Takahashi et al. 1997).

For homozygous dopamine D1 receptor knockouts (D1 KO mice), the conditioned place preference induced by cocaine is not affected, as compared with WT and heterozygous D1 KO mice. Nevertheless, the locomotor activity that is typically produced by administering cocaine is affected, since this increase in locomotion is not produced in homozygous D1, as compared to WT and heterozygous KO. Therefore, the authors propose that D1 receptors are involved in the locomotor effect of cocaine but does not play a significant role in the reinforcing effect of this drug (Miner et al. 1995). Nevertheless, with intravenous self-administration of cocaine, the D1 KO mice fail to acquire self-administration of this drug (Caine et al. 2007), indicating that D1 receptors are key to the long-term reinforcing effect of cocaine.

D2 KO mice self-administer more cocaine than WT, even at moderate and high doses (Caine et al. 2002). One CPP study reported that the reinforcing properties of cocaine significantly decrease in D2 KO mice as compared to WT, and D2 KO mice can only exhibit conditioned place preference with high doses of cocaine (Welter et al. 2007). But since these data do not agree with all the pharmacological studies that indicate that D2 receptors are important to the reward effect from this drug and from other psychostimulants, it is believed that D2 KO mice may show strong reward effects, such as increases in other DA receptors.

The dopamine D4 receptor has been shown to have significant involvement in drug abuse and addiction, especially with psychostimulants. One widely-studied polymorphism is that of the D4 receptor gene that produces various repeat alleles, known as D4L (D4 long, with over 7 repeats) or D4S (D4 short, with less than 7 repeats). The D4L polymorphism has primarily been associated with a high risk of substance abuse, impulsivity, and risk-taking behavior (Mallard et al. 2016, Ptacek, Kuzelova, and Stefano 2011).

A high prevalence of the D4L polymorphism has been reported in humans who consume methamphetamine (Chen et al. 2004). It has been found that methamphetamine and cocaine are stronger stimulants of locomotor activity in D4 KO mice than in WT (Katz et al. 2003, Rubinstein et al. 1997). No direct modulation of the reinforcing effect of cocaine has been found in mice with complete deletion of D4 (homozygous D4 KO mice) or with partial deletion (heterozygous D4 KO mice), given that their behavior in terms of intravenous self-administration of cocaine is similar to that of WT (Thanos, Habibi, et al. 2010). Nor have differences been found in conditioned place preference for cocaine for D4 KO mice, although they exhibit greater conditioned place preference than WT with low amphetamine doses (Thanos, Bermeo, et al. 2010). With regard to the CPP test and the role of D4 receptors in cocaine-seeking behavior and extinction and reinstatement, all have been found to have similar acquisition of place preference for cocaine, regardless of genotype (D4 KO mice or WT) and sex (male or female). However, extinction of place preference behavior for cocaine does not occur in female D4 KO mice, and reinstatement of preference does not occur in male D4 KO mice when a priming dose of cocaine is administered after extinction (Ananth et al. 2019). This suggests that the D4 receptor is involved in extinction and reinstatement but not in the acquisition of place preference for cocaine.

While the serotonergic system has been found to be significantly involved in the consumption of psychostimulants, mice that lack the serotonin transporter (SERT KO mice) exhibit cocaine-induced CPP behavior (Sora et al. 1998), just like DAT KO mice. While both SERT and DAT transporters have been shown to be involved in the reinforcing effects of stimulants, transporter knockouts do not seem to show any decrease in the reinforcing effects produced by these drugs. Nonetheless, more recent studies show that double knockouts (DAT/SERT KO mice) do not exhibit place preference for cocaine, suggesting that both transporters are involved in the reinforcing effects of this psychostimulant (Sora et al. 2001). On the other hand, it has been proposed that the reinforcing effects of cocaine are more specifically mediated by DAT than by SERT. In a line of DAT KO mice in which DA in the NAcc does not increase after administering cocaine (Shen et al. 2004), those mice fail to acquire reliable intravenous self-administration of cocaine, unlike the SERT KO mice, which do acquire it. This seems to indicate that DAT is key to mediating the reinforcing effects of this drug, and SERT is not (Thomsen, Hall, et al. 2009).

In 5-HT1B receptor KO mice, the administration of cocaine increases locomotor activity and their motivation to self-administer cocaine. Therefore, the absence of this receptor increases vulnerability to the consumption of this drug (Rocha, Scearce-Levie, et al. 1998).

The glutamatergic system is involved in drug reward. Glutamatergic neurons located in the prefrontal cortex activate dopaminergic neurons in the NAcc and ventral tegmental area (VTA). In NR1-deficient mice, NMDA receptor subunit NR1 expression is only 5%, compared to 100% at normal levels (Mohn et al. 1999), producing a NMDA receptor hypofunction model. With acute administration of amphetamine, locomotor activity does not increase for these mice, as compared to WT (Miyamoto et al. 2004), while it does increase for metabotropic glutamatergic receptors (GluR1) knockout mice (Mao, Conquet, and Wang 2001).

## NICOTINE

Heritability of nicotine addiction has been estimated to range from 31 to 60% (Bidwell et al. 2016). Nicotine is the main addictive component in tobacco and it acts on the nicotinic acetylcholine receptors (nAChRs). nAChRs are ligand-gated ion channels composed of five membrane subunits. The diversity of these receptors is due to the possible combinations of nine α subunits (α2-α10) and three β subunits (β2-β4) (Gotti et al. 2009). Important advances have been made as a result of the recent use of knockout mice to study addiction to nicotine. The genetic modification of these animals has made it possible to knock out a single subunit and re-express it, and even insert a cluster with a genetic variation associated with a high risk of dependency to tobacco and lung cancer in humans, such as CHRNA5-A3-B4. This represents great progress given that there is only a small variety of selective drugs that can specifically inhibit or activate the large variety of receptors that exist.

Independently, the β2 and α7 subunits are the ones that are most widely expressed in the brain (Gotti et al. 2009), while together, these subunits are the most abundant heteromeric nAChRs in the brain (McGranahan et al. 2011). In β2 KO mice, the expected increase in extracellular DA in the ventral striatum is not produced after systemic administration of nicotine. And the response of these knockouts to nicotine is reduced with an intravenous self-administration schedule that initially supplies cocaine and later substitutes that with nicotine (Picciotto et al. 1998). Studies comparing β2 KO and WT mice show that β2 KO mice do not acquire chronic intravenous self-administration of nicotine (Orejarena et al. 2012) or conditioned place preference for nicotine (Walters et al. 2006). After the administration of nicotine, the re-expression of the β2 subunit in the VTA of rescued KO mice is sufficient for restoring the release of extracellular DA in NAcc (Maskos et al. 2005). It can also restore acute administration of nicotine (Pons et al. 2008) and the acquisition and maintenance of chronic intravenous self-administration of nicotine (Orejarena et al. 2012). This shows that the presence of the β2 subunit in the VTA is important for nicotine reinforcement.

With regard to the α4 subunit and heteromeric α4β2-nAChRs, complete extinction of CPP for nicotine is observed when deleting only the α4 subunit in the dopaminergic neurons, and therefore, the α4 subunit in the dopaminergic system is necessary for nicotine reward. Also using this same animal model, an anxiety model (elevated plus maze) has shown that the anxiolytic effects of nicotine are mediated by the α4 subunit, and the elimination of α4β2-nAChRs in the dopaminergic neurons decreases sensitivity to the anxiolytic effects of nicotine (McGranahan et al. 2011). With regard to acute intravenous administration of nicotine, the KO of the α4 subunit does not produce self-administration of nicotine, nevertheless, its re-expression in the VTA is sufficient for restoring nicotine administration in these knockout mice (Pons et al. 2008).

With an acute nicotine administration schedule, it has been found that the KO of the α7 does not change either the reinforcement of nicotine or CPP for nicotine (Pons et al. 2008, Walters et al. 2006), indicating that the α7 subunit does not mediate the reinforcing effect of this drug. However, in α7 KO mice, nicotine does increase the release of DA in NAcc for a longer period of time (Besson et al. 2012). Since α7 KO mice do not exhibit the attention deficit typically present in nicotine withdrawal, these animals have been used to study nicotine withdrawal-induced inattention (Higa et al. 2017). The α7 subunit has recently been identified as a targeted therapy for treating nicotine addiction given that various pharmacological studies have shown that the activation of α7-nAChRs decreases motivation for nicotine use (Brunzell, McIntosh, and Papke 2014).

In humans, a single nucleotide polymorphism (SNP) in CHRNA5-A3-B4 has been found in heavy smokers, which is also related with a high risk of lung cancer (Ware, van den Bree, and Munafo 2011, Wen et al. 2016). And a different polymorphism, of the CHRNA5 (rs16969968) gene, has been found to double the risk of tobacco dependency (Berrettini et al. 2008, Grucza et al. 2008). Some of the contributions that have been made to the study of these genes by using genetically modified animals are described below.

β4-nAChRs are involved in the development of nicotine withdrawal and in the reinforcing effects of nicotine. The elimination of β4 in KO mice decreases intravenous self-administration of nicotine, as compared to WT (Harrington et al. 2016), while the overexpression of β4 in transgenic mice produces strong aversion to nicotine, which can be reversed by the expression of the α5 (D398N) variant in the medial habenula (Frahm et al. 2011). In β4 KO mice, DA neurons are more sensitive to lower doses of nicotine, as compared to WT mice, which agrees with the findings described. Furthermore, the re-expression of β4 in the interpeduncular nucleus (IPN) is sufficient for completely restoring intravenous self-administration of nicotine (Harrington et al. 2016), suggesting that the β4 subunit in the IPN is involved in maintaining the self-administration of nicotine. Lastly, β4 KO mice exhibit few somatic signs of withdrawal after chronic administration of nicotine (Salas, Pieri, and De Biasi 2004).

The α5 KO mice can self-administer high doses of nicotine, even at levels at which WT mice exhibit aversion. The re-expression of α5 in the medial habenula reverses this effect. Nicotine activates the peduncular-habenula pathway through α5-containing nicotinic receptors, thereby inhibiting motivation and limiting nicotine consumption (Fowler et al. 2011). Furthermore, these α5 subunit knockouts exhibit conditioned place preference with low doses of nicotine, as do WT mice. But unlike WT mice, they also show CPP with high doses of nicotine, which under normal conditions results in aversion in WT (Jackson et al. 2010). The deletion of the α5 subunit seems to diminish the adverse effects of high doses of nicotine, and the α5 subunit in the IP has recently been shown to be responsible for mediating aversion to nicotine (Morton et al. 2018).

Transgenic mice that overexpress the human CHRNA5-A3-B4 cluster are more vulnerable to nicotine consumption. After acute administration of nicotine, TgCHRNA5-A3-B4 mice exhibit increased vulnerability to nicotine, with high activation of the medial habenula and reduced activation of dopaminergic neurons in the VTA. Furthermore, their acquisition of nicotine increases when using an intravenous administration schedule, and their breaking point is higher when using a progressive-ratio schedule, as compared to WT. This indicates that reinforcement and motivation for seeking nicotine increases in TgCHRNA5-A3-B4 mice (Gallego et al. 2012). In transgenic mice, the overexpression of the human CHRNA5-A3-B4 cluster also produces hippocampal changes, resulting in cognitive deficits in this animal model. TgCHRNA5-A3-B4 mice exhibit significant damage to short-term novelty recognition memory, which can be reversed with chronic administration of nicotine. According to Molas et al. (2014), this suggests that chronic nicotine consumption by humans could be a compensatory strategy for restoring cognitive function in individuals with altered expression of CHRNA5-A3-B4 (Molas et al. 2014).

## Alcohol

Estimates by studies of twins (raised in the same families or in different adopted families) show that alcohol dependency has a heritability factor of roughly 50% (Heath et al. 1997, True et al. 1999, Verhulst, Neale, and Kendler 2015). Ethanol activates $GABA_A$ receptors, releases dopamine and opioid peptides, inhibits glutamate receptors, and interacts with the serotonergic system (Anton 1996, Fitzgerald and Nestler 1995).

$GABA_A$ receptors are composed of five subunits, including alpha (α), beta (β), gamma (ϒ), delta (δ), épsilon (ε), pi (π), theta (θ) and rho (ρ). The $GABA_A$ receptors and their subunits have been widely studied with alcohol consumption and abuse models that use genetically modified mice. With a two-bottle free-choice paradigm, KO of the α1-$GABA_A$ subunit significantly reduces preference for ethanol, while no change has been found with the KO of the β2-$GABA_A$ subunit. Nevertheless, both knockouts show a significant reduction in saccharin consumption, as compared to WT. And while both α1 and β2 KO mice exhibit conditioned place preference for ethanol, CPP is stronger in α1 KO and WT mice than in β2 KO mice. The α1 KO mice also develop a stronger conditioned taste aversion than β2 KO and WT mice. With regard to chronic alcohol consumption, β2 KO mice consume more and α1 KO consume less than WT (Blednov et al. 2003). With regard to α1-$GABA_A$ receptor subunit knockin mice, with insensitivity to the reinforcing effects of ethanol and normal sensitivity to GABA, increased anxiolytic effects and quicker recovery from the motor-impairing effects produced by ethanol were found, with no changes in preference, locomotor stimulation, cognitive impairment, or ethanol consumption (Werner et al. 2006).

Knockin mice with a mutation in the α2-$GABA_A$ receptor subunit, making them specifically insensitive to the reinforcement effect of ethanol while still having normal sensitivity to GABA, do not develop the typical conditioned taste aversion to ethanol and are not sensitive to the motor-stimulating effects of ethanol. Multiple tests have shown that ethanol consumption increases for mice with a mutation of the α2-$GABA_A$ receptor subunit, which is likely due to the lack of decreased aversion to ethanol (Blednov et al. 2011). These effects, which are produced by changes in the function of the α2-subunit, produce significant changes in alcohol consumption behavior and support the findings in humans that the Gabra2 ($GABA_A$ receptor α2-subunit) polymorphism is associated with alcoholism (Pierucci-Lagha et al. 2005).

Using a two-bottle free-choice paradigm, male ρ1-$GABA_A$ receptor subunit KO mice consume less ethanol and recover more quickly from acute motor incoordination produced by ethanol. Meanwhile, female mice with a ρ1-$GABA_A$ receptor subunit KO exhibit less sensitivity to ethanol-induced conditioned taste aversion (Blednov et al. 2014). With regard to δ-$GABA_A$ receptor subunit KO mice, these consume less ethanol and have less withdrawal symptoms after chronic administration of alcohol, as compared to WT (Mihalek et al. 2001). These data suggest that the ρ1- and δ-subunits participate in modulating consumption and in some of the effects produced by ethanol.

It has been suggested that the glutamatergic system is involved in craving and relapse, given the significant neuroplastic changes that occur after chronic consumption of drugs. With KO of the AMPA receptor GluR-

C subunit (GluR-C KO), operant self-administration of ethanol, or home-cage drinking, does not change compared to WT mice, and therefore, no effect on the consumption of alcohol has been observed. Nevertheless, after a period of alcohol withdrawal, GluR-C KO mice exhibit a reduction in cue-induced reinstatement and in the alcohol deprivation effect, as compared with WT, suggesting the involvement of the GluR-C subunit in alcohol seeking and relapse (Sanchis-Segura et al. 2006).

With regard to the dopaminergic system and alcohol consumption, the involvement of dopamine D2 receptors has been found. In both male and female mice, the deletion of the D2L (long) dopamine receptor increases ethanol consumption, which is attributable to an overexpression of D2S (short) dopamine receptors (Bulwa et al. 2011). In D3 KO mice, alcohol consumption is very low with two-bottle choice tests and binge-like ethanol-drinking paradigms, as compared to WT, and reward associated with alcohol consumption is nearly eliminated in D3 KO mice (Leggio et al. 2014). Alcohol consumption in mice is modulated by the overexpression and knockdown of NAcc dopamine D3-receptors. D3 knockdown mice exhibit less voluntary alcohol consumption, while the overexpression of the D3 receptor increases consumption (Bahi and Dreyer 2014). D3 KO mice have also been shown to be resistant to ethanol sensitization (Harrison and Nobrega 2009), making them more vulnerable to ethanol consumption. These data suggest the importance of the D3 receptor for mediating the reinforcing effects of ethanol consumption. Both male and female mice with DAT knockdown in the NAcc exhibit decreased ethanol preference and consumption, indicating that the expression of DAT in this nucleus contributes to mediating the reward from ethanol (Bahi and Dreyer 2019). Studies of DAT KO mice have also reported high sensitization to ethanol during induction and long-term expression phases, indicating that a lack of DAT facilitates sensitization to ethanol (Morice et al. 2010).

Lastly, a polymorphism of the aldehyde dehydrogenase-2 enzyme (ALDH2) in humans has be shown to be directly related with alcohol consumption. The ALDH2 polymorphism inhibits the enzyme's ability to metabolize alcohol, which produces an adverse reaction with the consumption of small amounts of alcohol (Chen et al. 2014). Just like humans with this polymorphism, ALDH2 KO mice avoid consuming ethanol (Isse et al. 2002, Fernandez et al. 2006), indicating that this enzyme is an important target for alcoholism treatment.

## CONCLUSION

Genetically modified mice are used to study and identify genes that function to predict the risk of developing certain types of addiction, and genes that function to protect against addiction. This information can be used to guide pharmacological prevention strategies and to treat addiction. Current genetic technology makes it possible not only to study the effects of the deletion and overexpression of specific genes, but also the effects of these strategies on specific tissue, making the findings increasingly more precise.

The different animal models that are used to study addiction can demonstrate specific aspects of the different phases of addiction. For example, acute self-administration models are more closely related with the initial effects produced by a drug (reinforcing effects) and are helpful for studying initial consumption of a substance, but not for studying dependence. On the other hand, chronic self-administration models are better for reproducing continuous drug use, including abuse and addiction, and also for studying withdrawal and relapse. Altogether, the diversity of the animal models that are available for studying addiction, as well as the diversity of genetically-modified animals, have shown us that the genes involved in acute drug consumption are not necessarily the same ones that are important for chronic consumption, withdrawal, or relapse.

## ACKNOWLEDGMENTS

The authors would like to Thank Sergio Broseta for figures design. This work received support from DGAPA-PAPIT-UNAM Grant IN215218 and

IA205218 to OPG and MMD respectively and the Programa de Fortalecimiento de la Calidad en Instituciones Educativas P/PFCE-2018-23MSU0140Z-08 to WVHM and LNJ.

## REFERENCES

American Psychiatric Association. 2013. *DSM-5: Diagnostic and statistical manual of mental disorders*. 5th ed ed. Washington: American Psychiatric Publishing.

Ananth, M., E. M. Hetelekides, J. Hamilton, and P. K. Thanos. 2019. "Dopamine D4 receptor gene expression plays important role in extinction and reinstatement of cocaine-seeking behavior in mice." *Behav Brain Res* no. 365:1-6. doi: 10.1016/j.bbr.2019.02.036.

Anton, R. F. 1996. "Neurobehavioural basis for the pharmacotherapy of alcoholism: current and future directions." *Alcohol Alcohol* no. 31 Suppl 1:43-53.

Bahi, A., and J. L. Dreyer. 2014. "Lentiviral vector-mediated dopamine d3 receptor modulation in the rat brain impairs alcohol intake and ethanol-induced conditioned place preference." *Alcohol Clin Exp Res* no. 38 (9):2369-76. doi: 10.1111/acer.12503.

Bahi, A., and J. L. Dreyer. 2019. "No effect of sex on ethanol intake and preference after dopamine transporter (DAT) knockdown in adult mice." *Psychopharmacology (Berl)* no. 236 (4):1349-1365. doi: 10.1007/s00213-018-5144-9.

Berrettini, W., X. Yuan, F. Tozzi, K. Song, C. Francks, H. Chilcoat, D. Waterworth, P. Muglia, and V. Mooser. 2008. "Alpha-5/alpha-3 nicotinic receptor subunit alleles increase risk for heavy smoking." *Mol Psychiatry* no. 13 (4):368-73. doi: 10.1038/sj.mp.4002154.

Besson, M., V. David, M. Baudonnat, P. Cazala, J. P. Guilloux, C. Reperant, I. Cloez-Tayarani, J. P. Changeux, A. M. Gardier, and S. Granon. 2012. "Alpha7-nicotinic receptors modulate nicotine-induced reinforcement and extracellular dopamine outflow in the mesolimbic system in mice."

*Psychopharmacology (Berl)* no. 220 (1):1-14. doi: 10.1007/s00213-011-2422-1.

Bidwell, L. C., R. H. Palmer, L. Brick, J. E. McGeary, and V. S. Knopik. 2016. "Genome-wide single nucleotide polymorphism heritability of nicotine dependence as a multidimensional phenotype." *Psychol Med* no. 46 (10):2059-69. doi: 10.1017/S0033291716000453.

Blednov, Y. A., J. M. Benavidez, M. Black, C. R. Leiter, E. Osterndorff-Kahanek, D. Johnson, C. M. Borghese, J. R. Hanrahan, G. A. Johnston, M. Chebib, and R. A. Harris. 2014. "GABAA receptors containing rho1 subunits contribute to in vivo effects of ethanol in mice." *PLoS One* no. 9 (1):e85525. doi: 10.1371/journal.pone.0085525.

Blednov, Y. A., C. M. Borghese, M. L. McCracken, J. M. Benavidez, C. R. Geil, E. Osterndorff-Kahanek, D. F. Werner, S. Iyer, A. Swihart, N. L. Harrison, G. E. Homanics, and R. A. Harris. 2011. "Loss of ethanol conditioned taste aversion and motor stimulation in knockin mice with ethanol-insensitive alpha2-containing GABA(A) receptors." *J Pharmacol Exp Ther* no. 336 (1):145-54. doi: 10.1124/jpet.110. 171645.

Blednov, Y. A., D. Walker, H. Alva, K. Creech, G. Findlay, and R. A. Harris. 2003. "GABAA receptor alpha 1 and beta 2 subunit null mutant mice: behavioral responses to ethanol." *J Pharmacol Exp Ther* no. 305 (3):854-63. doi: 10.1124/jpet.103.049478.

Brunzell, D. H., J. M. McIntosh, and R. L. Papke. 2014. "Diverse strategies targeting alpha7 homomeric and alpha6beta2* heteromeric nicotinic acetylcholine receptors for smoking cessation." *Ann N Y Acad Sci* no. 1327:27-45. doi: 10.1111/nyas.12421.

Budygin, E. A., M. S. Brodie, T. D. Sotnikova, Y. Mateo, C. E. John, M. Cyr, R. R. Gainetdinov, and S. R. Jones. 2004. "Dissociation of rewarding and dopamine transporter-mediated properties of amphetamine." *Proc Natl Acad Sci USA* no. 101 (20):7781-6. doi: 10.1073/pnas.0401418101.

Bulwa, Z. B., J. A. Sharlin, P. J. Clark, T. K. Bhattacharya, C. N. Kilby, Y. Wang, and J. S. Rhodes. 2011. "Increased consumption of ethanol and sugar water in mice lacking the dopamine D2 long receptor." *Alcohol* no. 45 (7):631-9. doi: 10.1016/j.alcohol.2011.06.004.

Caine, S. B., S. S. Negus, N. K. Mello, S. Patel, L. Bristow, J. Kulagowski, D. Vallone, A. Saiardi, and E. Borrelli. 2002. "Role of dopamine D2-like receptors in cocaine self-administration: studies with D2 receptor mutant mice and novel D2 receptor antagonists." *J Neurosci* no. 22 (7):2977-88. doi: 20026264.

Caine, S. B., M. Thomsen, K. I. Gabriel, J. S. Berkowitz, L. H. Gold, G. F. Koob, S. Tonegawa, J. Zhang, and M. Xu. 2007. "Lack of self-administration of cocaine in dopamine D1 receptor knock-out mice." *J Neurosci* no. 27 (48):13140-50. doi: 10.1523/JNEUROSCI.2284-07.2007.

Carboni, E., C. Spielewoy, C. Vacca, M. Nosten-Bertrand, B. Giros, and G. Di Chiara. 2001. "Cocaine and amphetamine increase extracellular dopamine in the nucleus accumbens of mice lacking the dopamine transporter gene." *J Neurosci* no. 21 (9):RC141: 1-4.

Chen, C. H., J. C. Ferreira, E. R. Gross, and D. Mochly-Rosen. 2014. "Targeting aldehyde dehydrogenase 2: new therapeutic opportunities." *Physiol Rev* no. 94 (1):1-34. doi: 10.1152/physrev.00017.2013.

Chen, C. K., X. Hu, S. K. Lin, P. C. Sham, W. Loh el, T. Li, R. M. Murray, and D. M. Ball. 2004. "Association analysis of dopamine D2-like receptor genes and methamphetamine abuse." *Psychiatr Genet* no. 14 (4):223-6.

Chen, R., M. R. Tilley, H. Wei, F. Zhou, F. M. Zhou, S. Ching, N. Quan, R. L. Stephens, E. R. Hill, T. Nottoli, D. D. Han, and H. H. Gu. 2006. "Abolished cocaine reward in mice with a cocaine-insensitive dopamine transporter." *Proc Natl Acad Sci USA* no. 103 (24):9333-8. doi: 10.1073/pnas.0600905103.

dela Pena, I., R. Gevorkiana, and W. X. Shi. 2015. "Psychostimulants affect dopamine transmission through both dopamine transporter-dependent and independent mechanisms." *Eur J Pharmacol* no. 764:562-70. doi: 10.1016/j.ejphar.2015.07.044.

Fernandez, E., W. Koek, Q. Ran, G. A. Gerhardt, C. P. France, and R. Strong. 2006. "Monoamine metabolism and behavioral responses to ethanol in mitochondrial aldehyde dehydrogenase knockout mice."

*Alcohol Clin Exp Res* no. 30 (10):1650-8. doi: 10.1111/j.1530-0277. 2006.00200.x.

Fitzgerald, L. W., and E. J. Nestler. 1995. "Molecular and cellular adaptations in signal transduction pathways following ethanol exposure." *Clin Neurosci* no. 3 (3):165-73.

Fowler, C. D., and P. J. Kenny. 2012. "Utility of genetically modified mice for understanding the neurobiology of substance use disorders." *Hum Genet* no. 131 (6):941-57. doi: 10.1007/s00439-011-1129-z.

Fowler, C. D., Q. Lu, P. M. Johnson, M. J. Marks, and P. J. Kenny. 2011. "Habenular alpha5 nicotinic receptor subunit signalling controls nicotine intake." *Nature* no. 471 (7340):597-601. doi: 10.1038/nature 09797.

Frahm, S., M. A. Slimak, L. Ferrarese, J. Santos-Torres, B. Antolin-Fontes, S. Auer, S. Filkin, S. Pons, J. F. Fontaine, V. Tsetlin, U. Maskos, and I. Ibanez-Tallon. 2011. "Aversion to nicotine is regulated by the balanced activity of beta4 and alpha5 nicotinic receptor subunits in the medial habenula." *Neuron* no. 70 (3):522-35. doi: 10.1016/j.neuron. 2011.04.013.

Gallego, X., S. Molas, A. Amador-Arjona, M. J. Marks, N. Robles, P. Murtra, L. Armengol, R. D. Fernandez-Montes, M. Gratacos, M. Pumarola, R. Cabrera, R. Maldonado, J. Sabria, X. Estivill, and M. Dierssen. 2012. "Overexpression of the CHRNA5/A3/B4 genomic cluster in mice increases the sensitivity to nicotine and modifies its reinforcing effects." *Amino Acids* no. 43 (2):897-909. doi: 10.1007/ s00726-011-1149-y.

Giros, B., M. Jaber, S. R. Jones, R. M. Wightman, and M. G. Caron. 1996. "Hyperlocomotion and indifference to cocaine and amphetamine in mice lacking the dopamine transporter." *Nature* no. 379 (6566):606-12. doi: 10.1038/379606a0.

Gotti, C., F. Clementi, A. Fornari, A. Gaimarri, S. Guiducci, I. Manfredi, M. Moretti, P. Pedrazzi, L. Pucci, and M. Zoli. 2009. "Structural and functional diversity of native brain neuronal nicotinic receptors." *Biochem Pharmacol* no. 78 (7):703-11. doi: 10.1016/j.bcp.2009. 05.024.

Grucza, R. A., J. C. Wang, J. A. Stitzel, A. L. Hinrichs, S. F. Saccone, N. L. Saccone, K. K. Bucholz, C. R. Cloninger, R. J. Neuman, J. P. Budde, L. Fox, S. Bertelsen, J. Kramer, V. Hesselbrock, J. Tischfield, J. I. Nurnberger, Jr., L. Almasy, B. Porjesz, S. Kuperman, M. A. Schuckit, H. J. Edenberg, J. P. Rice, A. M. Goate, and L. J. Bierut. 2008. "A risk allele for nicotine dependence in CHRNA5 is a protective allele for cocaine dependence." *Biol Psychiatry* no. 64 (11):922-9. doi: 10.1016/j.biopsych.2008.04.018.

Harrington, L., X. Vinals, A. Herrera-Solis, A. Flores, C. Morel, S. Tolu, P. Faure, R. Maldonado, U. Maskos, and P. Robledo. 2016. "Role of beta4* Nicotinic Acetylcholine Receptors in the Habenulo-Interpeduncular Pathway in Nicotine Reinforcement in Mice." *Neuropsychopharmacology* no. 41 (7):1790-802. doi: 10.1038/npp.2015.346.

Harrison, S. J., and J. N. Nobrega. 2009. "Differential susceptibility to ethanol and amphetamine sensitization in dopamine D3 receptor-deficient mice." *Psychopharmacology (Berl)* no. 204 (1):49-59. doi: 10.1007/s00213-008-1435-x.

Heath, A. C., K. K. Bucholz, P. A. Madden, S. H. Dinwiddie, W. S. Slutske, L. J. Bierut, D. J. Statham, M. P. Dunne, J. B. Whitfield, and N. G. Martin. 1997. "Genetic and environmental contributions to alcohol dependence risk in a national twin sample: consistency of findings in women and men." *Psychol Med* no. 27 (6):1381-96.

Higa, K. K., A. Grim, M. E. Kamenski, J. van Enkhuizen, X. Zhou, K. Li, J. C. Naviaux, L. Wang, R. K. Naviaux, M. A. Geyer, A. Markou, and J. W. Young. 2017. "Nicotine withdrawal-induced inattention is absent in alpha7 nAChR knockout mice." *Psychopharmacology (Berl)* no. 234 (9-10):1573-1586. doi: 10.1007/s00213-017-4572-2.

Isse, T., T. Oyama, K. Kitagawa, K. Matsuno, A. Matsumoto, A. Yoshida, K. Nakayama, K. Nakayama, and T. Kawamoto. 2002. "Diminished alcohol preference in transgenic mice lacking aldehyde dehydrogenase activity." *Pharmacogenetics* no. 12 (8):621-6.

Jackson, K. J., M. J. Marks, R. E. Vann, X. Chen, T. F. Gamage, J. A. Warner, and M. I. Damaj. 2010. "Role of alpha5 nicotinic acetylcholine receptors in pharmacological and behavioral effects of nicotine in mice." *J Pharmacol Exp Ther* no. 334 (1):137-46. doi: 10.1124/jpet.110.165738.

Kahlig, K. M., F. Binda, H. Khoshbouei, R. D. Blakely, D. G. McMahon, J. A. Javitch, and A. Galli. 2005. "Amphetamine induces dopamine efflux through a dopamine transporter channel." *Proc Natl Acad Sci USA* no. 102 (9):3495-500. doi: 10.1073/pnas.0407737102.

Katz, J. L., A. L. Chausmer, G. I. Elmer, M. Rubinstein, M. J. Low, and D. K. Grandy. 2003. "Cocaine-induced locomotor activity and cocaine discrimination in dopamine D4 receptor mutant mice." *Psychopharmacology (Berl)* no. 170 (1):108-14. doi: 10.1007/s00213-003-1513-z.

Koob, G. F., and N. D. Volkow. 2010. "Neurocircuitry of addiction." *Neuropsychopharmacology* no. 35 (1):217-38. doi: 10.1038/npp.2009.110.

Koob, G. F., and N. D. Volkow. 2016. "Neurobiology of addiction: a neurocircuitry analysis." *Lancet Psychiatry* no. 3 (8):760-73. doi: 10.1016/S2215-0366(16)00104-8.

Leggio, G. M., G. Camillieri, C. B. Platania, A. Castorina, G. Marrazzo, S. A. Torrisi, C. N. Nona, V. D'Agata, J. Nobrega, H. Stark, C. Bucolo, B. Le Foll, F. Drago, and S. Salomone. 2014. "Dopamine D3 receptor is necessary for ethanol consumption: an approach with buspirone." *Neuropsychopharmacology* no. 39 (8):2017-28. doi: 10.1038/npp.2014.51.

Mallard, T. T., J. Doorley, C. L. Esposito-Smythers, and J. E. McGeary. 2016. "Dopamine D4 receptor VNTR polymorphism associated with greater risk for substance abuse among adolescents with disruptive behavior disorders: Preliminary results." *Am J Addict* no. 25 (1):56-61. doi: 10.1111/ajad.12320.

Mao, L., F. Conquet, and J. Q. Wang. 2001. "Augmented motor activity and reduced striatal preprodynorphin mRNA induction in response to acute amphetamine administration in metabotropic glutamate receptor 1 knockout mice." *Neuroscience* no. 106 (2):303-12.

Maskos, U., B. E. Molles, S. Pons, M. Besson, B. P. Guiard, J. P. Guilloux, A. Evrard, P. Cazala, A. Cormier, M. Mameli-Engvall, N. Dufour, I. Cloez-Tayarani, A. P. Bemelmans, J. Mallet, A. M. Gardier, V. David, P. Faure, S. Granon, and J. P. Changeux. 2005. "Nicotine reinforcement and cognition restored by targeted expression of nicotinic receptors." *Nature* no. 436 (7047):103-7. doi: 10.1038/ nature03694.

Matsuda, I., and A. Aiba. 2004. "Receptor knock-out and knock-in strategies." *Methods Mol Biol* no. 259:379-90. doi: 10.1385/1-59259-754-8:379.

McGranahan, T. M., N. E. Patzlaff, S. R. Grady, S. F. Heinemann, and T. K. Booker. 2011. "alpha4beta2 nicotinic acetylcholine receptors on dopaminergic neurons mediate nicotine reward and anxiety relief." *J Neurosci* no. 31 (30):10891-902. doi: 10.1523/JNEUROSCI.0937-11.2011.

Medvedev, I. O., R. R. Gainetdinov, T. D. Sotnikova, L. M. Bohn, M. G. Caron, and L. A. Dykstra. 2005. "Characterization of conditioned place preference to cocaine in congenic dopamine transporter knockout female mice." *Psychopharmacology (Berl)* no. 180 (3):408-13. doi: 10.1007/s00213-005-2173-y.

Meisch, R. A. 2001. "Oral drug self-administration: an overview of laboratory animal studies." *Alcohol* no. 24 (2):117-28.

Mihalek, R. M., B. J. Bowers, J. M. Wehner, J. E. Kralic, M. J. VanDoren, A. L. Morrow, and G. E. Homanics. 2001. "GABA(A)-receptor delta subunit knockout mice have multiple defects in behavioral responses to ethanol." *Alcohol Clin Exp Res* no. 25 (12):1708-18.

Miner, L. L., J. Drago, P. M. Chamberlain, D. Donovan, and G. R. Uhl. 1995. "Retained cocaine conditioned place preference in D1 receptor deficient mice." *Neuroreport* no. 6 (17):2314-6.

Miyamoto, S., J. N. Snouwaert, B. H. Koller, S. S. Moy, J. A. Lieberman, and G. E. Duncan. 2004. "Amphetamine-induced Fos is reduced in limbic cortical regions but not in the caudate or accumbens in a genetic model of NMDA receptor hypofunction." *Neuropsychopharmacology* no. 29 (12):2180-8. doi: 10.1038/sj.npp.1300548.

Mohn, A. R., R. R. Gainetdinov, M. G. Caron, and B. H. Koller. 1999. "Mice with reduced NMDA receptor expression display behaviors related to schizophrenia." *Cell* no. 98 (4):427-36. doi: 10.1016/s0092-8674(00)81972-8.

Molas, S., T. Gener, J. Guell, M. Martin, I. Ballesteros-Yanez, M. V. Sanchez-Vives, and M. Dierssen. 2014. "Hippocampal changes produced by overexpression of the human CHRNA5/A3/B4 gene cluster may underlie cognitive deficits rescued by nicotine in transgenic mice." *Acta Neuropathol Commun* no. 2:147. doi: 10.1186/s40478-014-0147-1.

Morice, E., C. Denis, B. Giros, and M. Nosten-Bertrand. 2004. "Phenotypic expression of the targeted null-mutation in the dopamine transporter gene varies as a function of the genetic background." *Eur J Neurosci* no. 20 (1):120-6. doi: 10.1111/j.1460-9568.2004.03465.x.

Morice, E., C. Denis, B. Giros, and M. Nosten-Bertrand. 2010. "Evidence of long-term expression of behavioral sensitization to both cocaine and ethanol in dopamine transporter knockout mice." *Psychopharmacology (Berl)* no. 208 (1):57-66. doi: 10.1007/s00213-009-1707-0.

Morton, G., N. Nasirova, D. W. Sparks, M. Brodsky, S. Sivakumaran, E. K. Lambe, and E. E. Turner. 2018. "Chrna5-Expressing Neurons in the Interpeduncular Nucleus Mediate Aversion Primed by Prior Stimulation or Nicotine Exposure." *J Neurosci* no. 38 (31):6900-6920. doi: 10.1523/JNEUROSCI.0023-18.2018.

Nagy, A. 2000. "Cre recombinase: the universal reagent for genome tailoring." *Genesis* no. 26 (2):99-109.

Orejarena, M. J., A. Herrera-Solis, S. Pons, U. Maskos, R. Maldonado, and P. Robledo. 2012. "Selective re-expression of beta2 nicotinic acetylcholine receptor subunits in the ventral tegmental area of the mouse restores intravenous nicotine self-administration." *Neuropharmacology* no. 63 (2):235-41. doi: 10.1016/j.neuropharm.2012.03.011.

Picciotto, M. R., M. Zoli, R. Rimondini, C. Lena, L. M. Marubio, E. M. Pich, K. Fuxe, and J. P. Changeux. 1998. "Acetylcholine receptors containing the beta2 subunit are involved in the reinforcing properties of nicotine." *Nature* no. 391 (6663):173-7. doi: 10.1038/34413.

Pich, E. M., and M. P. Epping-Jordan. 1998. "Transgenic mice in drug dependence research." *Ann Med* no. 30 (4):390-6.

Pierucci-Lagha, A., J. Covault, R. Feinn, M. Nellissery, C. Hernandez-Avila, C. Oncken, A. L. Morrow, and H. R. Kranzler. 2005. "GABRA2 alleles moderate the subjective effects of alcohol, which are attenuated by finasteride." *Neuropsychopharmacology* no. 30 (6):1193-203. doi: 10.1038/sj.npp.1300688.

Pons, S., L. Fattore, G. Cossu, S. Tolu, E. Porcu, J. M. McIntosh, J. P. Changeux, U. Maskos, and W. Fratta. 2008. "Crucial role of alpha4 and alpha6 nicotinic acetylcholine receptor subunits from ventral tegmental area in systemic nicotine self-administration." *J Neurosci* no. 28 (47):12318-27. doi: 10.1523/JNEUROSCI.3918-08.2008.

Ptacek, R., H. Kuzelova, and G. B. Stefano. 2011. "Dopamine D4 receptor gene DRD4 and its association with psychiatric disorders." *Med Sci Monit* no. 17 (9):RA215-20. doi: 10.12659/msm.881925.

Rocha, B. A., F. Fumagalli, R. R. Gainetdinov, S. R. Jones, R. Ator, B. Giros, G. W. Miller, and M. G. Caron. 1998. "Cocaine self-administration in dopamine-transporter knockout mice." *Nat Neurosci* no. 1 (2):132-7. doi: 10.1038/381.

Rocha, B. A., K. Scearce-Levie, J. J. Lucas, N. Hiroi, N. Castanon, J. C. Crabbe, E. J. Nestler, and R. Hen. 1998. "Increased vulnerability to cocaine in mice lacking the serotonin-1B receptor." *Nature* no. 393 (6681):175-8. doi: 10.1038/30259.

Rubinstein, M., T. J. Phillips, J. R. Bunzow, T. L. Falzone, G. Dziewczapolski, G. Zhang, Y. Fang, J. L. Larson, J. A. McDougall, J. A. Chester, C. Saez, T. A. Pugsley, O. Gershanik, M. J. Low, and D. K. Grandy. 1997. "Mice lacking dopamine D4 receptors are supersensitive to ethanol, cocaine, and methamphetamine." *Cell* no. 90 (6):991-1001. doi: 10.1016/s0092-8674(00)80365-7.

Salas, R., F. Pieri, and M. De Biasi. 2004. "Decreased signs of nicotine withdrawal in mice null for the beta4 nicotinic acetylcholine receptor subunit." *J Neurosci* no. 24 (45):10035-9. doi: 10.1523/JNEUROSCI. 1939-04.2004.

Sanchis-Segura, C., T. Borchardt, V. Vengeliene, T. Zghoul, D. Bachteler, P. Gass, R. Sprengel, and R. Spanagel. 2006. "Involvement of the AMPA receptor GluR-C subunit in alcohol-seeking behavior and relapse." *J Neurosci* no. 26 (4):1231-8. doi: 10.1523/JNEUROSCI. 4237-05.2006.

Seiden, L. S., K. E. Sabol, and G. A. Ricaurte. 1993. "Amphetamine: effects on catecholamine systems and behavior." *Annu Rev Pharmacol Toxicol* no. 33:639-77. doi: 10.1146/annurev.pa.33.040193.003231.

Shen, H. W., Y. Hagino, H. Kobayashi, K. Shinohara-Tanaka, K. Ikeda, H. Yamamoto, T. Yamamoto, K. P. Lesch, D. L. Murphy, F. S. Hall, G. R. Uhl, and I. Sora. 2004. "Regional differences in extracellular dopamine and serotonin assessed by in vivo microdialysis in mice lacking dopamine and/or serotonin transporters." *Neuropsychopharmacology* no. 29 (10):1790-9. doi: 10.1038/sj.npp. 1300476.

Sora, I., F. S. Hall, A. M. Andrews, M. Itokawa, X. F. Li, H. B. Wei, C. Wichems, K. P. Lesch, D. L. Murphy, and G. R. Uhl. 2001. "Molecular mechanisms of cocaine reward: combined dopamine and serotonin transporter knockouts eliminate cocaine place preference." *Proc Natl Acad Sci USA* no. 98 (9):5300-5. doi: 10.1073/pnas. 091039298.

Sora, I., C. Wichems, N. Takahashi, X. F. Li, Z. Zeng, R. Revay, K. P. Lesch, D. L. Murphy, and G. R. Uhl. 1998. "Cocaine reward models: conditioned place preference can be established in dopamine- and in serotonin-transporter knockout mice." *Proc Natl Acad Sci USA* no. 95 (13):7699-704. doi: 10.1073/pnas.95.13.7699.

Spanagel, R. 2017. "Animal models of addiction." *Dialogues Clin Neurosci* no. 19 (3):247-258.

Spielewoy, C., G. Biala, C. Roubert, M. Hamon, C. Betancur, and B. Giros. 2001. "Hypolocomotor effects of acute and daily d-amphetamine in mice lacking the dopamine transporter." *Psychopharmacology (Berl)* no. 159 (1):2-9. doi: 10.1007/s0021301 00901.

Takahashi, N., L. L. Miner, I. Sora, H. Ujike, R. S. Revay, V. Kostic, V. Jackson-Lewis, S. Przedborski, and G. R. Uhl. 1997. "VMAT2 knockout mice: heterozygotes display reduced amphetamine-conditioned reward, enhanced amphetamine locomotion, and enhanced MPTP toxicity." *Proc Natl Acad Sci USA* no. 94 (18):9938-43. doi: 10.1073/pnas.94.18.9938.

Thanos, P. K., C. Bermeo, M. Rubinstein, K. L. Suchland, G. J. Wang, D. K. Grandy, and N. D. Volkow. 2010. "Conditioned place preference and locomotor activity in response to methylphenidate, amphetamine and cocaine in mice lacking dopamine D4 receptors." *J Psychopharmacol* no. 24 (6):897-904. doi: 10.1177/02698811091 02613.

Thanos, P. K., R. Habibi, M. Michaelides, U. B. Patel, K. Suchland, B. J. Anderson, J. K. Robinson, G. J. Wang, D. K. Grandy, and N. D. Volkow. 2010. "Dopamine D4 receptor (D4R) deletion in mice does not affect operant responding for food or cocaine." *Behav Brain Res* no. 207 (2):508-11. doi: 10.1016/j.bbr.2009.10.020.

Thomsen, M., F. S. Hall, G. R. Uhl, and S. B. Caine. 2009. "Dramatically decreased cocaine self-administration in dopamine but not serotonin transporter knock-out mice." *J Neurosci* no. 29 (4):1087-92. doi: 10.1523/JNEUROSCI.4037-08.2009.

Thomsen, M., D. D. Han, H. H. Gu, and S. B. Caine. 2009. "Lack of cocaine self-administration in mice expressing a cocaine-insensitive dopamine transporter." *J Pharmacol Exp Ther* no. 331 (1):204-11. doi: 10.1124/jpet.109.156265.

True, W. R., H. Xian, J. F. Scherrer, P. A. Madden, K. K. Bucholz, A. C. Heath, S. A. Eisen, M. J. Lyons, J. Goldberg, and M. Tsuang. 1999. "Common genetic vulnerability for nicotine and alcohol dependence in men." *Arch Gen Psychiatry* no. 56 (7):655-61. doi: 10.1001/archpsyc. 56.7.655.

Uhl, G. R. 2004. "Molecular genetic underpinnings of human substance abuse vulnerability: likely contributions to understanding addiction as a mnemonic process." *Neuropharmacology* no. 47 Suppl 1:140-7. doi: 10.1016/j.neuropharm.2004.07.029.

Uhl, G. R., G. F. Koob, and J. Cable. 2019. "The neurobiology of addiction." *Ann N Y Acad Sci*. doi: 10.1111/nyas.13989.

Ujike, H., M. Harano, T. Inada, M. Yamada, T. Komiyama, Y. Sekine, I. Sora, M. Iyo, T. Katsu, A. Nomura, K. Nakata, and N. Ozaki. 2003. "Nine- or fewer repeat alleles in VNTR polymorphism of the dopamine transporter gene is a strong risk factor for prolonged methamphetamine psychosis." *Pharmacogenomics J* no. 3 (4):242-7. doi: 10.1038/sj.tpj.6500189.

van den Bree, M. B., E. O. Johnson, M. C. Neale, and R. W. Pickens. 1998. "Genetic and environmental influences on drug use and abuse/dependence in male and female twins." *Drug Alcohol Depend* no. 52 (3):231-41.

Verhulst, B., M. C. Neale, and K. S. Kendler. 2015. "The heritability of alcohol use disorders: a meta-analysis of twin and adoption studies." *Psychol Med* no. 45 (5):1061-72. doi: 10.1017/S0033291714002165.

Walters, C. L., S. Brown, J. P. Changeux, B. Martin, and M. I. Damaj. 2006. "The beta2 but not alpha7 subunit of the nicotinic acetylcholine receptor is required for nicotine-conditioned place preference in mice." *Psychopharmacology (Berl)* no. 184 (3-4):339-44. doi: 10.1007/s00213-005-0295-x.

Ware, J. J., M. B. van den Bree, and M. R. Munafo. 2011. "Association of the CHRNA5-A3-B4 gene cluster with heaviness of smoking: a meta-analysis." *Nicotine Tob Res* no. 13 (12):1167-75. doi: 10.1093/ntr/ntr118.

Welter, M., D. Vallone, T. A. Samad, H. Meziane, A. Usiello, and E. Borrelli. 2007. "Absence of dopamine D2 receptors unmasks an inhibitory control over the brain circuitries activated by cocaine." *Proc Natl Acad Sci USA* no. 104 (16):6840-5. doi: 10.1073/pnas.0610790104.

Wen, L., K. Jiang, W. Yuan, W. Cui, and M. D. Li. 2016. "Contribution of Variants in CHRNA5/A3/B4 Gene Cluster on Chromosome 15 to Tobacco Smoking: From Genetic Association to Mechanism." *Mol Neurobiol* no. 53 (1):472-484. doi: 10.1007/s12035-014-8997-x.

Werner, D. F., Y. A. Blednov, O. J. Ariwodola, Y. Silberman, E. Logan, R. B. Berry, C. M. Borghese, D. B. Matthews, J. L. Weiner, N. L. Harrison, R. A. Harris, and G. E. Homanics. 2006. "Knockin mice with ethanol-insensitive alpha1-containing gamma-aminobutyric acid type A receptors display selective alterations in behavioral responses to ethanol." *J Pharmacol Exp Ther* no. 319 (1):219-27. doi: 10.1124/jpet.106.106161.

Zhuang, X., R. S. Oosting, S. R. Jones, R. R. Gainetdinov, G. W. Miller, M. G. Caron, and R. Hen. 2001. "Hyperactivity and impaired response habituation in hyperdopaminergic mice." *Proc Natl Acad Sci USA* no. 98 (4):1982-7. doi: 10.1073/pnas.98.4.1982.

In: Laboratory Animals and Neurosciences ISBN: 978-1-53618-462-4
Editors: B. Hernandez Godinez et al. 

*Chapter 7*

# PARTICIPATION OF HIPPOCAMPAL SEROTONIN DURING THE POSTICTAL PERIOD ON MOTOR RECOVERY IN AN ANIMAL MODEL WITH EPILEPSY

***Jose Luis Cortes Altamirano[1,2], Alberto Avila Luna[1], Luis Enrique Ruiz Sosa[1], Cindy Bandala[1,4], Samuel Reyes Long[1,4] and Alfonso Alfaro-Rodriguez[1,*]***

[1]División de Neurociencias, Instituto Nacional de Rehabilitación "Luis Guillermo Ibarra Ibarra", CDMX, México

[2]Department of Chiropractic, State University of the Valley of Ecatepec (UNEVE), Ecatepec de Morelos, Estado de México, México

[3]Laboratorio de Cromatografía y Microdiálisis, Servicio de Neurorrehabilitación, Instituto Nacional de Rehabilitación, CDMX, México

[4]Escuela Superior de Medicina, Instituto Politécnico Nacional, CDMX, México

* Corresponding Author's E-mail: alfa1360@yahoo.com.mx.

## Abstract

Animal models have generated a great advance in biological and health sciences, both in the understanding of the pathology and for its treatment. In chronic neurological diseases such as epilepsy a series of morphological and neurochemical changes are triggered, which are expressed as cognitive and/or motors deficits. The systemic administration of pentylenetetrazol (PTZ) produces a model of epilepsy, causing neurochemical changes and neuronal death at the hippocampal level. Serotonin (5-HT) has been related to motor aspects, coordinated and controlled by the cerebellum. It has been demostrated the association between the hippocampus and the cerebellum, which led to the approach of knowing what is the relationship between the hippocampal 5-HT and motor alterations induced by PTZ. Methods: 18 Wistar male rats (300 ± 10 g) were used, assigned to 2 groups: control (n = 9, saline solution) and experimental (n = 9, PTZ). Counting of myoclonic shakes and evaluation of motor behaviour were recorded during 3 hours post injection of PTZ (90 mk/kg). The hippocampus was dicected from each rat for the determination of 5-HT by high performance liquid chromatography. Results: The PTZ produced an increase in the total levels of hippocampal 5-HT and the presence of myoclonic shakes, as well as a marked motor deficit in the experimental group, without finding a correlation between them. Conclusion: Acute administration of PTZ at doses of 90 mg/kg possibly leads to two effects: the sensitization of the hippocampus manifested by the increase of 5-HT, and the transient global effects manifested by the motor deficit.


**Keywords**: pentylenetetrazol, serotonin, hippocampus, myoclonic jerks, motor deficit

## Introduction

### Animal Models

The advancement of knowledge at every discipline is supported by looking for the answers of different problems which have been confronted (i.e., research projects). In the biomedical research, it has been demonstrated the importance of the animals use, mostly in physiology, pathology, therapeutics, and pharmacology. One of the main factors in the development of medicine is animal testing.

This triggered the necessity to identify which are the animals who could have relevance in the comparative perspective to demonstrate more about the human body (Cohen et al., 2017).

For many years, the animal models have been used in human diseases in different research areas, being part of the development in biomedicine. They are useful in research projects like diagnostic and therapeutics tests as well as to control the pharmaceutics products. The Pan American Health Organization (PAHO) mentioned that "the country's who have increased the control of human and animal diseases are the ones who have established entities to improve the development of science in laboratory animals." Nevertheless, this progress has to be associated with the obedience of the legal ethics laws. That is the reason why the Science of Laboratories Animals was created so they could help the scientific community in order to succeed all the challenges they have faced with animal test (Rodríguez-Yunta, 2007).

The researchers who evaluate animal models take account of three types of validation. Construct validity means that a test measures what it claims. Therefore, in animal models, it means that everything that causes symptoms in animals it also contributes to human diseases. It is easy to obtain this validity when the condition is caused by only one gene, however most of them are more complicated. Validity means that a test seems to measure what it needs (e.g., the symptoms in an animal model reflect those in a human body). The predictive validity is how a test could predict a future outcome. In an animal model, the animal has to react to the drugs as a human would do. For example, in some cases antidepressants are evaluated as a result of their effects in "swimming forced test" which measures how much time the mouse tries to go out of the tank before it gives up. As well, there are not effective drugs which are useful as positive controls for autism. Even when drugs exist, either the symptoms or the mechanisms capturated by an individual behaviour trial, is not possible to pick up all the relevant information (Monya, 2011).

Animal models in human diseases are used to study the causes of therapeutics and preventives methods of human diseases as well as the development of new drugs (Nomura et al., 1987). There different kind of animal models, they variety depends on the disease and conditions such as neurologic diseases (Barnes, 1986) and convulsive epilepsy models (Chadwick, 1994). Animal models have allowed a crucial development in the comprehension and understanding in this kind of pathologies and biologic mechanisms in order to roll out new therapeutic strategies for a better patients quality of life (Rangasamy et al., 2017).

## Epilepsy

Humanity has long suffered from epilepsy, and even today it remains one of the most difficult diseases to understand and overcome (Cuan et al., 2017). Epilepsy is considered one of the most common chronic neurological disease of today, causing progressive neuronal degeneration (Zhu et al., 2017), which is characterized mainly by recurrent epileptic seizures (Zorsi et al., 2019). Epileptic seizures are transient events of signs and/or symptoms evoked by excessive abnormal neuronal activity (decrease or increase) (Moshe et al., 2015; Johnson et al., 2018).

Epilepsy is frequently associated with some type of neuronal damage such as head trauma, stroke, anozia or hypoxia, as well as synaptic reorganization, brain tumors, infectious diseases or idiopathic. There are several types of epileptic seizures, which can be broadly divided into generalized seizure and focal seizure, this type of seizures is directly associated with the affected brain area.

In this chapter, emphasis will be placed on myoclonic-type seizure, originated by cortical discharges that produce brief, unique, mild to severe jerks, mainly in the arms or head (Hernán et al., 2016; Villaba et al., 2016).

## PTZ-Induced Epilepsy Animal Model

Animal models have made great strides in the treatmente of epilepsy (Cuan et al., 2017). Systemic administration of pentylenetetrazol (PTZ) produces an epilepsy model, which has been widely used for the development of new antiepileptic drugs for decades (White 1998; Sarkisian 2001; Meldrum 2002; Vesna et al., 2003; Cuan et al., 2017). PTZ is an antagonist of GABAA receptors in the central nervous system (Macdonald and Barker 1977; Kulkarni et al., 1995; Huang et al., 2001; Gáll et al., 2017). Histological changes after PTZ administration are neuronal death and induction of massive degenerative processes in all regions of the hippocampal formation (Franke and Kittner, 2001; Ahmadi et al., 2017). PTZ modulates the activity of monoaminergic systems. (Becker et al., 2000). The reduction of noradrenaline (NA), dopamine (DA) and the increase of serotonin (5-HT) has been associated with the development of seizure (Shouse 2001) and motor disorders (Yonekawa et al., 1980). Seizure disorders may be indicators of the association between the serotonergic system and the hippocampus (Okada et al., 1999; Syndler et al., 2002).

It has been reported that after acute administration of some drugs such as PTZ and kainic acid (KA), animals show a complex pattern of behavior known as "myoclonic head shaking" that have been related to the serotonergic system (Osorio-Rico et al., 2003; Alfaro-Rodriguez et al., 2009) and are commonly observed as a phase prior to limbic-type seizures in the hippocampus and/or amygdala (Velísek and Mares 2004). Myoclonic shakes can be mediated by selective activation of 5-HT2A and 5-HT1A receptors (Colasanti et al., 1975; Renyi et al., 1992; Schreiber 1995). These data indicate that observed changes in behavior may be due to modification in the synthesis and release of 5-HT caused by alteration of synaptic processes that may occur as a consequence of neuronal loss (Szyndler et al., 2002).

## Epilepsy and Its Relationship to the Hippocampus

The hippocampus is involved in the region that regulates emotions and is probably also involved in the comorbidity of epilepsy (Peng et al., 2018). Both electrophysiologically and pathologically, the hippocampus is the most studied structure in temporal lobe epilepsy. The electroencephalogram (EEG) of epileptic animals shows clear signs of interictal activity, although these develop earlier in other areas, such as the perirrinal and piriform cortex (Kairiss et al., 1984). It has been reported that by losing volume of interneurons in the hippocampus of a brain with epilepsy, the balance between excitation and inhibition signals is altered, causing hyperexcitability (Zhu et al., 2019).

The most typical alteration of the epileptic hippocampus is sclerosis (Eadie et al., 2016), characterized by reinnervation of the dentate gyrus granules by mossy fibers and neuronal death in the hilus, areas of CA3 and CA1 and the superficial layers of the entorhinal cortex (Nadler et al., 1980; Qian et al., 2019). Despite this evidence, reinnervation by mossy fibers is thought to be a mechanism for amplifying discharges. In vitro records have shown that these aberrant glutamatergic circuits are functional and favor neuronal synchronization (Scharfma et al., 2003). Responses have been detected in discharges in the dentate gyrus and greater activation of granule dendrites (Otsu et al., 2000). Reinvervated circuits are glutamatergic in nature. Another of the alterations associated with reinnervation by mossy fibers is related to glutamatergic kainate receptors, which play a fundamental role in the presynaptic and postsynaptic control of excitability. The expression of subunit KA1 is permanently increased in the CA3 region, but not in the dentate gyrus of rats subjected to kindling (Hikiji et al., 1993).

Another of the most important alterations in the epileptic hippocampus is the inhibition of the GABAergic cell population (Zhu et al., 2019). It has been described that the glutamatergic disconnection of interneurons from the hilus causes a disinhibition of the dentate gyrus and the CA3 region that facilitates the generation of discharges (Sloviter, 1991). However, other studies have shown that the decrease in inhibition progressively recovers in parallel with the reinnervation by mossy fibers (Sloviter, 1992).

## BASIC CONCEPTS OF SEROTONIN

Seretonin is an indoleamine which can not cross the blood-brain barrier easily. Nevertheless, it was discovered in the brain, so researchers thought that it was where it is synthesized there (Goodman and Gilman, 2019). Neurons take the amino acid L-Tryptophan from blood by facilitated diffusion mechanism and then is converted into serotonin (Baumgarten et al., 2000; O´Mahony et al., 2015). Serotonin, also known as 5-Hydroxytryptamine (5-HT) is synthesized by a pathway of two stages from an essential amino acid, tryptophan. This molecule is involved in a variety of sensory, motor and conductual process in differents functions and pathologies that make it the target of multiplies research with different perspectives (Thomas et al., 2004). Nowadays, 5-HT has reached a new height due its relation with multiple functions (e.g., sensorimotor activity) (Glennon, 1990).

### Neuroanatomy of the Serotonergic System

Fluxe, in 1965 mediate histoimmunofluorescence identified the nuclei of serotonergicc neurons, observing nine nuclei of neurons that constitute the serotonergic system, located in the midline in the region of the brain stem (Fluxe 1968; Steinbush et al., 1981). According to their embryonic origin Jacobs and Azmitia (1992) classified these nuclei in two groups. The upper nucleus from the midbrain is made up of four subgroups: Linear Caudal Nucleus (LCN), Medial Raphe Nucleus (MRN), Dorsal Raphe Nucleus (DRN) and Lemniscus Nucleus (LN). This group of nuclei preserves almost the entire brain, including areas such as the hippocampus and cerebellum (Azmitia, 1999). Likewise, serotonergic efferent fibers in the thalamus have benn found to be associated with limbic functions. The cerebral cortex receives serotonergic fibers from the MRN and DRN, the vesicular and somatosensory area receives axons from the DRN and the motor and frontal parte receive DRN afferences (Jacobs and Azmitia, 1992).

On the other hand, previosu studies show that the activation of serotonergic neurons in the medial rafe nucleus have a suppressive effect on GABAergic synchronization mechanisms in the hippocampus (Varga et al., 2002). The ascending serotonergic systema plays an important role in the control of brain functions including learning and memory (Jacobs and Azmitia 1992).

GABAergic control is mediated by the large local population of GABAergic neurons in the dorsal rafe nucleus and medial rafe nucleus and by strong GABAergic projections from different areas (Gervasoni et al., 2000). Including the hippocampus (Kinney et al., 1995).

Similarly, it is suggested that GABAergic neurons may also participate in another type of regulation in the medial rafe nucleus that provide a slower rate of serotonin release (Varga et al., 2002). GABAergic interneurons, in addition to the activation of GABAA receptors, activate GABAB receptors, which in turn leads to slowing the hyperpolarization of serotonergic neurons producing an effect similar to 5-HT1A receptors (Abella et al., 2000). It is well known that the discharges of these neurons are controlled by the locally released 5-HT acting on the somato-dendrytic part of the 5-HT1A receptors (Pan et al., 1993).

Moreover, two lines of research have demonstrated the association cerebellum/hippocampus through emotions in humans: studies of lesions (Schmahmann 2004), and studies of functional neuroimaging (Reiman et al., 1997; Paradiso et al., 2003). The anatomical connections of the cerebellum with the regions involved in the regulation of emotion and the perception of relevant social-emotional material are revealing. The cerebellum is bidirectional linked to regions that innervate the social perception is relevant, including the posterior parietal cortex and the prefrontal regions (Middleton and Strick 2001; Dum and Strick 2003; Kelly and Strick 2003). It has been proposed that the cerebellum is adequate to regulate emotions as well as connections with limbic regions, including the amygdala, hippocampus and septal nucleus (Anand et al., 1959; Annoni et al., 2003; Schmahmann 2004). In addition, reciprocal connections link the cerebellum to areas of the brainstem that contain neurotransmitters involved in cognitive and motor aspects, such as 5-HT, NA and DA (Dempesy et al., 1983; Marcinkiewicz et al., 1989).

The animal model of epilepsy with PTZ not only produces behavioral and neurochemical changes, but also produces cognitive changes, similar to those observed in human epilepsy, particularly in that type of epilepsy involving the temporal lobe. Therefore, it is proposed that the systemic injection of PTZ in the rat will be a good biological, model for the study of epilepsy, in order to understand if the hippocampal 5-HT presents participation in the alteration of motor activity controlled and coordinated by the cerebellum. The main objective of this study was to determine the concentration of hippocampal 5-HT during the PTZ-induced postictal period and to correlate biochemical data with motor changes and myoclonic shakes.

## Materials and Methods

### Animals

Male Wistar rats (n = 18) weighing 300 ± 10 g were used. The rats were housed in cages and kept in light/dark cycles of 12 hrs at a temperature of 22°C. Water and feed were supplied ad libitum. The rats were handled with strict adherence to the technical specifications for the production, care and use of laboratory animals (NOM-062-ZOO-1999).

### Habituation of Rats

All rats were accustomed to laboratory conditions and used to the evaluation of motor function through two motor tests such as: Footprint printing, which evaluates the gait method described by González-Piña et al., (2005) and the paradigm of the balance bar, which evaluates motor coordination, using the criteria suggested by Brailowsky et al., (1986) and Bueno-Nava et al., (2010).

## Distribution of the Groups

Once accustomed, the animals wew randomly distributed in 2 groups: Control (n = 9, saline solution 1ml/kg subcutaneously); Experimental (n = 9, PTZ 90 mg/kg subcutaneously). All records were made between 9:00 am and 13:00 hrs to avoid variation of 5-HT due to the circadian cycle.

## Obtaining the Samples

Inmediately after registration, each animal was decapitated for extraction from the hippocampus. The tissue was immersed in Teflon tubes with antioxidant solution composed of 0.4 N perchloric acid with 0.1% (w/v) sodium metabisulfite. Subsequently the samples were centrifuged for 20 minutes at 14,000 rpm and 4°C. The supernatant was filtered and placed in eppendorf tubes to be injected to the High-Performance Liquid Chromatography (HPLC) system coupled to the electrochemical detector.

## Biochemical Analysis

The hippocampal samples from each group were biochemically analyzed. Levels of 5-HT were determined by HPLC coupled to the electrochemical detector ("ESA") coulochem III. An Alltech brand HPLC pump (model 626) and an Alltech furnace (model 631) and a 50 μL loop were used. A specific column for catecholamines ("adsorbosphere catecholamine" of 100 x 4.6 mm and 3 μm particle size) was used. The mobile phase consisted of an aqueous solution of phosphates (0.1 M, pH = 3.2) containing (per liter), 835 mL HPLC-grade deionized water, 165 mL of HPLC-grade methanol, 4 g monobasic sodium phosphate (NaH2PO4), 0.6 g sodium octyl sulfate, 160 mg EDTA. The quantification of 5-HT was established under the following detection conditions: for the analytical cell (ESA 5011A), potentials = 200 mV, 200 nA = E1 and E2 = -200 mV, 5nA, with a flow of 1.6 mL/min and 40°C. The calibration curves for monoamines were constructed with known concentratios of the standards prepared according to the protocol of Bueno-Nava et al., (2010). The peaks were integrated with the SI EZCrom program (version 3.2.1).

### Data Analysis

The data obtained were expressed with means + standard error. The results of motor behavior and myoclonic head jerks were analyzed with the U of Mann-Whitney test, while for statistical analysis of the 5-HT results a one-way ANOVA test was conducted. In all cases, significance levels were established with a $p<0.05$. Pearson correlations were used to examine the relationships between hippocampal 5-HT and motor behavior. For the analysis of descriptive statistics and statistical inference the SAS program for Windows (version 8) was used.

## Results

### PTZ Effect from Head's Myoclonic Seizures

After the systemic administration of PTZ (dose: 90mg/kg) by subcutaneous injection, animals presented myoclonic seizures which were quantify every 5 minutes during 3 hours that the register last. It reached the highest number during the first hour and it started to decrease gradually almost until the end of the register. In the same way, in head myoclonic seizures researches found significant differences in the group which was administrated with PTZ at the end of each hour comparing the experimental group with control group (Table 1).

**Table 1. Effect of the drug agonist for GABAA receptors Pentilentetrazol (PTZ), on the motor behavior of the rat**

| PTZ (90 mg/kg) | Hr. 1 | Hr. 2 | Hr. 3 |
|---|---|---|---|
| *Myoclonic Shakes* | 120.22 ± 15.31*** | 30.89 ± 10.94*** | 6.22 ± 2.39** |
| *Length of stride* | -37.70 ± 3.37**** | -29.52 ± 2.05**** | -23.52 ± 2.86*** |
| *Stride width* | 30.32 ± 11.26* | 41.08 ± 8.09*** | 34.15 + 5.89* |
| *Stride angle* | 93.98 + 16.31**** | 72.31 + 11**** | 57.73 + 11.13* |
| *Motor coordination* | 456.25 ± 19.90**** | 284.38 ± 51.09**** | 137.50 ± 37.20* |

Values were expressed with mean ± standard error. The results were analyzed with the U Mann-Whitney test significant difference compared with the control group: *P < 0.02, **P < 0.003, ***P < 0.001, ****P < 0.0005.

## Walking Evaluation

After PTZ administration, it was produced a prominent increase in the percent of the stride width deficit during 3 hours of the register which presented meaningful differences when the first, second and third hour were evaluated with control group (Table 1).

It presented a tendency in the deficit stride width recovery at the third hour. On the other hand, the percent of the stride width, during whole evaluation both groups presented meaningful differences. The stride width higher percentage was observed in the second hour and then a recovery tendency was presented in the experimental group at the first, second and third hour (Table 1).

Furthermore, it was observed an increase in angle stride in both groups where meaningful differences were presented between experimental group and control group during 3 hours. As well, a recovery tendency took place at the end of the record at first, second and third hour (Table 1).

## Assessment of Motor Coordination

The experimental group presented a motor deficit increase an amount of 456%, 284% and 137% at the first, second, and third hour respectively in contrast with the control group at the first, second and third hour (Table 1).

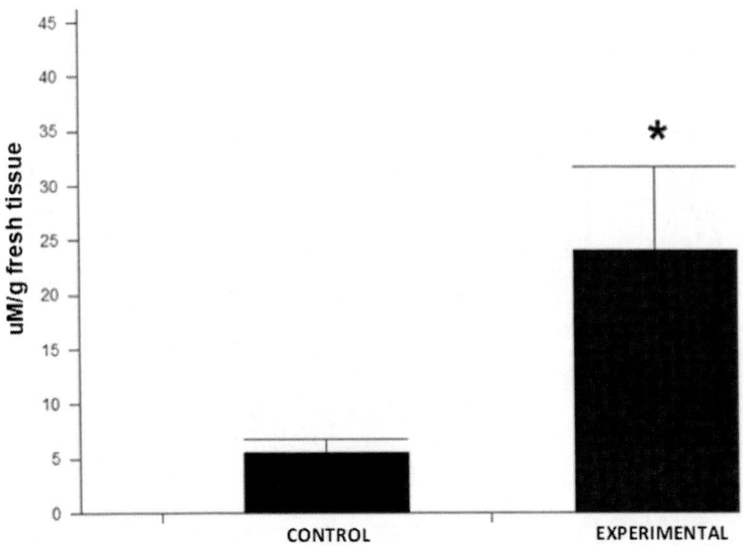


Figure 1. Total 5-HT content in the hippocampus of rat.

## Total Content of 5-HT Hippocampal

In the hippocampus, the concentration of 5-HT was increased in the experimental group at hour 3 after subcutaneous administration of 90 mg/kg PTZ compared to the control group with a significant difference ($p = .014$) (Figure 1).

## Correlation between Hippocampal 5-HT and Myoclonic Head Shakes, Gait and Coordination

The correlation between the total content of hippocampal 5-HT and the total number of myoclonic head jerks was sought, however, there was no such correlation at the third hour after PTZ administration. Similarly, there was no significant correlation in both the length, width and angle of the stride and the total 5-HT hippocampal content as well as in motor coordination.

# DISCUSION

According to this study, an increase in total levels of 5-HT in the hippocampus and a decrease in motor function in the adult rat were observed, as well as the presence of myoclonic head shakes after acute PTZ administration in a group of adult rats producing brain damage and neurochemical changes, such as those described by Cockerell et al. (1995). 5-HT projects almost all brain areas and participates in sensory, motor and behavioral processes (Pérez-García et al., 2006). In this study, acute administration at doses of 90 mg/kg of PTZ caused an imbalance of the serotonergic system, resulting in aberrant behavior as described by Adamec et al., (2006), translated into an increase of 5-HT at the hippocampal level in rats treated with this drug. This result is consistent with studies conducted by Gholipour et al. (2009) describing an increase in serotonergic neurotransmission in the hippocampus after induction of seizures.

Our results suggest that increased levels of 5-HT in the hippocampus of PTZ-treated rats may be a compensatory response to neuronal excitability after PTZ-induced brain damage. It has been previously demonstrated that direct lesions on serotonergic neurons can produce a compensatory response such as serotonergic reorganization in the dentate area after lesions of the middle raphe nucleus (Haring 1991).

In this study, the increase in hippocampal 5-HT occurred independently of changes in rat motor behavior after PTZ administration. During the convulsive process produced by PTZ not only the glutamatergic and GABAergic systems are involved, but also the monoaminergic systems (klynchuk 200). PTZ is a GABA antagonist, which second to the disinhibition of excitation processes in the brain also modulates the activity of monoaminergic systems (Becker et al., 200). On the other hand, the acute systemic administration of PTZ caused a marked transient brain dysfunction reflected in motor deficit. The hippocampus has cellular elements that receive inputs and send outputs to important areas of the bridge and cerebral cortex. Newman and Reza (1979) hypothesized that there are relationships between the hippocampus and the cerebellum. The pattern of electrical activity developed by the hippocampus is closely related to the performance of movements that occur during arousal and other behavioral changes. None of the proposals that have been made claim that the hippocampus participates in the feedback of muscle activity, but emphasize the possibility of a direct influence on motor control systems.

Assuming that the output of the hippocampus can modulate the motor control circuits, it is reasonable to suggest that the hippocampus itself guides the signals of the cerebellum for its normal operations. In turn, the hippocampus is involved in providing the information required for the cerebellum, just as proprioceptive information is used to correct movements in the locomotor system. There are fast and slow connections that operate in both directions. The postulated connection of the hippocampus is via the pontine, reticular nucleus and olive grove and the return connection is through the fastigial nucleus and thalamus (Newman and Reza, 1979). Although a relationship between the hippocampus and cerebellum has been described, in this study contemplating neurochemical aspects through 5-HT, it was not possible to show a relationship between these two structures. Although the somas of serotonergic neurons are found in the nuclei or the raphe in the midbrain, their fibers are projected throughout the CNS including the hippocampus and cerebellum (Azmitia and Whitaker-Azmitia 1991). In addition, these neurons tend to sprout after damage caused either by direct chemical injury (Zhou et al., 1995).

In some morphological studies, PTZ has been shown to cause the loss of neurons in many brain structures. Neuronal necrosis is found in the areas of the hippocampus CA1, CA3, and the dentate gyrus regions (Franke and Kittner 2001). Therefore. It is possible in the motor context that this alteration is due to a deterioration of the acquisition and/or retention of contextual signals, caused by damage in the hippocampus.

Goldstein (2003) notes that tests used to evaluate sensorimotor functions after cortical injury, such as the balance bar and footprint impression, may provide a complete assessment of motor deficit-related injury. A study by Hruska et al., (1979) proposes the measurement of the footprint based on the length, width, and angle of the stride as quantitative aspects of normal rat locomotion. The footprint test is specific to certain types of deficits that are not observable on the balance bar (Hruska et al., 1979; Goldstein 2003). Specifically, our results indicate that the length, width and angle of the stride increased considerably after PTZ administration. Presumably, these results were induced by the loss of neurons and/or errors or damage to brain-cerebellum connectivity, in addition to the monoaminergic imbalance. Similarly, the balance bar is a test that can qualitatively measure the motor coordination of the rat (Hruska 1979). It has been reported that focal cortical damage in rats induces a temporary motor deficit (Gonzáles-Piña et al., 2005; Goldstein 2006; Bueno-Nava et al., 2008).Together, the reciprocal connections that link the hippocampus with the cerebellum and with the areas of the brain stem derive from the participation of neurotransmitters that intervene in cognitive and motor aspects, such as serotonin, NA and DA (Dempesy et al., 1983; Marcinkiewicz et al., 1989). The results of the present work revealed that the administration of PTZ significantly increased the motor deficit during the three hours of recording. The data in this study may indicate that observed changes in motor behavior may be due to modification in the synthesis and release of monoamines, caused by alteration of synaptic regulatory processes, which may occur as a result of neuronal loss, gliosis, or neuronal breakouts as described by Szyndler et al. (2002). However, the return to basal motor conditions is evident in both motor behavior and myoclonic jerks after PTZ administration from the second hour, so it can be speculated that there may be mechanism that lead to a spontaneous restoration of monoamine levels, thus decreasing the degree of motor deficit.

Although there was no direct correlation between hippocampal serotonin and motor deficit, presumably there is an indirect involvement between serotonin and motor changes, acting as a neuromodulator, since serotonin changes the concentration of other monoamines directly involved in motor aspects such as NA and DA.

## CONCLUSION

The increase in hippocampal serotonin occurs independently of the rat's motor changes. Acute administration of PT at doses of 90 mg/kg produces two effects: sensitization of the hippocampus, reflected by increased serotonin and convulsive activity, and the transient global effects reflected in the cerebellum and motor deficit. Although physiological and behavioral studies have demonstrated the relationship between hippocampus and cerebellum, this biochemical study through the measurement of the 5-HT hippocampus failed to relate these two structures. However, it was possible to show the behavior of the phenomenon under study, without ruling out the possible participation of the hippocampal 5-HT in the motor alteration.

## REFERENCES

Abellan, M.T., Jolas, T., Aghajanian, G.K., Artigas, F. (2000). Dual control of dorsal raphe serotonergic neurons by GABAB receptors. Electrophysiological and microdialysis studies. *Synapse*. 36, 21-34. Doi:

10.1002/(SICI)1098-2396(200004)36:1<21::AID-SYN3>3.0.CO;2-D.

Adamec, R., Burton, P., Blundell, J., Murphy, D.L., Holmes, A. (2006). Vulnerability to mild predator stress in serotonin transporter knockout mice. *Behav Brain Res.* 170, 126–140. Doi: 10.1016/j.bbr.2006.02.012.

Ahmadi Mahboubeh, Dufour Jean-Philippe, Seifritz Erich, Mirnajafi-Zadeh Javad, Saab Bechara J. (2017). The PTZ kindling mouse model of epilepsy exhibits exploratory drive deficits and aberrant VTA dopamine neuron activity in both familiar and novel space. *Behavioural Brain Research.* 330, 1-7. Doi: 10.1016/j.bbr.2006.02.012.

Akaike, A., Tanaka, H., Tojo, S., Fukumoto, S., Imamura, S., Takigawa, M. (2001). Kainic acidinduced dorsal and ventral hippocampal seizures in rats. *Brain Res.* 900, 65–71. Doi: 10.1016/s0006-8993(01)02252-1.

Alfaro-Rodríguez, A., González-Piña, R., Arch-Tirado, E., Carrasco-Portugal, M., Pérez-Guillé, B., Soriano-Rosales, R.E., Padilla-Martin, K., Uribe-Escamilla, R., Labra-Ruiz, N. (2009). Neuroprotective effects of carbamazepine on sllep patterns and body shakes in kainic acid-treated rats. *Chemico-Biological Interactions* 180, 376–382. Doi: 10.1016/j.cbi.2009.04.007.

Alfaro-Rodríguez, A., González-Piña, R., Bueno-Nava, A., Arch-Tirado, E., Avila-Luna, A., Uribe-Escamilla, R., Vargas-Sánchez, J. (2011). Effects of oxcarbazepine on monoamines content in hippocampus and head and body shakes and sleep patterns in kainic acid-treated rats. *Metabollic Brain Dis.* 26, 213-220. Doi: 10.1007/s11011-011-9254-x.

Anand, B.K., Malhotra, C.L., Singh, B., Dua S. (1959). Cerebellar projections to limbic system. *Journal of Neurophysiology.* 22,451–457. Doi: 10.1152/jn.1959.22.4.451.

Annoni, J.M., Ptak, R., Caldara-Schnetzer, A.S., Khateb, A., Pollermann, B.Z. (2003). Decoupling of Autonomic and cognitive emotional reactions after cerebellar stroke. *Annals of Neurology.* 53,654–658. Doi: 10.1002/ana.10549.

Aronica, E.M., Gortler, J.A., Paupard, M.C., Grooms, S.Y., Bennett, M.V., Zukin, R.S. (1997). Status epilepticus-induced alterations in metabotropic glutamate receptor expression in young and adult rats. *J. Neurosci.* 17, 8588–8595. Doi: 10.1523/JNEUROSCI.17-21-08588. 1997.

Azmitia, E.C., Whitaker-Azmitia, P.M. (1991). Awakening the sleeping giant: anatomy and plasticity of the brain serotonergic system. *J Clin Psychiatry.* 52, 4–16. PMID:1752858.

Becker, A., Grecksch, G., Thiemann, W., Hollt, V. (2000). Pentylene-tetrazol-kindling modulates stimulated dopamine release in the nucleus accumbens of rats. Pharmacol. *Biochem. Behav.* 66, 425–428. Doi:10.1016/s0091-3057(99)00264-6.

Ben-Ari, Y., Tremblay, E., Riche, D., Ghilini, G., Naquel, R. (1981). Electroencephalographic, clinical and pathological alterations following systemic administration of kainic acid, bicuculine or pentetrazole: metabolic mapping using the deoxyglucose method with special reference to the pathology of epilepsy, *Neuroscience.* 6, 1361–1391. Doi: 10.1016/0306-4522(94)90098-1.

Brailowsky, S., Knight, R.T., Blood, K. (1986). Gamma-aminobutyric acid-induced potentiation of cortical hemiplegia. *Brain Res.* 362,322-330. Doi: 10.1016/0006-8993(86)90457-9.

Bueno-Nava, A., González-Piña, R., Alfaro-Rodriguez, A., Nekrassov-Protasova, V., Durand-Rivera, A., Montes, S., Ayala-Guerrero F. (2010). Recovery of motor déficit, cerebellar serotonin and lipid peroxidation levels in the cortex of injured rats. *Neurochem Res* 10,1538-1545.doi: 10.1007/s11064-010-0213-4.

Bueno-Nava, A., Montes, S., De la Garza-Montano, P., Alfaro-Rodriguez, A., Ascencion- Ortiz, González-Pina, R. (2008). Reversal of noradrenergic depletion and lipid peroxidation in the pons after brain injury correlates with motor function recovery in rats. *Neurosci Lett* 443,32–36. Doi: 10.1016/j.neulet.2008.07.046.

Cockerell, O.C., Johnson, A.L., Sander, J.W., Hart, Y.M., Shorvon, S.D. (1995). Remission of epilepsy: results from the National General Practice Study of Epilepsy. *Lancet* 346, 140-144. Doi: 10.1016/s0140-6736(95)91208-8.

Cohén. (2017). Aging across the tree of life: The importance of a comparative perspective for the use of animal models in aging. *BBA-Molecular Basis Of Disease,* 1-2. Doi: 10.1016/j.bbadis.2017.03.002.

Colasanti, B.K., Jane, E., Kosa., Charles, R., Craig. (1975). Appearance of Wet Dog Shake Behavior during Cobalt Experimental Epilepsy in the Rat and Its Suppression by Reserpine. *Psychopharmacologia (Berl.).* 44, 33-36. Doi: 10.1007/bf00421180.

Dempesy, C.W., Tootle, D.M., Fontana, C.J., Fitzjarrell, A.T., Garey, R.E., Heath, R.G. (1983). Stimulation of the paleocerebellar cortex of the cat: increased rate of synthesis and release of catecholamines at limbic sites. *Biological Psychiatry.*18, 127–132. PMID:6830922.

Dum, R.P., Strick, P.L. (2003). An unfolded map of the cerebellar dentate nucleus and its projections to the cerebral cortex. *Journal of Neurophysiology.* 89,634–639.doi: 10.1152/jn.00626.2002.

Emily L. Johnson. (2018). Seizures and Epilepsy. *Medical clinics.* 103, 309-324.doi: 10.1016/j.mcna.2018.10.002.

Eadie, M.J. (2016). Epilepsy, Ammon´s horn sclerosis, and Camille Bouchet. Journal of the History of the Neurosciences. *Basic and Clinical Perspectives.* 26, 231-237. Doi: 10.1080/0964704X.2016.1224141.

Franke, H., Kittner, H. (2001). Morphological alterations of neurons and astrocytes and changes in emotional behavior in pentylenetetrazol-kindled rats. *Pharmacol. Biochem. Behav.* 70, 291–303. Doi: 10.1016/s0091-3057(01)00612-8.

Gáll, Z., Koncz, S., Gáll, O., Kolcsár, M. (2017). Lacosamide reduces seizure severity but increases seizure frequency in PTZ-Kindled rats. *Acta Medica Marisiensis.* 63(4), 173-177. Doi: 10.1515/amma-2017-0037.

Gervasoni, D., Peyron, C., Rampon, C., Barbagli, B., Chouvet, G., Urbain, N., Luppi, P.H. (2000). Role and origin of the GABAergic innervations of dorsal raphe serotonergic neurons. *J. Neurosci.* 20, 4217-4225. Doi: 10.1523/JNEUROSCI.20-11-04217.2000.

Gholipour, T., Ghasemi, M., Razi, K., Ghaffarpour, M., Dehpour, A. (2009). Seizures susceptibility alteration through 5-HT (3) receptor: modulation by nitric oxide. *Seizure.* 19, 17-22.doi: 10.1016/j.seizure.2009.10.006.

Giroud, M., Dumas, R., Dauvergne, M., D'Athis, P., Rochette, L., Beley, A. (1990). 5- Hydroxyindoleacetic acid and homovanillic acid in cerebrospinal fluid of children with febrile convulsions. *Epilepsia.* 31,178–81. Doi: 10.1111/j.1528-1167.1990.tb06303.x.

Goldstein, L.B. (2003). Model of recovery of locomotor ability after sensorimotor cortex injury in rats. *ILAR J* 44, 125–129. Doi: 10.1093/ilar.44.2.125.

Goldstein, L.B. (2006). Neurotransmitters and motor activity: effects on functional recovery after brain injury. *NeuroRx.* 3,451–457. Doi: 10.1016/j.nurx.2006.07.010.

Gonzálcz-Piña, R., Bueno-Nava, A., Montes, S. (2005). Pontine norepinephrine content after motor cortical ablation in rats. *Proc. West. Pharmacol. Soc.* 48,73-76. PMID: 16416666.

Haring, J.H. (1991) Reorganization of the area dentata serotoninergic plexus after lesions of the median raphe nucleus. *J Comp Neurol.* 306,576–584. Doi: 10.1002/cne.903060404.

Hernán, P. (2016). *Búsqueda de nuevos anticonvulsivos a partir de métodos computacionales* (tesis de doctorado). Universidad Nacional de la Plata, Buenos Aires, Argentina. [*Search for new anticonvulsants using computational methods* (doctoral thesis).]

Hruska, R.E., Kennedy, S., Silbergeld, E.K. (1979). Quantitative aspects of normal locomotion in rats. *Life Sci* 25,171–180. Doi: 10.1016/0024-3205(79)90389-8.

Huang, R.Q., Bell-Horner, C.L., Dibas, M.I., Covey, D.F., Drewe, J.A., Dillon, G.H. (2001). Pentylenetetrazole-induced inhibition of recombinant gamma-aminobutyric acid type A (GABA(A)) receptors: mechanism and site of action. *J Pharmacol Exp Ther.* 298, 986-995. PMID:11504794.

Isaac, M. (2005). Serotonergic 5-HT2C receptors as a potential therapeutic target for the design antiepileptic drugs. *Curr. Top. Med. Chem.* 5, 59–67. Doi: 10.2174/1568026053386980.

Jacobs, B.L., Azmitia, E.C. (1992). Structure and function of the brain serotonin system. *Physiolo Rev.* 72,165-229. doi: 10.1152/physrev. 1992.72.1.165.

Brunton, L.L., Hilal-Dandan, R., Knollmann, B.C. Goodman & Gilman. *The pharmacological bases of therapeutics.* Thirteenth edition. McGraw-Hill. *España.* 2019. P. 351.

Kandel, E.R., Schuartz, J.H., Jessell, T.M. *Neuroscience principles*. Fourth edition. McGraw-Hill. España. 2001. P 893.

Kelly, R.M., Strick, P.L. (2003). Cerebellar loops with motor cortex and prefrontal cortex of a nonhuman primate. *Journal of Neuroscience.* 23,8432–8444.

Kinney, G.G., Kocsis, B., Vertes, R.P. (1995). Injections of muscimol into the median raphe nucleus produce hippocampal theta rhythm in the urethane anesthetized rat. *Psychopharmacology.* 120, 244-248.doi: 10.1007/bf02311170.

Klynchuk, L.E. (2000). Long-term amygdala kindling in rats as a model for the study of interictal emotional in temporal lobe epilepsy. *Neurosci. Biobehav. Rev.* 24, 691–704. PMID:10974352.

Kulkarni, S.K., George, B. (1995). Pentylenetetrazol-induced kindling in animals: protective effect of BR-16A. *Indian J Exp Biol.* 33,424-427. PMID:7590948.

Liu, H., Mazarati, A.M., Katsumori, H., Sankar, R., Wasterlain, C.G. (1999). Substance P is expressed in hippocampal principal neurons during status epilepticus and plays a critical role in the maintenance of status epilepticus. *Proc. Natl. Acad. Sci. U.S.A.* 96, 5286–5291. Doi: 10.1073/pnas.96.9.5286.

Macdonald, R.L., Barker, J.L. (1977). Pentylenetetrazol and penicillin are selective antagonists of GABA-mediated post-synaptic inhibition in cultured mammalian neurones. *Nature.* 267, 720-721. Doi: 10.1038/267720a0.

Marcinkiewicz, M., Morcos, R., Chretien, M. (1989). CNS connections with the median raphe nucleus: retrograde tracing with WGA-apoHRP-Gold complex in the rat. *Journal of Comparative Neurology.* 289,11–35. Doi: 10.1002/cne.902890103.

Meldrum, B. (1991). Excitotoxicity and epileptic brain damage. *Epilepsy Res.* 10, 5561. Doi: 10.1016/0920-1211(91)90095-W.

Meldrum, B. (2002). Do preclinical seizure models preselect certain adverse effects of antiepileptic drugs. *Epilepsy Res.* 50, 33-40. 10.1016/S0920-1211(02)00066-9.

Middleton, F.A., Strick, P.L. (2001). Cerebellar projections to the prefrontal cortex of the primate. *Journal of Neuroscience.* 21,700–712. Doi: 10.1523/JNEUROSCI.21-02-00700.2001.

Mikati, M.A., Abi-Habib, R.J. Sabban, M.E., Dbaibo, G.S., Kurdi, R.M., Kobeissi, M., Farhat, F., Asaad, W. (2003). Hippocampal programmed cell death after status epilepticus: evidence for NMDA-receptor and ceramide-mediated mechanisms. *Epilepsia.* 44, 282–291. Doi: 10.1046/j.1528-1157.2003.22502.x.

Moshé, S.L., Emilio Perucca, Philippe Ryvlin, Torbjöm Tomson. (2015). Epilepsy: new advances. *The Lancet, Seminar.* 385, 884-898. Doi: 10.1016/S0140-6736(14)60456-6.

Newman, P., Reza, H. (1979). *Functional relationships between the hippocampus and the cerebellum: an electrophysiological study of the cat.* From the Department of Physiology, School of Medicine. Great Britain. 287, 405-426. Doi: 10.1113/jphysiol.1979.sp012667.

Nickels, J.L., Schneider, W.N., Dombovy, M.L., Wong, T.M. (1994). Clinical use of amantadine in brain injury rehabilitation. *Brain Inj.* 8, 709-18. Doi: 10.3109/02699059409151025.

NORMA Oficial Mexicana NOM-062-ZOO-1999. *Technical specifications for the production, care and use of laboratory animals.*

Okada, M., Hirano, T., Mizuno, K., Kawata, Y., Wada, K., Mizuno, K., Kondo T., Kaneko S. (1999). Biphasic effects of zonisamide on serotonergic system in rat hippocampus. *Epilepsy Res.* 34, 187–197. Doi: 10.1016/S0920-1211(98)00109-0.

Osorio-Rico, L., Mancera-Flores, M., Ríos, C. (2003). Changes in brain serotonin turnover, body and head shakes in kainic acid-treated rats, *Pharmacol. Toxicol.* 92, 143-147. Doi: 10.1034/j.1600-0773.2003.920307.x.

Pan, Z.Z., Wessendorf, M.W., Williams, J.T. (1993). Modulation by serotonin of the neurons in rat nucleus raphe magnus in vitro. *Neuroscience.* 54,421-429. Doi: 10.1016/0306-4522(93)90263-F.

Paradiso, S., Robinson, R.G., Boles-Ponto L.L., Watkins, G.L., Hichwa, R.D. (2003). Regional cerebral blood flow changes during visually induced subjective sadness in healthy elderly persons. *Journal of Neuropsychiatry and Clinical Neurosciences.* 15,35–44. PMID: 12556569.

Peng, W., Mao, L., Yin, D., Sun, W., Wang, H., Zhang, Q., Wang, J., Chen, C., Zeng, M., Ding, J., Wang, X. (2018). Functional network changes in the hippocampus contribute to depressive symptoms in epilepsy. *Seizure: European Journal of Epilepsy.* 60, 16-22. Doi: 10.1016/j.seizure.2018.06.001.

Perea, M.V., Ladera, V., Morales, F., (1999). Valor predictivo de los tests breves sobre la situación cognitiva en traumatismos craneoencefálicos. *Rev Neurol.* 29,1099-103. [Predictive value of brief tests on the cognitive situation in head injuries. *Rev Neurol*]

Pérez-García, G., liy-Salmerón, G., Meneses, A. (2006). *Receptores serotonérgicos y memoria. revista mexicana de análisis de la conducta.* 32,241-269. ISSN: 0185-4534. [*Serotonergic receptors and memory. Mexican magazine of behavior analysis*.]

Qin, Y.L., Carter, C.S., Silk, E.M., Stenger, V.A., Fisell, K., Goode, A., Anderson, J.R. (2004). The change of the brain activation patterns as children learn algebra equation solving. *Proceeding of the National Academy of Sciences of the United States of America,* 101, 5686-5691. Doi: 10.1073/pnas.0401227101.

Reiman, E.M., Lane, R.D., Ahern, G.L., Schwartz, G.E., Davidson, R.J., Friston, K.J., et al. (1997). Neuroanatomical correlates of externally and internally generated human emotion. *American Journal of Psychiatry.* 154,918–925. PMID: 9210741.

Renyi, L., Angeby-Moller, K., Ensler, K., Evenden, J. (1992). The non-competitive NMDA receptor antagonist MK-801 counteracts the long-lasting attenuation of the hypothermic response induced by acute doses of 8-OH- DPAT in the rat. *Neuropharmacology* 31,1265–1268. Doi: 10.1016/0028-3908(92)90055-T.

Rubio-Donnadieu F. (1997). Aspectos generales y clasificación de la epilepsia, in *Epilepsia* (Feria Velasco A., Martínez de Muñoz D., and

Rubio Donnadieu F., eds.), pp. 1-24. Cognos Editores S.A. de C.V., México, D.F. [General aspects and classification of epilepsy, in *Epilepsy*]

Sampathkumar Rangasamy, Mohan J. Narayanan, Isabelle Schrauwen, Alysson R. Muotri and Vinodh Narayanan. (2017). Celullar and Animal Models of Neurologic Disease. *Swaiman's Pediatric Neurology.* 6, 114-122.

Sarkisian, M.R. (2001). Overview of the Current Animal Models for Human Seizure and Epileptic Disorders. *Epilepsy Behav.* 2, 201-216. Doi: 10.1006/ebeh.2001.0193.

Schmahmann, J.D. (2004). Disorders of the cerebellum: ataxia, dysmetria of thought, and the cerebellar cognitive affective syndrome. *Journal of Neuropsychiatry and Clinical Neurosciences.* 16,367–378. Doi: 10.1176/jnp.16.3.367.

Schreiber, R., Brocco, M., Audinot, V., Gobert, A., Veiga, S., Millan, M.J. (1995). [1 (2,5-Dimethoxy-4-iodophenyl)-2-aminopropane]-induced head-twitches in the rat are mediated by 5-hydroxytryptamine(5-HT)2A receptors: modulation by novel 5-HT2A/2C antagonists, D1 antagonists and 5-HT1A agonists. *J Pharmacol Exp Ther,* 273,101–112. PMID: 7714755.

Shouse, N.M., Staba, R.J., Ko, P., Saquib, S.F., Farber, R.P., (2001). Monoamines and seizures: microdialysis findings in locus ceruleus and amygdala before and during amygdale kindling. *Brain Res.* 892 176–192. Doi: 10.1016/S0006-8993(00)03292-3.

Statnick, M.A., Maring-Smith, M.L., Clough, R.W., Wang, C., Dailey, J.W., Jobe, P.C., Browning, R.A. (1996). Effect of 5,7-dihydroxytryptamine on audiogenic seizures in genetically epilepsy-prone rats. *Life Sci.* 59, 1763–1771. Doi: 10.1016/0024-3205(96)00519-X.

Syndler, J., Wierzba-Bobrowicz., Maciejak, P., Siemiatkowski., Rok, P., Lehner, M., Czlonkowska, A.I., Bidzinsk,i A., Wislowska, A., Zienowicz, M., Plaznik A. (2002). Pentylenetetrazol-kindling of seizures selectively decreases [3H]-citalopram binding in the CA-3 area of rat hippocampus. *Neurosci Lett.* 335, 49-53. Doi: 10.1016/ S0304-3940(02)01141-2.

Szyndler, J., Paulina, R., Piotr, M., Jerzy, W., Agnieszka, I., Czl C., Halina S., Aleksandra, W., Ma, l Cgorzata Zienowicz., Mal Cgorzata Lehner., Andrzej, Bidzin´ski., Wojciech, Kostowski., Adam, P. (2002). Effects of pentylenetetrazol-induced kindling of seizures on rat emotional behavior and brain monoaminergic systems. *Pharmacology, Biochemistry and Behavior.* 73, 851–861. Doi: 10.1016/S0091-3057(02)00912-7.

Takeda, K., Nakata, K., Takahashi, S., Chikuma, T., Kato, T. (1998). Effect of pentylenetetrazol treatment on cholecystokinin mRNA and peptide levels in rat hippocampus and cortex. *Brain Res.* 779, 320–323. 10.1016/S0006-8993(97)01179-7.

Varga, V., Sik, A., Freund, T.F., Kocsis, B. (2002). GABAB receptors in the median raphe nucleus: distribution and role in the serotonergic control of hippocampal activity. *Neuroscience.* 109,119-132. Doi: 10.1016/S0306-4522(01)00448-1.

Velísek, L., Mares, P. (2004). Hippocampal afterdischarges in rats. I. Effects of antiepileptics. Physiol. Res. 53, 453-46. PMID:15312006.

Vesna, E., Gordana, Ž., Jadranka, V., Ante S. (2003). Pentylenetetrazol-induced seizures and kindling: changes in free fatty acids, superoxide dismutase, and glutathione peroxidase activity. *Neurochemistry International.* 42,.173–178. Doi: 10.1016/S0197-0186(02)00070-0.

Villaba, M. (2016). *Síntesis de sulfamidas con acción anticonvulsiva* (tesis doctoral). Universidad Nacional de la Plata, Buenos Aires, Argentinca. Doi: 10.35537/10915/53069. [*Synthesis of sulfonamides with anticonvulsant action* (doctoral thesis).]

de Zorzi, V.N., F. Haupenthal, A.S. Cardoso, et al.,(2019). Galangin prevents increased susceptibility to pentylenetetrazol-stimulated seizures by prostaglandin E2. *Neuroscience.* 1-3. Doi: 10.1016/j. neuroscience.2019.06.002.

White, H.S. (1998). *Chemoconvulsants, in Neuropharmacology methods in epilepsy research* (Peterson S.L. and Albertson T.E., eds.), pp. 27-40. CRC Press.

Qian, X., Z-R. Wang, J-J. Zheng, J-Q. Ding, J-G. Zhong, T-Y. Zhang, W. Li, M, Zhang. (2019). Baicalein improves cognitive deficits and hippocampus impairments in temporal lobe epilepsy rats. *Brain Research.* 1714, 111-118. Doi: 10.1016/j.brainres.2019.02.028.

Xinjuan Zhu, Jingde Dong, Bing Han, Rongrong Huang, Aifeng Zhang, Zhengrong Xia, Huanhuan Chang, Jie Chao and Honghong Yao. (2017). Neuronal Nitric Oxide Synthase Contributes to PTZ Kindling Epilepsy-Induced Hippocampal Endoplasmic Reticulum Stress and Oxidative Damage. *Frontiers In Cellular Neuroscience.* 11, 1-14. Doi: 10.3389/fncel.2017.00377.

Ye Cuan, Xirui He, Yuhui Zhao, Jiajun Yang, Yajun Bia, Yin Sun, Qiang Zhang, Zefeng Zhao, Xiaoyang Wei, Xiaohui Zheng. (2017). Anticonvulsant Activity of Halogen-Substituted Cinnamic Acid Derivatives and Their Effects on Glycosylation of PTZ-Induced Chronic Epilepsy in Mice. *MPDI Molecules* 23, 76, 1-8. Doi: 10.3390/molecules23010076.

Yonekawa, W.D., Kupferberg, H.J., Woodbury, D.M. (1980). Relationship between pentylenetetrazol-induced seizures and brain pentylenetetrazol levels in mice. *J. Pharmuc. e-up. Ther.* 214, 589-593. PMID:7400961.

Zhou, F.C., Azmitia, E.C., Bledsoe, S. (1995). Rapid serotonergic fiber sprouting in response to ibotenic acid lesion in the striatum and hippocampus. *Brain Res Dev Brain Res.* 84,89–98. Doi: 10.1016/0165-3806(94)00158-V.

Zhu, X., Yao, Y., Li, X., Dong, J., Zhang, A. (2019). Alteration of GABAergic signaling is associated with anxiety-like behavior in temporal lobe epilepsy mice. *Progress in Neuropsychopharmacology & Biological Psychiatry.* 93, 141-148. Doi: 10.1016/j.pnpbp. 2019.03.020.

In: Laboratory Animals and Neurosciences ISBN: 978-1-53618-462-4
Editors: B. Hernandez Godinez et al.© 2020 Nova Science Publishers, Inc.

*Chapter 8*

# EVALUATION PROBES IN COGNITIVE DYSFUNCTION IN RODENT MODELS BASED ON DIETARY-INDUCED OBESITY

***Verónica Salas-Venegas*[1,2]**
***and Norma E. López-Díazguerrero*[2,*]**
[1]Posgrado en Biología Experimental,
Universidad Autónoma Metropolitana-Iztapalapa,
Ciudad de México, México
[2]Departamento de Ciencias de la Salud,
Laboratorio de Bioenergética y Envejecimiento Celular,
Universidad Autónoma Metropolitana-Iztapalapa,
Ciudad de México, México

## ABSTRACT

The association between obesity and cognitive function deterioration has become relevant in recent years, due to the increase in overweight and

* Corresponding Author's E-mail: norm@xanum.uam.mx.

obese people. Obesity is usually associated with chronic low-grade systemic inflammation and is part of a set of disorders called "metabolic syndrome." It is known that obesity-associated inflammatory response affects different brain structures such as the hypothalamus, the hippocampus, the cortex, the brainstem, and the amygdala. These alterations contribute to the neuroinflammation process and cognitive dysfunctions. Animal models based on dietary-induced obesity are essential to understand the factors involved in the central nervous system pathophysiology of obesity, particularly in regions involved in learning and memory. Morris Water Maze and Barnes Maze that are well-validated techniques to assess spatial learning and memory in rodents, have provided valuable information related to the effect of obesity on cognitive impairment.

**Keywords**: obesity, hypothalamus, hippocampus, cytokines, neuroinflammation, Morris Water Maze, Barnes Maze

## Introduction

The incidence of obesity is a growing problem worldwide due to high-calorie intake and a sedentary lifestyle. It is determined when the body mass index (BMI) is 30 $kg/m^2$ or more. It is known that obesity involves metabolic alterations and comorbidities (Lainez et al., 2019; Nguyen et al., 2014), in addition to compromising cognitive ability (Jurdak et al., 2008). Obesity leads to the establishment of a chronic systemic inflammatory state of low grade due to an increase in circulating cytokines, free fatty acids, and the activation of immune cells (Miller & Spencer, 2014). This systemic inflammation can reach other regions such as the brain and initiate a local inflammatory process known as "neuroinflammation" (Moreno-Navarrete et al., 2017; Miller & Spencer, 2014) that generates glial activation and synaptic remodeling with repercussions on cognition.

Rodent models in neuroscience can be useful to understand the consequences of obesity and its effects on cognitive impairment. These animal models show many of the metabolic abnormalities observed in human obesity, including elevated blood glucose levels and lipids, insulin resistance, and high blood pressure (Jurdak et al., 2008). Cognitive tests in rodents allow the evaluation of memory and learning processes during obesity and are dependent on brain regions such as the cortex and the hippocampus (Douglass et al., 2017). These tests assume that the animal learns to solve maze using positive or negative environmental factors. In the Barnes maze test, the rodent is placed on the surface of a platform where he must learn and remember the location of an escape box (a safe, dark shelter located beneath the surface of the platform). The second part of the test (reverse learning) consists of changing the position of the shelter, which allows assessing the cognitive flexibility to re-learn a new location (Gawel et al., 2019). Another test is the Morris water maze (MWM), which is a spatial learning test that is based on distal cues to navigate from start locations around the perimeter of an open swimming arena to locate an escape platform, guided by distant tracks (Vorhees & Williams, 2006). The Morris water maze is a test of spatial learning for rodents that relies on distal cues to navigate around the perimeter of an open swimming arena to locate a submerged escape platform. The test trials that assess cognitive impairment in rodents allow a better approach to the implications of memory and learning processes generated by different types of diets for the induction of obesity. Also, they enable dissecting the pathways involved in this condition, and can even suggest various interventions (medications, exercise) to reduce cognitive impairment.

## Obesity, Metabolic Syndrome and Cognitive Impairment

Nutritional changes, and especially the increase in fat and carbohydrate intake in the last 30 years, have resulted in the current epidemic of obesity and disorders such as metabolic syndrome. Obesity is a risk for a wide range of diseases that include insulin resistance, type 2 diabetes, dyslipidemia, cardiovascular disease, neurodegenerative disorders, among others. Likewise, obesity is characterized by the combined result of dysfunction of the center of satiety at the cerebral level, imbalance of intake, and use of energy. Obesity has also been considered a process of chronic systemic inflammation of low grade. The incidence of obesity, classified by the body mass index (BMI) > 30 kg/m2 (BMI = is the weight in kilograms divided by the square of height in meters), is continuously increasing throughout the world population. This condition is attributed to unhealthy diets (i.e., excessive consumption of high fat, high sugar, and high salt foods and beverages) and physical inactivity (Nguyen et al., 2014). Moreover, different studies in humans and murine models in recent decades have revealed that the interaction between genes and environmental factors also impacts food intake and energy homeostasis favoring the development of obesity (Friedman et al., 2004).

In addition to weight gain, obesity is associated with a set of disorders called "metabolic syndrome." The development of metabolic syndrome is associated with an increase in cognitive impairment and an increased risk of dementia. Some of the different mechanisms through metabolic syndrome and cognitive impairment can be associated, are neuroinflammation, increased adipose tissue, and insulin resistance (Yaffe et al., 2007). Therefore, to prevent obesity and to find new treatments, it is vital to develop animal models that might share the characteristics of human obesity and its comorbidities.

In humans, to be diagnosed with this syndrome, the individuals must have at least three of the following criteria:

1. Abdominal obesity measured by the size of waist circumference (88 cm for women and 102 cm for men).
2. Plasma triglycerides ≥ 1.7 mmol/L.
3. High-density lipoprotein (HDL) greater than 1.30 mmol/L for women and 1.04 mmol/L for men.
4. Blood pressure ≥ 130/85 mm Hg
5. Fasting glucose level exceeding 6.1 mmol/L (Guillemot-Legris & Muccioli., 2017).

## SATIETY REGULATION

The central nervous system (CNS) is a crucial regulator in the control of the energy state and the glucose levels of the organism. The hypothalamus is the master regulator and integrator of the energy homeostasis of the whole body (Myers & Olson, 2012). In particular, the arcuate nucleus (ARC) of the hypothalamus is essential for the regulation of feeding and metabolism. ARC is adjacent to the median eminence (ME) that facilitates the transport of hormonal and nutrient signals to be detected by this nucleus. In this way, the integration of peripheral hormonal and nutritional metabolic signals by the ARC, as well as the neuronal inputs, realize a coordinated feedback response (Rodríguez et al., 2010). In the ARC, there are two types of neurons with different functions: 1) orexigenic neurons, that express neuropeptide Y (appetite stimulant) (NPY) as well as the agouti-related peptide (AgRP) AgRP/NPY; and 2) anorexigenic neurons, that express the propeptide-opiomelanocortin (POMC) (appetite suppressant) and are therefore called POMC neurons (Timper & Brüning, 2017).

POMC neurons project to the paraventricular hypothalamic nucleus (PVN) neurons, and also to the dorsomedial hypothalamus (DMH), the lateral hypothalamus (LH) and the ventromedial hypothalamus (VMH). Neurons within the PVN control the flow of sympathetic outflow to peripheral organs and secrete different regulatory neuropeptides (Roh et al., 2016). The destruction of PVN generates excessive food intake and obesity, highlighting the role of PVN neurons for the inhibitory control of food intake. Also, VMH damage produces hyperphagia and obesity (Shimizu et al., 1987). The POMC and AgRP/NPY neurons receive activating glutamatergic feedback input from other hypothalamic nuclei such as VMH and PVN. PVN neurons receive inhibitory signaling from LH neurons that promote feeding. This process conducts a tunned food intake regulation (Waterson & Horvath, 2015).

The POMC and AgRP neurons from the ARC, develop insulin and leptin resistance in response to a high-fat diet that may be the result of overactivation of signal transducers and activator of transcription-3/suppressor of cytokine signaling-3 (STAT3/SOCS3), an intracellular pathway that is activated by leptin (Vaisse et al., 1998). Chronic activation of STAT3, due to elevated leptin levels resulting from increased adiposity, generates an increased activation of SOCS3 that inhibits STAT3 signaling, resulting in leptin and insulin resistance (Ernst et al., 2009).

## FROM OBESITY TO NEUROINFLAMMATION

Obesity is associated with chronic low-grade inflammation, not only at a systemic level but also in the CNS (Miller & Spencer, 2014). An apparent cause of inflammation in diet-induced obesity models is the diet itself. A high-fat diet in the short term can cause hypothalamic neuroinflammation, even before the weight gain (Marques et al., 2016).

It is reported that the increment in the amount of saturated fatty acids circulating can cross the blood-brain barrier (BBB) and induce an inflammatory response of the hypothalamic neurons, causing the activation of the microglia (Thaler & Scwartz, 2010). This response is associated with the capacity of fatty acids to activate the innate immune system through its binding to Toll-like receptors (TLR) (Könner & Brüning, 2011). The binding of fatty acids to TLR4 can activate two different transcription factors: Nuclear factor κB (NF-κB) and activator protein 1 (AP-1), that in turn regulate the expression of pro-inflammatory mediators such as interleukin 1β (IL-1β), interleukin 6 (IL-6), tumor necrosis factor-alpha (TNFα), chemokine ligand chemokines 2 (CCL2), and chemokine 10 with CXC motif (CXCL10) (Guillemot-Legris & Muccioli, 2017).

Besides the hypothalamus, the hippocampus is the best-studied structure of the CNS in the context of obesity-induced neuroinflammation. Inflammatory signaling mediated by IKKB / NF-kB can be found in the hippocampus of animals with high-fat diets (Lu et al., 2011). In obesity, the neuroinflammation in the hippocampus is characterized by increased expression of cytokines involved in the pro-inflammatory process, like IL-1β, IL-6, and TNF-α, and enzymes such as cyclooxygenase 2 (COX2) and inducible nitric oxide synthase (iNOS) (Guillemot-Legris & Muccioli, 2017).

The cerebral cortex is another structure that presents changes during obesity. Animals fed with high-fat diets showed an increased BBB permeability and activation of the NF-kB pathway, which conducts to the expression of pro-inflammatory cytokines (IL-1b, IL-6, TNF-α) and chemokines such as CCL2 and CXCL10 (Carlin et al., 2016). Also, cortical astrocytes and microglia are activated as well as a lower in synaptic density (Wang et al., 2016). It has also been found that cortical astrocytes and microglia are activated, resulting in a lower synaptic density because, during neuroinflammation, the microglia engulf damaged synapses and causes structural remodeling (Lainez & Coss., 2019). Microglial cells can detect changes in the environment and activate in a pro-inflammatory (M1) or anti-inflammatory (M2) phenotype. The M1 profile microglia secretes cytokines such as IL-1b, IL-6, IL-18, TNF-α, while the M2 microglia secretes IL-6, the brain-derived neurotrophic factor (BDNF) and TGF-β. It is important to note that during obesity, a persistence of microglia with the M1 phenotype has been observed (Maldonado-Ruiz et al., 2017).

## Consequences of Obesity in Cognitive Impairment

Since studies in animal models allow precise control of the diet, it has been shown that there is a detrimental effect of diet-induced obesity on cognitive function, mainly in working memory and learning (Nguyen et al., 2014). A study conducted in male Wistar rats by Mc Neilly et al., in 2011 demonstrated that the consumption of a high-fat diet (45%) generated obesity, insulin resistance, and a decrease in short-term memory and executive functioning.

At a cellular level, it is known that microglia and astrocytes, which are the main population of brain cells that express TLR4, can be activated directly by inflammatory mediators like proinflammatory cytokines, prostaglandins, and nitric oxide, that increase during obesity (Könner & Brüning., 2011). After only one week on a high-fat diet, the microglia changes towards an activated morphology and reactive gliosis (Thaler et al., 2012). In this state, the microglia can significantly impact the phenomena of synaptic and neuronal plasticity (Miller & Spencer, 2014). During obesity, synaptic remodeling is present. The activation of microglia favors the phagocytosis of synaptic elements, such as dendritic spines, which are primary sites of excitatory synapses related to synaptic plasticity and cognitive function (Cope et al., 2018). This process is particularly aggressive; therefore, chronic microglial activation can lead to extensive synaptic remodeling (Miyamoto et al., 2013).

Inflammatory cytokines derived from CNS (mainly from microglia and astrocytes), as well as systemic, can also influence neuronal health. Cytokines are essential for an appropriate inflammatory response. However, an excess of proinflammatory cytokines also participates in the development of neurodegenerative diseases. For example, IL-6 may have a neurotrophic role in response to neuronal damage, but in higher amounts, it can induce neurodegeneration in several brain diseases. TNFα also promotes cell survival, depending on the time and degree of expression. Still, for a long time or at high concentrations, it can also mediate neurodegeneration by increasing glutamate production. Recent evidence suggests that prolonged production of central proinflammatory cytokines contribute to neurodegeneration (Miller & Spencer, 2014).

## Obesity Models in Rodents

Due to the high interest in the study of these alterations, appropriate and useful animal models have been sought to conduct research related to pathogenesis and therapies to combat these metabolic disorders.

Animal obesity models must have similarities to human characteristics to be considered adequate. A rodent study model must allow the study of biological phenomena, animal behavior, and induced or spontaneous pathological processes.

The obesity animal models provide adequate information about the establishment and development of diseases and their comorbidities. Currently, the search for answers about the physiological dysfunctions during obesity in an animal model is increasingly demanding (Fernandes et al., 2016).

The animal obesity models can be divided into two categories, 1) models using gene manipulation, and 2) models exposed to obesogenic environments, like hypercaloric diets.

Obesity has a multifactorial origin, where environmental or behavioral factors influence such as the ingested diet; therefore, diet-induced models of obesity are preferred. These models more realistically represent the development and establishment of obesity, unlike animal models with genetic alterations for the induction of obesity. For this reason, animal models of diet-induced obesity are preferably used. In these models, body fat accumulates over a relatively long period, although the harmful metabolic consequences are evident in a few days. Comparing to the models of gene manipulation, the gradual increase of weight over time in the models of diet-induced obesity is better represented, as it happens in the human population as a consequence of an energy imbalance over several years (Friedman et al., 2004; Guillemot-Legris & Muccioli, 2017).

Considering rodent models, the use of rats has several advantages compared to mice:

- The rat size facilitates the performance of surgical procedures as well as the administration of drugs through different routes.
- Rats are also much easier to handle than mice and have less stress from human contact.
- A larger volume of biological samples can be obtained in rats for biochemical tests (blood, urine, tissues).
- For imaging studies, the rat brain offers a better spatial resolution.

Although the brains of rats and mice show high anatomical similarity, there are significant functional differences that must be considered. For example, serotonin is a neurotransmitter primarily involved in emotional regulation, cognition, and impulsivity. The distribution of the serotonin 5-HT6 receptor subtype is different between species. This receptor has a crucial role in the perception of rewards, habit formation, cognitive flexibility, and motor functioning. It is also involved in most psychiatric disorders (Hirst et al., 2003). Rats and humans have elevated levels of 5-HT6 messenger RNA and receptor in the dorsal and ventral striatum, but mice present lower levels of the receptor in the same regions (Ellenbroek & Youn, 2016).

If the research has to evaluate brain processes such as memory and learning, it is essential to consider that rats and mice have differences in processes such as neurogenesis, which contributes to synaptic plasticity in different regions such as the hippocampus. In a study conducted by Snyder et al., (2009), it was shown that the rate of neurogenesis in the hippocampus of adult rats was higher than in adult mice. In another study, a mature neuronal marker profile was found two weeks earlier in rats than mice and twice as likely to escape cell death. The neurons from rats were also ten times more likely to activate during learning circuits, unlike mice neurons. Therefore, this study revealed substantial differences in neuronal plasticity between rats and mice, which was not limited to the hippocampus, but also extended to cortical regions (Snyder et al., 2009).

## Diets Used to Induce Obesity

Different types of diets can be used for the generation of an obesity model (Table 1); the choice of the kind of diet will depend on the variables that are going to be evaluated in the research.

High percentages in diets of sucrose, dextrose, fructose, fat, or their combinations generate weight gain, adiposity, dyslipidemia, and arterial hypertension. Cafeteria diets show a notable increase in metabolic dysfunction due to voluntary hyperphagia. In murine models, it has been shown that a high-fat diet is more efficient to induce obesity, and a diet high in salt or high in fructose is more efficient in causing hypertension (Higa et al., 2014). Hypercaloric or hyperlipidemic diets have been used as models of induction of obesity in animals, due to their similarity with the metabolic responses caused in human obesity (Guillemot-Legris & Muccioli, 2017).

**Table1. Different rodent diet composition (% kcal) (Higa et al., 2014).**

| | Chow | Western Diet (WD) | Cafeteria Diet (CD) | High Fat Diet (HFD) |
|---|---|---|---|---|
| **Kcal/g** | 3.78 | 4.67 | 4.23 | 5.17 |
| **Protein** | 22% | 17% | 14.8% | 20% |
| **Carbohydrate** | 55% | 43% | 56% | 20% |
| **Fat** | 4% | 41% | 18.7% | 60% |

# LEARNING AND MEMORY EVALUATION

A great diversity of laboratory tests can be used for the evaluation of spatial learning and memory in animal models. These tests are based on the ability of the animals to navigate in mazes and to learn how to solve them, using positive (food, water, shelter) or negative (immersion in water, intense light or noise) stimulus, which motivate them to find the exhaust box (Rosenfeld et al., 2014; Gawel et al., 2019). Some examples of those testes will be described below.

An important aspect to consider is that there are also other differences in learning between rats and mice. Mice often need longer habitations and training sessions to perform specific tasks than rats, which can lead to more stress and anxiety (Ellenbroek & Youn., 2016).

# BARNES MAZE (BM)

This test is based on the assumption that the rat placed on a platform must learn and remember the location of an exhaust box located below the surface of the platform, to shelter after receiving an aversive stimulus such as light (Figure 1). The different phases of the task allow measuring spatial learning, memory recovery, and cognitive flexibility (Gawel et al., 2019).

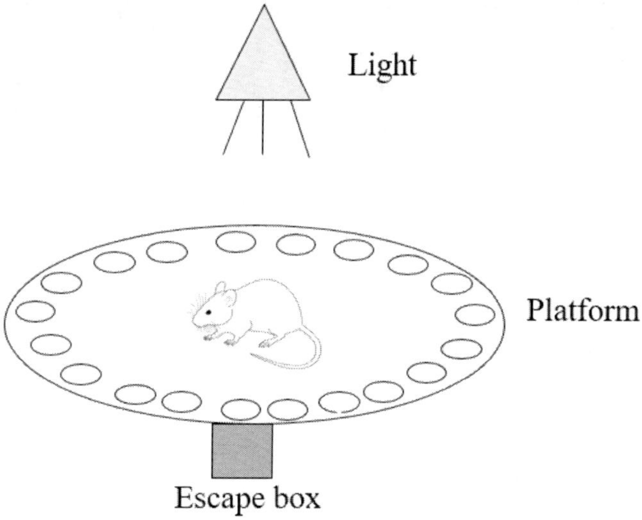


Figure 1. Schematic representation of the Barnes maze.

The test consists of different phases. The first phase is the *habituation* during which animals are introduced to the environment. Subsequently, is the *acquisition phase*, in which animals learn to find the location of the escape box. After some tests, the latencies (time required to reach the escape box) become shorter. The next phase is the *probe test* performed by removing the exhaust box from the hole and measuring the time spent in the vicinity of the hole. The probe test allows the evaluation of the spatial memory recovery that is associated with the function of the hippocampus. The next part of the test consists of *reverse learning*, for which the position of the exhaust box is changed, thus assessing cognitive flexibility when trying to learn a new location. This process is associated with the function of the frontal cortex (Pitts, 2018; Rosenfeld et al., 2014).

The first part of the BM, that is, the acquisition phase followed by the probe test, allows an evaluation of spatial learning and spatial memory, which is associated with the function of the hippocampus. While the second part of the task, reverse learning allows the evaluation of cognitive flexibility that is associated with frontal cortex function (Gawel et al., 2019).

## Barnes Maze Experimental Setup Plataform

The platform is circular (122 cm diameter), with 18 holes (9.5 cm diameter) located on the periphery of the platform. The platform is located 91 cm away from the ground to prevent rats from jumping. This structure can be made of solid wood, acrylic, or metal.

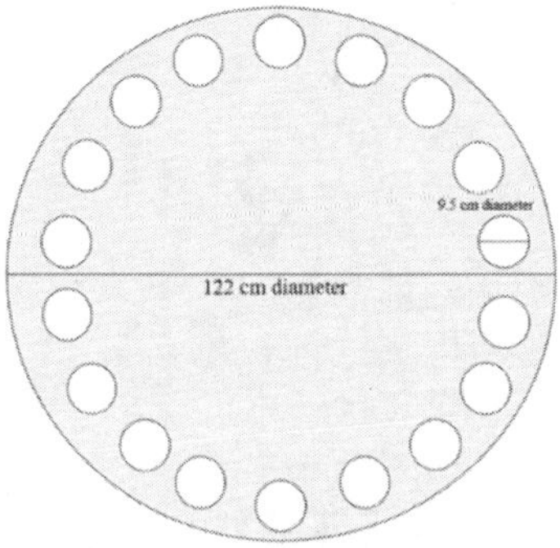


Figure 2. Platform.

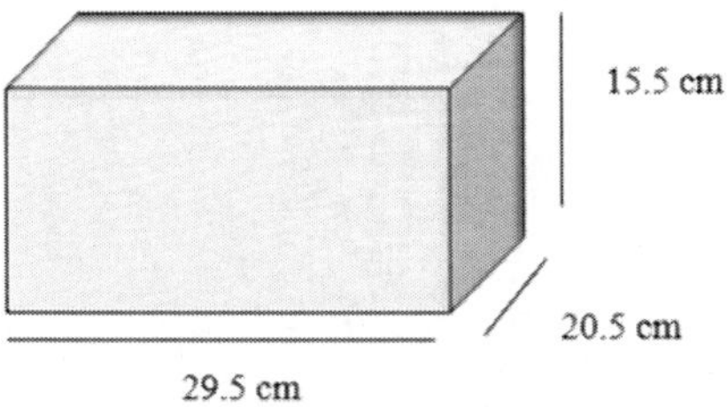


Figure 3. Escape box.

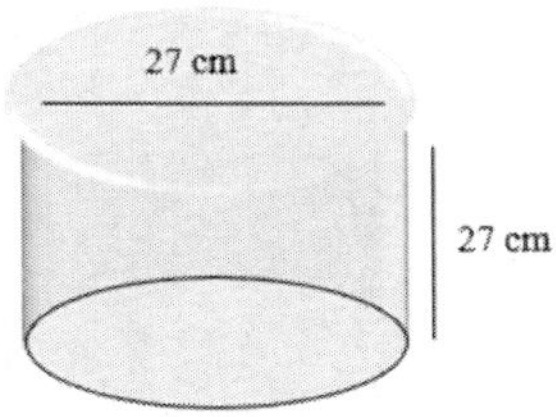


Figure 4. Start chamber.

The box dimentiosn are 29.5 x 20.5 x 15.5 cm. It can be made of wood, acrylic or metal. It is placed under one of the holes in the platform. It is usually black, taking advantage of rodents' preference to stay in dark environments, which motivates the rat to escape the surface of the platform.

A circular box that is usually used to protect the animal when starting the test. It is placed in the center of the platform. It can be acrylic or wood, painted in a dark color to prevent light from entering.

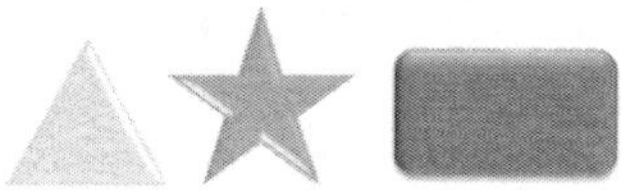

Figure 5. Distant cues.

Visual cues such as visible, colorful geometric shapes must be placed on the walls of the test room. They must be seen from the surface of the platform. These signals are at a distance between 50 to 200 cm from the platform.

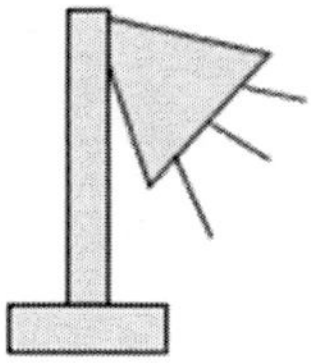

Figure 6. Lamp.

A 500W light source can be placed suspended on the platform. as a motivation for the animals to enter the escape box.

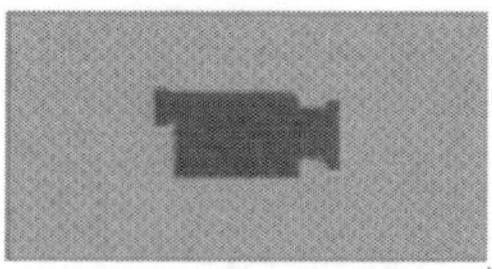

Figure 7. Camera.

The data can be acquired by using a recording camera placed on the platform to monitor and record the movements of the animal.

The animals are habituated to the platform and the escape box. The rat is placed in the center of the platform and allow to explore for one minute freely. Then, the rat is situated in the escape box for two minutes, as shown in Figure 8. The habituation must be carried out in dark conditions.

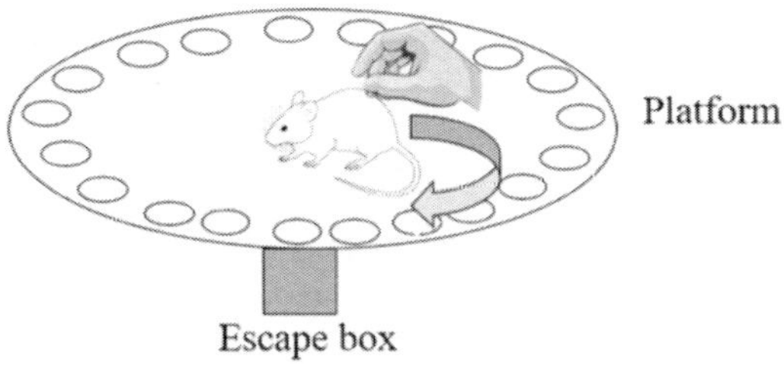


Figure 8. Habituation to the platform and escape box.

***Reversal Learning***

For this test, the hole containing the exhaust box must be rotated 180° from its original position and must be kept constant throughout the entire reversal learning test period. The steps described in the acquisition phase are followed for three successive days (6 trials per rat; 2 trials per day for Three Days).

***Reversal Probe Trial***

One day after the last reversal learning test, the steps described in the Acquisition probe trial are performed. The results obtained from the tests can be reported, as shown in Figure 9.

In a study conducted by Hsu et al., they reported that rats that consumed high amounts of sucrose and fructose (HFCS-55), had altered the acquisition of the space task in the Barnes Maze, compared to the controls (Figure 10). This study demonstrates that the consumption of added sugar impairs hippocampus-dependent spatial learning and memory in rats (Hsu et al., 2015).

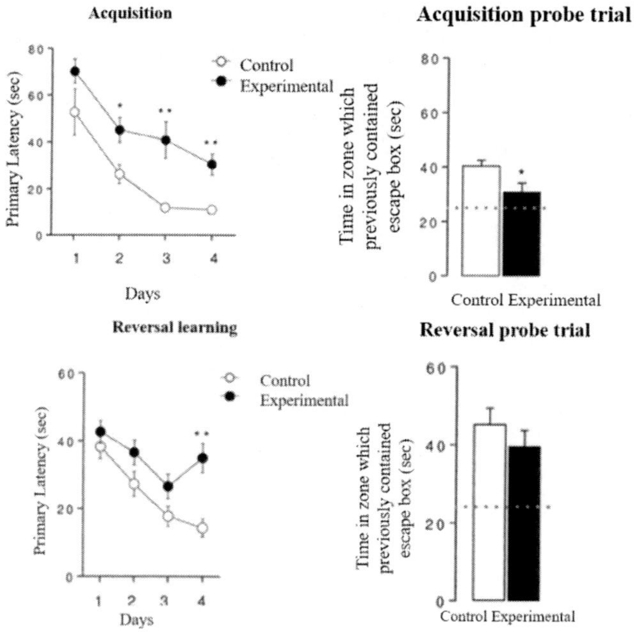


Figure 9. Graphical representation of the data obtained in the Barnes maze (Rosenfeld et al., 2014; Darcet et al., 2014).

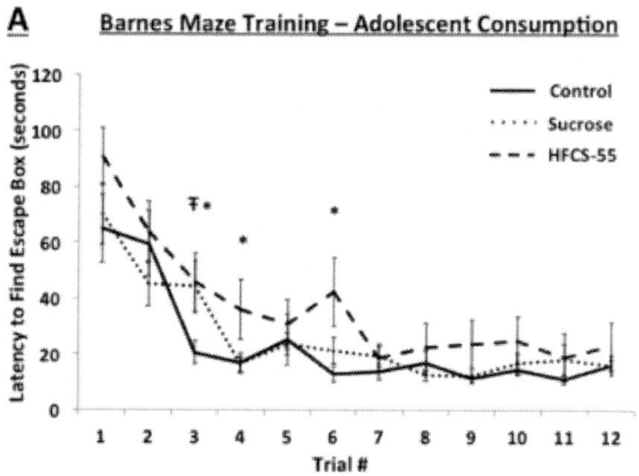


Figure 10. Latency to find the escape box (seconds) during 6-day Barnes maze training (Hsu et al., 2015).

## MORRIS WATER MAZE

The Morris water maze (MWM) is a test designed to assess rodent space learning, using distal cues for the animal to navigate from an initial point around the perimeter to locate a submerged escape platform in a pool, as shown in Figure 11.

Increasing the body mass of the rat is not an impediment to swimming to find the platform and escape the water, which makes it ideal for studies with animal obesity models.

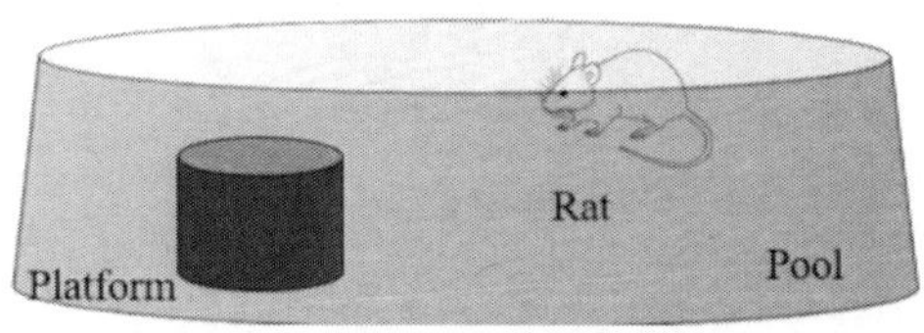


Figure 11. Schematic representation of the Morris water maze.

This maze was designed to evaluate spatial learning with high reliability in the results obtained. It is validated as a reference measure of memory and spatial navigation dependent on the hippocampus (Vorhees & Williams, 2006; Maei et al., 2009). The neurogenesis of the adult hippocampus contributes to the generation of new functional neurons in this brain structure that is of particular importance for the learning and memory processes (Lazarov & Hollands, 2016). Because the new neurons are exclusively in the dentate gyrus (DG) and are integrated only in the local circuits of the hippocampus, their functional contribution is closely related to aspects utterly dependent on the hippocampus of space learning (Garthe & Kempermann., 2013).

## MORRIS WATER MAZE EXPERIMENTAL SETUP

It is a circular tank of 120 cm in diameter and 50 cm high. This tank is filled with water with a height of 40 cm, and white non-toxic paint is added. Water temperature should be monitored during the test by keeping it at 28°C.

It consists of a circular platform of a 5 cm radius that is submerged 0.5 cm below the surface of the water.

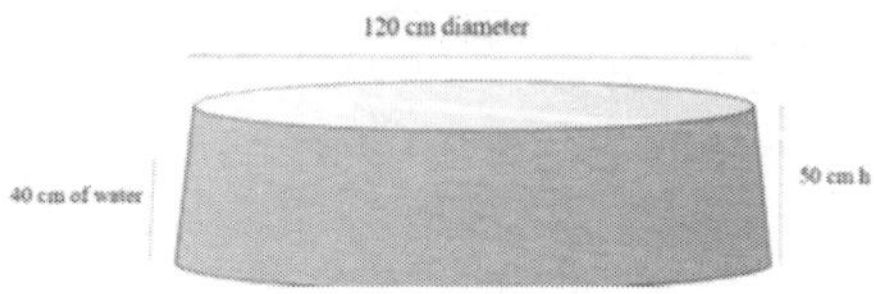


Figure 12. Pool.

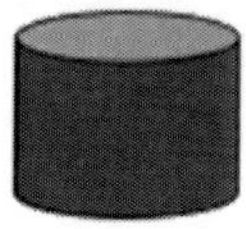

Figure 13. Platform.

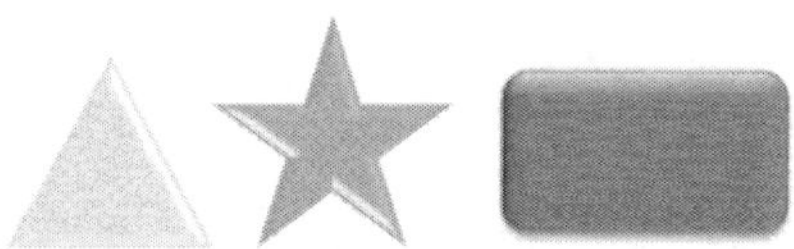

Figure 14. Visual cues.

The pool is surrounded a meter away by white curtains that contain different visual cues as geometric figures of different colors.

Data acquisition is by placing a recording camera on the platform to monitor and record the movements of the animal.

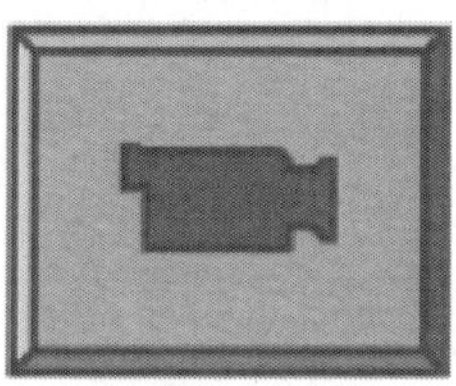

Figure 15. Camera.

The main component of the maze is the pool, where the escape platform is placed. During the training process, the platform must be placed on the water to be visible to the rat. After training, the escape platform is hidden below the surface of the water. The platform is not visible because the water is opaque by the addition of non-toxic paint (Nunez, 2008).

## MORRIS WATER MAZE TEST

### Pre-Training

The rat is placed on the platform for 20 seconds to familiarize it with its presence in the maze. The water pool is divided into four positions: north, south, east, and west. The animal is gently submerged, dipping the tail first. The animal is allowed to swim for 60s to find the platform. Once the rat finds the platform, the stopwatch stops. If the rat does not arrive in the following 60s, it is gently taken and guided to the platform and left there for 15s. Two more tests must be performed for each rat. Upon completion of the three trials, the rat is dried with a towel.

Each rat must perform 12 trials, 3 for each position (north, south, east, and west). Each test lasts 60 seconds, and there must be a 2-minute interval between each trial. The same starting address should not be used twice in a row. The rat is tracked until it reaches the platform, recording the time it takes. Latency is registered (the time it takes the rat to reach the platform). The distance traveled by the rat is quantified until the rat finds the platform. In case the rat did not reach the platform in the 60s, the rat should be guided to the platform and allowed to remain there for 10s (Vorhees & Williams, 2006). Once the trial is completed, the rat has to be dry entirely and return to its cage. The results obtained in the test can be reported as follow:

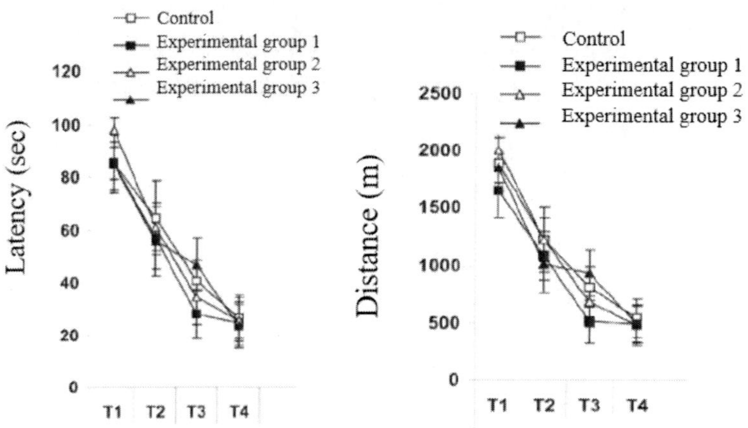


Figure 16. Graphical representation of the data collected in the Morris water maze test (Vorhees & Williams, 2006).

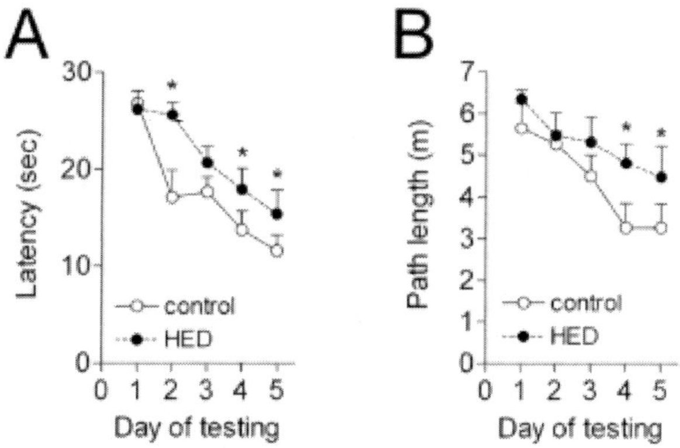


Figure 17. The high-calorie diet impairs hippocampus-dependent learning (Stranahan et al., 2008).

In a study by Stranahan et al., They fed rats with a diet high in saturated fats and simple sugars, in addition to supplementing their water with high fructose corn syrup. After eight months on a diet, the rats performed poorly in the Morris water maze compared to the rats in the control diet. In Figure 17, in graph A, it is observed that rats maintained on a high-calorie diet took longer to find a hidden platform in the water maze. Graph B shows that rats on a high-calorie diet also traveled a longer route to reach the platform. The preceding showed that excessive energy consumption impairs hippocampus-dependent memory (Stranahan et al., 2008).

## Conclusion

As mentioned throughout this chapter, obesity is a problem that is associated with different comorbidities, including cognitive impairment due to changes in the CNS. In obesity, the neuroinflammatory process increments the secretion of cytokines generating synaptic remodeling and neurodegeneration, which can alter the brain functions. The cortex and the hippocampus are mainly affected. A good model for the study of the effect of this condition on cognitive function is the animal model based on dietary-induced obesity. Some studies carried out on obese rats using probe trials such as the Morris Water Maze and the Barnes Maze have evidenced the adverse effects of obesity on memory and the learning process.

## References

Barrett, P., Mercer, J. G. & Morgan, P. J. (2016). Preclinical models for obesity research. *Disease models & mechanisms*, *9*(11), 1245-1255. https://doi.org/10.1242/dmm.026443.

Carlin, J. L., Grissom, N., Ying, Z., Gomez-Pinilla, F. & Reyes, T. M. (2016). Voluntary exercise blocks Western diet-induced gene expression of the chemokines CXCL10 and CCL2 in the prefrontal cortex. *Brain, behavior, and immunity*, *58*, 82-90. https://doi.org/10.1016/j.bbi.2016.07.161.

Cope, E. C., LaMarca, E. A., Monari, P. K., Olson, L. B., Martinez, S., Zych, A. D., & Gould, E. (2018). Microglia play an active role in obesity-associated cognitive decline. *Journal of Neuroscience*, *38*(41), 8889-8904. https://doi.org/10.1523/JNEUROSCI.0789-18.2018.

Darcet, F., Mendez-David, I., Tritschler, L., Gardier, A. M., Guilloux, J. P., & David, D. J. (2014). Learning and memory impairments in a neuroendocrine mouse model of anxiety/depression. *Frontiers in behavioral neuroscience*, *8*, 136. https://doi.org/10.3389/fnbeh.2014.00136.

Ellenbroek, B. & Youn, J. (2016). Rodent models in neuroscience research: is it a rat race?. *Disease models & mechanisms*, *9*(10), 1079-1087. https://doi.org/10.1242/dmm.026120.

Ernst, M. B., Wunderlich, C. M., Hess, S., Paehler, M., Mesaros, A., Koralov, S. B. & Alber, J. (2009). Enhanced Stat3 Activation in POMC Neurons Provokes Negative Feedback Inhibition of Leptin and InsulinSignaling in Obesity. *Journal of Neuroscience*, *29*(37), 11582-11593. https://dx.doi.org/10.1523%2FJNEUROSCI.5712-08.2009.

Fernandes, M. R., Lima, N. V. D., Rezende, K. S., Santos, I. C. M., Silva, I. S. & Guimarães, R. D. C. A. (2016). Animal models of obesity in rodents. An integrative review. *Acta cirurgica brasileira*, *31*(12), 840-844. https://dx.doi.org/10.1002%2F0471141755.ph0561s58.

Friedman, J. M. (2004). Modern science versus the stigma of obesity. *Nature medicine*, *10*(6), 563. https://doi.org/10.1038/nm0604-563.

Garthe, A., & Kempermann, G. (2013). An old test for new neurons: refining the Morris water maze to study the functional relevance of adult hippocampal neurogenesis. *Frontiers in neuroscience*, *7*, 63. https://doi.org/10.3389/fnins.2013.00063.

Gawel, K., Gibula, E., Marszalek-Grabska, M., Filarowska, J. & Kotlinska, J. H. (2019). Assessment of spatial learning and memory in the Barnes maze task in rodents—methodological consideration. *Naunyn-Schmiedeberg's archives of pharmacology*, *392*(1), 1-18. https://doi.org/10.1007/s00210-018-1589-y.

Guillemot-Legris, O. & Muccioli, G. G. (2017). Obesity-induced neuroinflammation: beyond the hypothalamus. *Trends in Neurosciences*, *40*(4), 237-253. https://doi.org/10.1016/j.tins.2017.02.005.

Higa, T. S., Spinola, A. V., Fonseca-Alaniz, M. H., Sant, F., & Evangelista, A. (2014). Comparison between cafeteria and high-fat diets in the induction of metabolic dysfunction in mice. *International journal of physiology, pathophysiology and pharmacology*, *6*(1), 47.

Hirst, W. D., Abrahamsen, B., Blaney, F. E., Calver, A. R., Aloj, L., Price, G. W. & Medhurst, A. D. (2003). Differences in the central nervous system distribution and pharmacology of the mouse 5-hydroxytryptamine-6 receptor compared with rat and human receptors investigated by radioligand binding, site-directed mutagenesis, and molecular modeling. *Molecular pharmacology*, *64*(6), 1295-1308. https://doi.org/10.1124/mol.64.6.1295.

Hsu, T. M., Konanur, V. R., Taing, L., Usui, R., Kayser, B. D., Goran, M. I., & Kanoski, S. E. (2015). Effects of sucrose and high fructose corn syrup consumption on spatial memory function and hippocampal neuroinflammation in adolescent rats. *Hippocampus*, *25*(2), 227-239. https://doi.org/10.1002/hipo.22368.

Könner, A. C. & Brüning, J. C. (2011). Toll-like receptors: linking inflammation to metabolism. *Trends in Endocrinology & Metabolism*, *22*(1), 16-23. https://doi.org/10.1016/j.tem.2010.08.007.

Lainez, N. M., & Coss, D. (2019). Obesity, Neuroinflammation, and Reproductive Function. *Endocrinology*, 160(11), 2719-2736. https://doi.org/10.1210/en.2019-00487.

Lazarov, O. & Hollands, C. (2016). Hippocampal neurogenesis: learning to remember. *Progress in neurobiology*, *138*, 1-18. https://doi.org/10.1016/j.pneurobio.2015.12.006.

Lu, J., Wu, D. M., Zheng, Y. L., Hu, B., Cheng, W., Zhang, Z. F. & Shan, Q. (2011). Ursolic acid improves high fat diet-induced cognitive impairments by blocking endoplasmic reticulum stress and IκB kinase β/nuclear factor-κB-mediated inflammatory pathways in mice. *Brain, behavior, and immunity*, *25*(8), 1658-1667. https://doi.org/10.1016/j.bbi.2011.06.009.

Maei, H. R., Zaslavsky, K., Teixeira, C. M. & Frankland, P. W. (2009). What is the most sensitive measure of water maze probe test performance?. *Frontiers in integrative neuroscience*, *3*, 4. https://dx.doi.org/10.3389%2Fneuro.07.004.2009.

Maldonado-Ruiz, R., Montalvo-Martínez, L., Fuentes-Mera, L., & Camacho, A. (2017). Microglia activation due to obesity programs metabolic failure leading to type two diabetes. *Nutrition & diabetes*, *7*(3), e254. https://doi.org/10.1038/nutd.2017.10.

Marques, C., Meireles, M., Norberto, S., Leite, J., Freitas, J., Pestana, D. & Calhau, C. (2016). High-fat diet-induced obesity Rat model: a comparison between Wistar and Sprague-Dawley Rat. *Adipocyte*, *5*(1), 11-21. https://doi.org/10.1080/21623945.2015.1061723.

McNeilly, A. D., Williamson, R., Sutherland, C., Balfour, D. J. & Stewart, C. A. (2011). High fat feeding promotes simultaneous decline in insulin sensitivity and cognitive performance in a delayed matching and non-matching to position task. *Behavioural brain research*, *217*(1), 134-141. https://doi.org/10.1016/j.bbr.2010.10.017.

Miller, A. A. & Spencer, S. J. (2014). Obesity and neuroinflammation: a pathway to cognitive impairment. *Brain, behavior, and immunity*, *42*, 10-21. https://doi.org/10.1016/j.bbi.2014.04.001.

Miyamoto, A., Wake, H., Moorhouse, A. J. & Nabekura, J. (2013). Microglia and synapse interactions: fine tuning neural circuits and candidate molecules. *Frontiers in cellular neuroscience*, *7*, 70. https://doi.org/10.3389/fncel.2013.00070.

Myers Jr, M. G. & Olson, D. P. (2012). Central nervous system control of metabolism. *Nature*, *491*(7424), 357. https://doi.org/10.1038/nature11705.

Nguyen, J. C., Killcross, A. S. & Jenkins, T. A. (2014). Obesity and cognitive decline: role of inflammation and vascular changes. *Frontiers in neuroscience*, *8*, 375. https://doi.org/10.3389/fnins.2014.00375.

Nunez, J. (2008). Morris water maze experiment. *JoVE (Journal of Visualized Experiments)*, (19), e897. https://dx.doi.org/10.3791%2F897.

Pitts, M. W. (2018). Barnes Maze Procedure for Spatial Learning and Memory in Mice. *Bio-protocol*, *8*(5). https://dx.doi.org/10.21769%2Fbioprotoc.2744.

Rodríguez, E. M., Blázquez, J. L. & Guerra, M. (2010). The design of barriers in the hypothalamus allows the median eminence and the arcuate nucleus to enjoy private milieus: the former opens to the portal blood and the latter to the cerebrospinal fluid. *Peptides*, *31*(4), 757-776. https://doi.org/10.1016/j.peptides.2010.01.003.

Roh, E., Song, D. K. & Kim, M. S. (2016). Emerging role of the brain in the homeostatic regulation of energy and glucose metabolism. *Experimental & molecular medicine*, *48*(3), e216. https://doi.org/10.1038/emm.2016.4.

Rosenfeld, C. S., & Ferguson, S. A. (2014). Barnes maze testing strategies with small and large rodent models. *JoVE (Journal of Visualized Experiments)*, (84), e51194. https://doi.org/10.3791/51194.

Shimizu, N., Oomura, Y., Plata-Salamán, C. R. & Morimoto, M. (1987). Hyperphagia and obesity in rats with bilateral ibotenic acid-induced lesions of the ventromedial hypothalamic nucleus. *Brain research*, *416*(1), 153-156. https://doi.org/10.1016/0006-8993(87)91508-3.

Snyder, J. S., Choe, J. S., Clifford, M. A., Jeurling, S. I., Hurley, P., Brown, A. & Cameron, H. A. (2009). Adult-born hippocampal neurons are more numerous, faster maturing, and more involved in behavior in rats than in mice. *Journal of Neuroscience*, *29*(46), 14484-14495. https://doi.org/10.1523/JNEUROSCI.1768-09.2009.

Stranahan, A. M., Norman, E. D., Lee, K., Cutler, R. G., Telljohann, R. S., Egan, J. M., & Mattson, M. P. (2008). Diet-induced insulin resistance impairs hippocampal synaptic plasticity and cognition in middle-aged rats. *Hippocampus*, *18*(11), 1085-1088. https://doi.org/10.1002/hipo.20470.

Thaler, J. P., & Schwartz, M. W. (2010). Minireview: Inflammation and obesity pathogenesis: the hypothalamus heats up. *Endocrinology*, *151*(9), 4109-4115. https://doi.org/10.1210/en.2010-0336.

Thaler, J. P., Yi, C. X., Schur, E. A., Guyenet, S. J., Hwang, B. H., Dietrich, M. O. & Nguyen, H. T. (2012). Obesity is associated with hypothalamic injury in rodents and humans. *The Journal of clinical investigation*, *122*(1), 153-162. https://doi.org/10.1172/JCI59660.

Timper, K. & Brüning, J. C. (2017). Hypothalamic circuits regulating appetite and energy homeostasis: pathways to obesity. *Disease models & mechanisms*, *10*(6), 679-689. https://doi.org/10.1242/dmm.026609.

Vaisse, C., Clement, K., Guy-Grand, B. & Froguel, P. (1998). A frameshift mutation in human MC4R is associated with a dominant form of obesity. *Nature genetics*, *20*(2), 113. https://doi.org/10.1038/2407.

Vorhees, C. V. & Williams, M. T. (2006). Morris water maze: procedures for assessing spatial and related forms of learning and memory. *Nature protocols*, *1*(2), 848. https://doi.org/10.1038/nprot.2006.116.

Wang, S., Huang, X. F., Zhang, P., Wang, H., Zhang, Q., Yu, S. & Yu, Y. (2016). Chronic rhein treatment improves recognition memory in high-fat diet-induced obese male mice. *The Journal of nutritional biochemistry*, *36*, 42-50. https://doi.org/10.1016/j.jnutbio.2016.07.008.

Waterson, M. J. & Horvath, T. L. (2015). Neuronal regulation of energy homeostasis: beyond the hypothalamus and feeding. *Cell metabolism*, *22*(6), 962-970. https://doi.org/10.1016/j.cmet.2015.09.026.

Yaffe, K., Haan, M., Blackwell, T., Cherkasova, E., Whitmer, R. A. & West, N. (2007). Metabolic syndrome and cognitive decline in elderly Latinos: findings from the Sacramento Area Latino Study of Aging study. *Journal of the American Geriatrics Society*, *55*(5), 758-762. https://doi.org/10.1111/j.1532-5415.2007.01139.x.

In: Laboratory Animals and Neurosciences ISBN: 978-1-53618-462-4
Editors: B. Hernandez Godinez et al. 

*Chapter 9*

# EFFECT OF ANTIEPILEPTICS ON CEREBRAL INJURIES INDUCED BY KAINIC ACID IN ANIMALS MODELS

***Alfonso Alfaro-Rodríguez***[1]***,***
***José Luis Cortes-Altamirano***[1,2]***, Samuel Reyes-Long***[1,2]***,***
***Cindy Bandala***[1,2]***, Herlinda Bonilla-Jaime***[3]***,***
***Rafael Reynoso-Robles***[4] ***and Angélica González-Maciel***[4,*]
[1]División de Neurociencias, Instituto Nacional de Rehabilitación, "Luis Guillermo Ibarra Ibarra," Ciudad de México, México
[2]Escuela Superior de Medicina, Instituto Politécnico Nacional, Ciudad de México, México
[3]Departamento de Biología de la Reproducción, Universidad Autónoma Metropolitana-Iztapalapa, Ciudad de México, México
[4]Laboratorio de Morfología Celular y Tisular, Instituto Nacional de Pediatría, Ciudad de México, México

* Corresponding Author's E-mail: agonzalezmaciel@yahoo.com.

## ABSTRACT

Animal models of experimentation have been an alternative for the study and analysis of the central nervous system (CNS). A strict design can help us understand functions as complex as memory and learning, inform us of the ability of the CNS to respond to external stimuli, to understand what is wrong in cases of illness and even try substances that can alleviate this. In this chapter we will briefly review the phenomenon of epilepsy, in which the neuronal excitation without the fine control of inhibition, can end in the death of neurons of brain regions related to memory and learning such as the hippocampus, or the cerebellum, responsible for movement. We will also review the use of antiepileptics to alleviate this pathology. We will refer to the experimental animal model in which using kainic acid can produce status epilepticus in rats, characterized by prolonged seizures. Finally, we will present results of experiments using this animal model; performed with the aim of know if the use of antiepileptics not only decreases the frequency and intensity of the seizures, but also if they are able to prevent neuronal damage from increasing, an aspect that in our opinion it has not been completely elucidated.


**Keywords**: animal models, kainic acid, Central Nervous System, Epilepsy, antiepileptics, neuronal damage

## INTRODUCTION

Animal models have been a valid and widely employed alternative for the study and analysis of the Central Nervous System (CNS). A strict and meticulous design can help researchers to understand complex phenomena such as memory, learning, also how the CNS respond to external stimuli and to assess what happens in case of a disease and even try substances in order to alleviate them. In this chapter we will briefly revise Epilepsy, a complex phenomenon in which neuronal excitation without the fine inhibitory control can finish in neuronal death in brain structures related with memory and learning like hippocampus and cerebellum (Löscher, 2011).

First a brief description of the brain structures of the CNS will be presented, then the employment of antiepileptic drugs will be revised, next the experimental model of Kainic acid will be discussed. Finally results of experiments employing this model will be presented, performed with the aim of knowing whether the administration of antiepileptic drugs not only diminish frequency and intensity of epileptic crisis, but also if they are capable of avoiding the appearance and further increase of neuronal damage, an aspect to which not a lot of importance has not been given.

## NERVOUS SYSTEM

The Nervous system is divided in Central and Peripheral (vegetative or autonomous). The brain and the spinal chord compose CNS, meanwhile peripheral nervous system (PNS) is conformed by motor nerves, (afferent and efferent), spinal ganglions and nerve endings. Brain can be divided into: anterior, medial and posterior. Anterior brain is conformed by cerebral cortex, thalamus, hypothalamus and hypophysis, medial by reticular formation (involved in sleep and wake cycle) and the posterior groups the brainstem (pons and oblongata medulla) and cerebellum (Clarke and Lemon, 2016).

In the brain the limbic system is found, and it is composed by different nuclei distributed along the brain itself. This system is responsible for the majority of the basic impulses of emotion and associated movements important for the survival of the organisms: fear, fury, sexual behavior, pain and anguish (Brailowsky, 1995).

The principal components of this system include sub-cortical structures like amygdala, hippocampus, hypothalamus, thalamic nuclei, mammillary bodies, and the septum pellucidum. In temporal lobe epilepsy it is very common to hear the patient report strange smells just before a crisis starts, this symptom are caused by the invasion and excessive neuronal activity of the structures of the limbic system like the amygdala and hippocampus; region which intervenes in emotions and function associated to memory (Schmidt-Rhaesa et al., 2015).

The hippocampus receives its name due to the similarity with a seahorse; it is found at the base of the temporal lobe and is connected to many cortical structures (Leuner Gould, 2010). It is a cylindrical curved structure whose ventral-dorsal axis forms a semicircle that surrounds the thalamus. Since the description performed by Santiago Ramón y Cajal, the hippocampus is divided into four regions, traditionally designated as CA1 – CA4 (from the Latin Cornu Ammone), the regions from the dentate gyrus (GD), subículum (S) and the entorinal cortex (EC). Three cell layers form all the hippocampus: polymorphic, pyramidal and molecular. It has been shown that it contributes to functions related to recent memory (recently acquired information). Patients not responding pharmacological treatment, undergo surgery to the hippocampus in order to diminish epileptic crisis, in them some deficiencies in memory have been observed, for example short-term memory (Clarke and Lemon, 2016).

## EPILEPSY

Epilepsy is defined as an alteration to the nervous system from different origins, which results from the increase of the excitatory mechanisms and the decrease from the inhibitory. It is characterized for an abnormal synchronization of the neuronal activity, which can be focalized or generalized (Luedke et al., 2019).

It is the second most frequent neurological disorder after the cerebrovascular accident. The most common symptom are periodical attacks which are short and recurring, in them the motor, sensitive and psychological function are heavily impaired. These attacks are known as epileptic convulsions, they originate from abnormal synchronic electrical discharges of millions of encephalic neurons, probably from abnormal and reverberant circuitry. The discharges stimulate other neurons in order to continue the stimulus along their currents. As a consequence, the patient suffering from an attack may contract muscles in an involuntary and abrupt manner, may see lights, hear noises or perceive smells without the actual stimuli. The electrical discharges can inhibit certain brain centers, for example: a decrease in the activity if the reticular formation, can result in unconsciousness (Banerjee et al., 2009)

Prevalence studies in Mexico, performed by the National Institute of Neurology and Neurosurgery, show that over a million people in the country have this disorder; 76% of them present their first epileptic crisis before adolescence, and the rest after the age of 25, which is known as late-epilepsy which etiology is mainly because of cysticercoids or a encephalic trauma (Rubio, 1999; García Martín and Serrano Castro, 2018). The concept in which the origin of the epileptic seizures is based is the presence of an organic injury or some functional alteration localized in certain brain structures. It is probable to identify the exact cause only if this relates with injuries resulting from a cranial traumatism, from birth or caused by tumors. In other instances, lesion cannot be evident but their existence is inferred with base in abnormal electroencephalographic registries.

Epilepsy is not only characterized by seizures, but also by sensory and cognitive alterations. It all depends in the site of the brain in which the abnormal neuronal group is located (French et al., 1998; Holmes, 2015). The crisis can affect the patient partially (focal or localized epilepsy) or totally (generalized epilepsy); in the latter convulsions may appear. Frequently, generalized epilepsies can be accompanied by lost of consciousness. Some types of epilepsies affect only the children, like the absence, and other impact only adults (Cruz-Cruz et al., 2017).

Epilepsy classification is a complex subject mainly because it is associated with several clinical manifestations. Given that this goes out of the objective of the present chapter, the different types of epilepsies will not be discussed.

## Epilepsy Origin

Neuronal activity is maintained in a dynamic, yet balanced state regulated by inhibitory and excitatory processes. Normally, a neuron receives excitatory and inhibitory information, and the temporal-spatial algebraic sum of this information dictates the neuron to initiate, or not, an action potential (Roberts, 1978; Banerjee et al., 2009). The equilibrium between the excitatory and the inhibitory states is regulated by a disinhibitory mechanism in which the excitatory afferences have an important role.

The presence of a great quantity of inhibitory neurons modulate the activity of the nervous tissue inhibiting its function; for this function to be expressed, the circuitry must free itself from the influence of the inhibitor neurons, and this determines the appearance of the disinhibitory phenomenon. The inhibition can disappear if the inhibited neuron becomes depolarized (excited), or if the inhibitory neuron is deactivated (disinhibition), or by a combination of both mechanisms. Next, in order to maintain equilibrium, the disinhibited neurons must be inhibited again. In the modulation of neuronal excitation, the role of excitatory neurons over the inhibitory is important fro the release of neurotransmitters (Banerjee et al., 2009).

Here, it is worth noticing the principal inhibitory neurotransmitters (NTs) in the CNS: the gamma-Aminobutyric acid (GABA) and glycine, and the excitatory: glutamate, aspartate and acetylcholine (Stiges, 1993). A great deal is currently known about epilepsy but a theory in which all the causing mechanisms are accounted is still missing. From the existent hypothesis, two stand out. One propose that a disinhibition process occurs in the neuronal tissue, and the other suggest that apart from this process, a potentiation of the synaptic transmission is established.

Considering the last paragraph, the neuronal disinhibition would result in release of the NTs glutamate, which would travel trough the presynaptic space and coupled to the kainate receptors (KQ) present in the postsynaptic membrane giving place to a sequence of events like the intracellular influx of monovalent ions, facilitating the removal of Mg2+ bloking the NMDA receptors-associated channels. Once these channels become free, the influx of Ca2+ initiates and with it, the activation of processes Calcium-dependent. In normal conditions, Ca2+ influx coupled to the NMDA receptor induces intracellular changes that promote the maintenance of the potentiation of the long-term synaptic transmission, and also the activation of the necessary enzymes to maintain it. There is also activation of transcription resulting in the synthesis of neuronal growth factor (NGF) and the formation of new synapses (Collingridge and Bliss, 1987; Lange et al., 2016).

During epileptogenic events, neurons present high voltage waves caused by big currents of Ca2+, which cause long-term depolarization and initiate burst action potentials. The massive influx of Ca2+ first results in the activation of lipases and proteases. In an attempt of restitute membrane electric potential it has been determined that an influx of Cl- and the recapture of Ca2+ by mitochondria and endoplasmic reticulum, and this cause osmotic damage in other organelles and consequently neuronal death (Rothman and Olney, 1990).

## Cerebral Injury Caused by Epilepsy

Besides the changes in cellular activity during epileptic events, which are involved in synaptic function, in the ionic and osmotic microenvironment and the metabolic equilibrium, changes in the blood flow in the brain ocuur (Niedermeyer, 1983; Beghi and Perucca, 1995; Boison, and Steinhäuser, 2018). It is probable that this changes combined are responsible for neuronal death found in epileptic patients.

In relation to the brain blood flow, it is known that during the beginning of the convulsive attack a rapid decrease in blood pressure exists, and at the same time produces a reduction in brain-vascular circulation, that is not completely compensated by the increase at the loading of arterial dilation. This event is transitory and quick and immediately after, an augment of blood pressure arises, and consequently the brain blood pressure, which carries metabolic changes that are conditioned by the anaerobic conditions caused by the difficulty of the oxygen to arrive, with subsequent hypoxic states (Boison, and Steinhäuser, 2018).

Hughling Jackson identified the association between hippocampal neuronal death and temporal lobe epilepsy over a hundred years ago. Subsequently several studies gave place to the description of the damage pattern in this structure, which was referred as hippocampal sclerosis (Trimble, 2017). In relation to the last, it has also been found that many structures are damage by generalized crisis this has been confirmed in tissue from animal model as well as patients. The brain structures damaged are the hippocampus, piriform cortex, cerebellum, cortex, thalamus, striate body; in one hemisphere or both (Vezzani e al., 2016).

In animal models under established chronic epilepsy, it has been determined that the complete blockade of the inhibition produced convulsions, which is why it has been suggested that the GABAergic system is susceptible to alterations. Experimentally, it has been proven that the GABAergic neurons are sensitive to hypoxia, and if it persists, degenerative changes and cellular lysis are initiated (Maljevic et al., 2019).

In this way, even though it has been established that convulsive crisis can originate brain lesions, it is generally accepted that one great generalized convulsion, hardly produces macroscopic or microscopic morphological lesions. It is in fact the repetition of the convulsive schemes and the related alterations, the ones that condition a great part of the neruomorphological changes found (Maljevic et al., 2019).

One of the alterations that characteristically present the association between seizures and brain lesions is the status epilepticus. In studies performed in pediatric hospitals and geriatric homes, severe brain damage has been found and even the death of the patients that presented an associated cardiorespiratory deficiency. The patients that survived presented severe brain damage and metal retardation or intellectual disability (Terrone et al., 2019).

It is worth noticing that the location of these lessions, corresponds to the topography of neuropathological alterations that present an increase in brain blood pressure independently to the appearance of seizures, like traumatisms (Terrone et al., 2019). However, it is generally accepted that the principal factors conditioning the location of such injuries are consequence of the hypoxia and the susceptibility that these regions present in the CNS.

## Epilepsy Treatment

Pharmacological treatment of Epilepsy cover a period of 140 years and in divided in two main stages. The first one initiated in 1857, with the introduction of potassium bromide by Sir Charles Locock, who characterized for the research of anticonvulsive drugs. The second stage (the last 50 years) has characterized for the search of pharmaceutical with more specificity to the types of epilepsy. This took to the discovery and further application of benzodiazepines, initially etosuximida, primidona y metabarbital were employed. Given that these drugs controlled an estimate of 70% of all convulsive crisis, research on antiepileptic drugs (AED) was relegated. It was necessary to emphasize that 30% of crisis that remained uncontrolled by this pharmacological scheme in order to resume intensive research, thankfully this was managed by the chapter "Epilepsy" of the National Institute of Neurological and Communicative Disorders and Strokes (NINCDS) and next the development of valproate, carbamazepine, clonazepam and more recently, vigabatrina, lamotrigina, felbamato, and lastly clobazam, gabapentin y come Calcium agonist like nimodipina y flunarizina (Panayiotopoulos, 2007).

## Antiepileptic Drug's Mechanism of Action

Focal or partial epileptogenic activity occurs in an area of the cortex, which exhibits excess in excitability. The initial discharge in an electroencephalogram (EEG) is a manifestation of the hyper excitability of the brain and it serves as a marker for an area of abnormal localized excitability. Interstitial discharges (IDs) occur when a group of pyramidal neurons synchronize and develop great depolarizing potentials. At the cellular level this has been named as paroxysmal depolarization (PD). PD is followed by a long hyper polarization, which is a cellular correlate of the slow wave that usually follows the spike of the EEG. The PD is generated by a combination of the synaptic currents, mediated by glutamate and aspartate, and voltage-dependent depolarizing currents, particularly Calcium. The hyperpolarization that comes after the PD, is believed to be produced by a combination of synaptic events, especially those mediated by GABA, via GABA receptors A and B, potassium voltage-dependent currents and calcium, potassium and probably chloride-dependent currents (Rogawski and Cavazos, 2015).

It is hypothesized that many types of generalized Epilepsy have their origins in genetics. They are characterized by short-wave discharges and bilateral EEG synchronized spikes. The discharges can be generated by thalamic-cortical rhythms. Under normal circumstances, the thalamic-cortical network generates low frequency oscillations, and the frequency of them depends on waking the individual. During epilepsy events, however, these neurons may be more synchronized and they can produce bigger and high-voltage waves in consequence of big voltage-dependent currents of Ca2+ that produce longer depolarizations that initiate explosions of action potentials. Next, these same neurons develop hyperpolarization (Rogawski and Cavazos, 2015).

Based on the brief description of the mechanisms of action in which the epileptogenic activity depends, several targets for the AED can be inferred. If all the seizures are associated with the surging of repeated action potentials (bursting) in neurons, then a target is to avoid this generation of action potentials, however this should be done considering that all the information in the brain is coded by trains of action potentials, which is why it is important to ensure that any drug administered by long periods of time, does not influence over normal cerebral activity. An additional target can be the voltage-dependent current involved in the maintenance of neuronal excitability. In addition, like synaptic inhibition plays an important role in all types of epilepsy, the drugs that increase the inhibition may be protective in many cases. In a similar way the drugs that avoid synaptic excitation can be employed for the suppression of the development of attacks and further propagation.

All the conventional AED currently available were developed without knowing its mechanism of action, next several test have been performed in the lab in order to elucidate the cellular mechanisms, and it appears to be that they exert their antiepileptic activity via one of the following mehcanisms:

1) Inhibition of the voltage-dependent Na+ currents.
2) Increase of GABA effect over the GABA-A receptors.
3) Suppression of the voltage-dependent Ca2+ currents.

The mechanisms of action of several of the new AED act in a similar manner that conventionals, however, some exert their effect by means of novel mechanisms. For example, lamotrigina (LTG) acts by suppressing voltage-dependent Na+ currents, however research suggest that it can also inhibit the release of glutamate, probably as a consequence of the blockade of NA+ channels. In the case of oxcarbamazepine (OXC), that has a similar mechanism of CBZ, it has been proven that it acts over voltage-dependent Na+ currents (Soares-da-Silva P, 2015). Contrary to CBZ, it has been shown that in striatum body, acts by blocking postsynaptic glutamate-excitatory potentials (EPSPs). This could depend on presynaptic mechanisms and it has been suggested that it could be related to the decrease in voltage-dependent Ca2+ currents; however, this has to be determined with further studies (Sitges, 2016). In general, it can be stated that the mechanism of action of several of the novel AEDs is known, still, this is not sufficient enough to explain all of the antiepileptic effects they possess, which is why research still continues in order to elucidate all the mechanisms involved (Rogawski and Cavazos, 2015).

## Characteristics of an Antiepileptic Drug

It is important to mention that the ideal AED should cover the following requisites: quick brain bioavailability in all kind of crisis, prolonged half-life, adequate elimination, little to no toxicity, and the capacity of not causing respiratory depression, it can be administered orally, and in case of emergency via parenteral. Also, and in special occasions, the clinical characteristics of the patients along with the specific traits of the epilepsy should be considered (Rubio, 1999; Rogawski and Cavazos, 2015).

Even though extensive research has been performed, to this day it has not been formerly stated if the administration of one or more (poly-pharmacology) AEDs could have effect over the cognitive development of patients under treatments (Rogawski and Cavazos, 2015).

Here, it is relevant to note that current research has focused mainly to determinate if the AED evaluated fulfills all the characteristics mentioned above, but little attention has been putted to the neuronal damage caused by previous seizures and if the AED help to decrease this damage.

In this sense, only a few experimental studies have been performed. It has been found that Diazepam (Ault et al., 1986) and Phenobarbital (Fandesen et al., 1990) partially prevent brain damage, additionally difenilhidantonia, carbamazepine combined with ether anesthesia, and bacoflen all have a significant protective effect against brain damage.

Thus, based on the fact that there are no studies in which the neuronal damage is monitored for increase or decrease by the effect of AEDs, our research team began studying about it, beginning by a morphologic analysis for two brain areas heavily impacted by epileptic seizures.

## Experimental Model

We boarded the problem following the strategy proposed by the University of Utah's Project for the Development of Antiepileptic Drugs (White et al., 1998), which consists in testing if a drug possesses the quality of protecting against the appearance of epileptic seizures. Following this protocol, the AED was administered before the seizures were induced, employing Kainic Acid (KA). In this way, it was considered that if the morphologic damage found after the seizures was direct consequence of the hypoxic states and of the cerebral edema, it is to be expected that if the AED is administered before, less or even no amount of damage will be found. This will be evaluated by contrasting with the damage caused by the administration of KA without the AED.

The morphological examination was performed in the hippocampus and cerebellum of rats, ten days after being treated with the following strategies: a) Intra peritoneal (i.p.) administration of saline solution (Control Group), b) Intra gastric administration of Carbamazepine/Oxcarbamazepine (CBZ/OXC, 80 mg/kg; 100 mg/kg), c) Administration of CBZ/OXC followed by administration of KA (10 mg/kg) one hour later, d) I.p. administration of KA (10 mg/kg).

As stated above, we employed of two AED, one of conventional use (CBZ) and one relatively recent (OXC), both employed for partial and general epileptic crisis (Rubio, 1999; Ambrósio et al., 2002). CBZ acts at synaptic level; it reduces brain levels of AMPc acts at noradrenergic level and facilitates the activation of inhibitory GABAergic circuits (Ambrósio et al., 2002).

The efficacy of OXC is similar of that of the CBZ. OXC and the metabolite monohidroxil (MHD) were tested in cortical neuron culture, and it was found that they suppress the firing of action potentials of high frequency and Sodium currents (Wamil et al., 1994). Further, it is known that OXC but not the MDH, can interact with Ca2+ channel type L in concentrations of 0.3 mM. Besides blocking Ca2+, they also inhibit K+ channels (McLean et al., 1994; Ambrósio et al., 2002). In order to induce convulsive crisis, several strategies have been boarded, some of which are the electric stimulation and the administration of pharmaceuticals in specific areas of the brain or administered via i.p.

We employed KA, because it is one of the most effective drugs to induce epileptic seizures with posterior damage to the hippocampus and cerebellum, similar in that found in humans with epilepsy of temporal lobe. The structural similarity of the KA with Glutamate, the main excitatory neurotransmitter in the brain, confers it an excitatory and toxic effect over the CNS. It has been proven that the administration of KA to rats via i.p. or subcutaneous, at doses 8-12 mg/kg, or intrathecally at 0.4-1-5 mg/ml of saline solution, is equally effective for inducing the appearance of continuous, spontaneous and recurring epileptic seizures, associated to a characteristic pattern of brain damage to that described in humans with temporal lobe epilepsy.

## Morphological Findings

Before going into further details, is important to mention that the behavior that the rats in the groups administered with saline solution and OXC and CBZ was normal. The rats treated with KA presented 30 minutes after its administration, the behavior described for animals with KA. The animals showed instability and a continuous movement across the cage. Their faces contract they start moving their head, began a chewing behavior, exhibit dog-like shakes and they start drooling. This behavior continues approximately for one hour and is followed by the generalized seizures. Three hours later after the administration of KA the seizures began declining and the rats leave exhausted.

When OXC and CBZ were administered, before the KA, a similar behavior was observed, the only change present was the time in which the crisis appear, for OXC, they expressed three hours later. The CBZ attenuated seizures attacks (Ayala-Guerrero et al, 2001; Ambrósio et al., 2002). In the hippocampus and cerebellum of control animals, a normal histology was found (Figures 1-2). In the case of the animals treated with OXC and CBZ, the results were similar (González-Maciel, et al., 2000: 2001). In the hippocampus of the animals treated only with KA a selective lesion already described for CA1. It consists of a necrosis of pyramidal neurons and after removal of the death neurons, this appears as a discontinuity of the laminae of pyramidal neurons of CA1. This lesion was found at the left, right and both hemispheres of the brain (Figure 1). The neuronal population affected by the KA at the cerebellum was that of Purkinje cells. In all the lobules we found a great quantity of necrosis or even absence of neurons (Figure 2). At the hippocampus and cerebellum of animals trated with OCX and CBZ followed by KA, the lesion of CA1 described before was found, however it is worth pointing out that this was much bigger in extension in comparison with the animals treated only with KA (González-Maciel, et al., 2000: 2001). Plus in this groups extensive areas of lesions were found, including great population of neuronal death, damage to the neuropil, both in the dentate gyrus, the medial thalamus and the piriform cortex (Figure 3). Our findings corroborated the presence of epileptic seizures induced by the administration of KA, and ion the same way the characteristic lesion in the hippocampus was found, described in temporal lobe epilepsy of humans (Ben-Ari, 1985; Bedner et al., 2015).

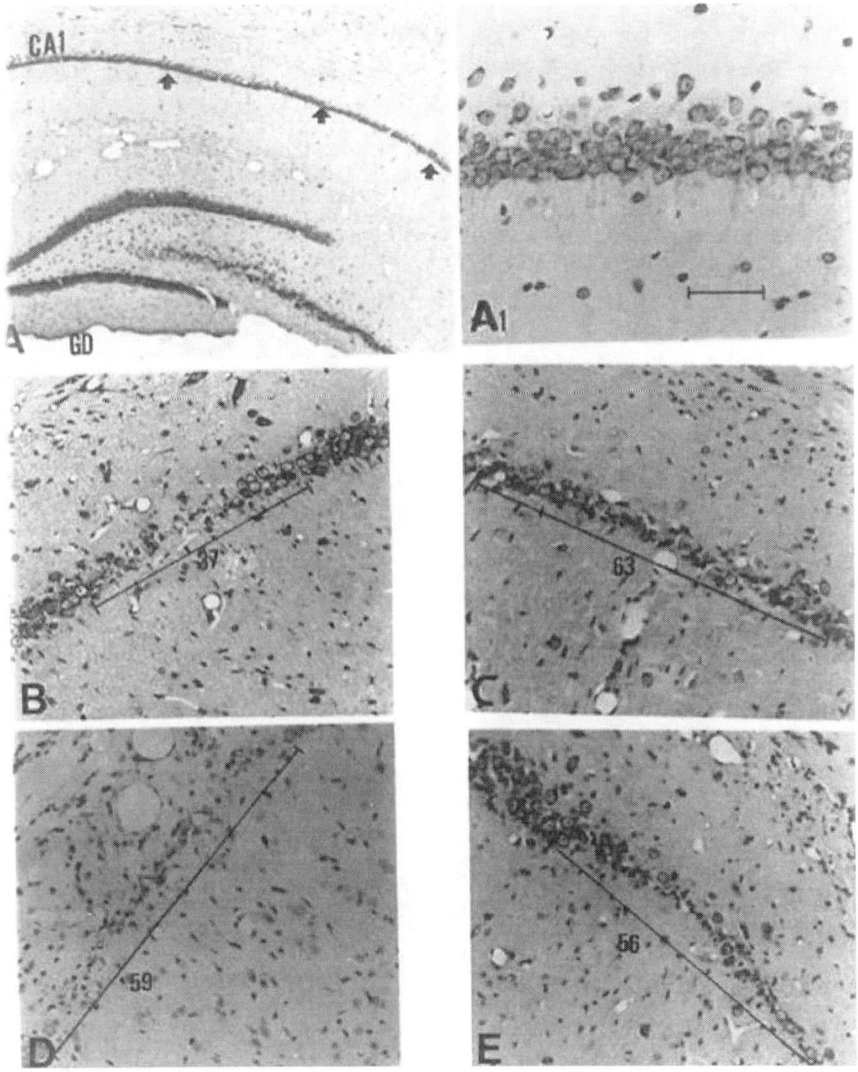


Figure 1. A) Microphotograph of a dorsal slice of a Control rat hippocampus, the arrows point to the areas of CA1 where the characteristic lesion induced by KA can be observed. In A1 can be appreciated an increase of the side of neurons of CA1 under control conditions, it is composed about 4 pyramidal cells. Note the loss of there neurons under experimental conditions were the lesion is of less extension of that in animals treated only with KA (B) and greater in animals treated with OXC and CBZ (C, D) or only CBZ (E). Stained with cresyl violet, bar scale A = 47 μm; A1 = 10 μm.

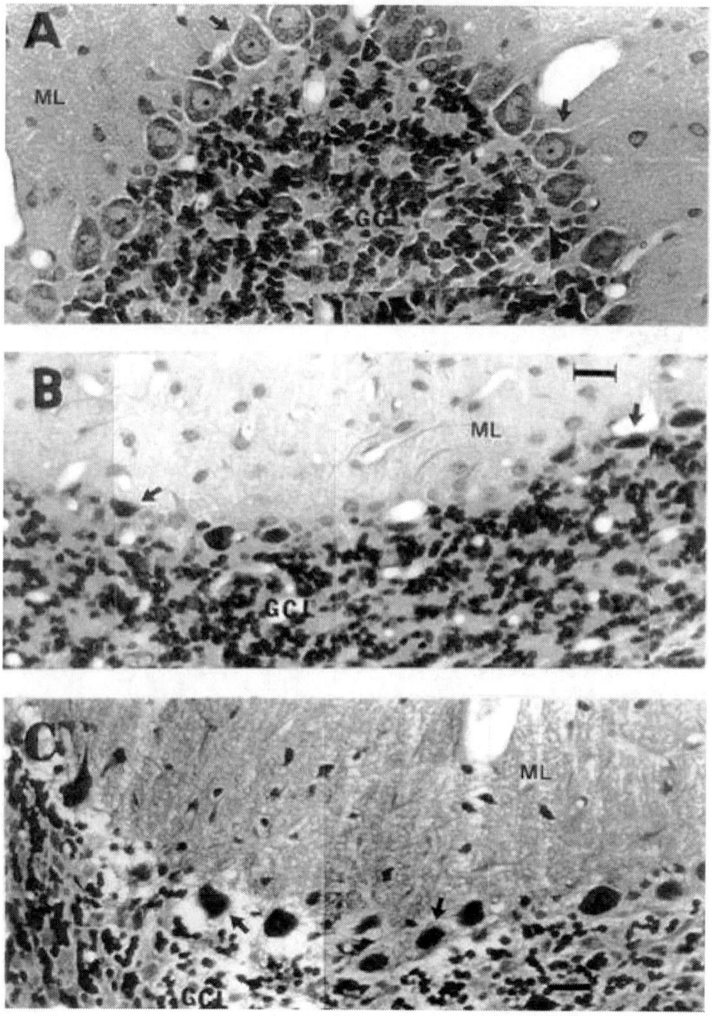


Figure 2. Sagittal slices of brains stained with cresyl violet. A) Control animal. B) Animal treated with KA. In Purkinje cells only remains of neurons can be found (arrows). C) In animals treated with OXC previous to KA, necrotic remains of Purkinje cells were found but also, extensive areas in the molecular layer (ML) and in the granular layer with neuropil damage. Bar scale 5 μm.

It is hard to explain the increase in brain damage of animals treated with the AEDs previous to the KA, for that, it could be proposed a synergism between the AEDs and KA, however it remains to elucidate totally the mechanisms of action of both OXC and CBZ but also the KA.

Because of the severity of the possibility of an AED to be neurotoxic and cause some kind of unknown neuronal damage, it is important for future research to consider that this drugs should not be capable of increasing the previously established neuronal damage by the epileptic seizures. The AED of current employment, need to be evaluated following the same strategy or even implementing new ones.

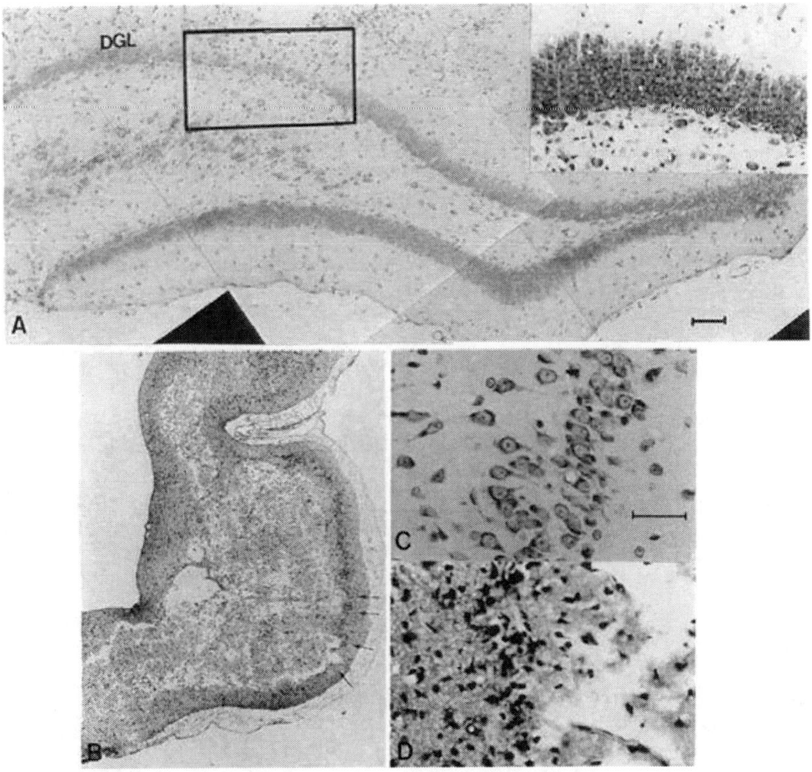


Figure 3. Microphotograph of animals treated with OXC previous to KA. A) In the dentate gyrus a decrease in granular cells was found at the dorsal gyrus dentate (DGL). In the insert it is shown an increase of an area equivalent to that of control animals; the stripe is composed approximately of eight granular cells. B) Necrotic neurons were found (arrows) and extensive neuropil damage at the piriform cortex (at greater zoom in D). C) A bigger zoom of the area pointed with arrows in the control animal. Bar scale A = 25 µm; B = 80µm; C, D = 10µm.

## Conclusion

In conclusion, CBZ/OXC partially inhibit seizures produced by the model with KA; but it was ineffective in inhibiting the neural damage induced by the administration of KA. However, only one dose was tested for CBZ and OXC, therefore, it cannot be excluded that other doses would have had another effect on the state and neurodegeneration. Finally, we will present results of experiments using this animal model; carried out in order to know if the use of antiepileptic drugs not only decreases the frequency and intensity of seizures, but also if they can prevent neuronal damage from increasing, an aspect that, in our opinion, has not been fully clarified.

## References

Ambrósio, A. F., Soares-da-Silva, P., Carvalho, C. M., Carvalho, A. P. (2002). Mechanisms of action of carbamazepine and its derivatives, oxcarbazepine, BIA 2-093, and BIA 2-024. *Neurochemical research,* 27(1-2), 121-130. DOI:10.1023/A:101481492.

Ault, B., Gruenthal, M., Armstrong, D. R., Nadler J. V. (1986). Efficacy of baclofen and Phenobarbital against the kainic acid limbic seizure-brain damage syndrome. *J Pharmac. Exp Ther.* 239 612 –617. ISSN 1521-0103.

Ayala-Guerrero, F., Vargas, L., Romero, R. M., Reynoso-Robles, R., González-Maciel A. (2001). Effect of oxcarbazepine on kainic acid-induced seizure. *Proc. West Pharmacol.* 44 173-175. PMID: 11793973.

Banerjee, P. N., Filippi, D., Hauser, W. A. (2009). The descriptive epidemiology of epilepsy—a review. *Epilepsy research,* 85(1), 31-45. doi.org/10.1016/j.eplepsyres.2009.03.003.

Banerjee, P. N., Filippi, D., Hauser, W. A. (2009). The descriptive epidemiology of epilepsy—a review. *Epilepsy research,* 85(1), 31-45. doi.org/10.1016/j.eplepsyres.2009.03.003.

Bedner, P., Dupper, A., Hüttmann, K., Müller, J., Herde, M. K., Dublin, P., Henneberger, C. (2015). Astrocyte uncoupling as a cause of human temporal lobe epilepsy. *Brain,* 138(5), 1208-1222. doi.org/10.1093/brain/awv067.

Beghi, E., Perucca, E. (1995). The Mangement of epilepsy in the 1990s. *Drug* 49 680-694. doi.org/10.2165/00003495-199549050-00004.

Ben-Ari, Y. (1985). Limbic seizure and brain damage produced by kainic acid: mechanisms and relevance to human temporal lobe epilepsy. *Neuroscience,* 14(2), 375-403. doi.org/10.1016/0306-4522(85)90299-4.

Boison, D., Steinhäuser, C. (2018). Epilepsy and astrocyte energy metabolism. *Glia,* 66(6), 1235-1243. doi.org/10.1002/glia.23247.

Brailowsky, S. (1995) The substances of dreams. *Neuropsychopharmacology.* La ciencia para todos (130), FCE, México, 355 pp.

Clarke, C., Lemon, R. (2016). Nervous system structure and function. *Neurology: A Queen Square Textbook,* 11-67. doi.org/10.1002/9781118486160.ch2.

Collingridge, G. L., Bliss, T. V. P. (1987) NMDA receptors- their role in long – term potentiation. *Trends Neurosci.* 10 288- 296. doi.org/10.1016/0166-2236(87)90175-5.

Cruz-Cruz, M., Gallardo-Elías, J., Paredes-Solís, S., Legorreta-Soberanis, J., Flores-Moreno, M., Andersson, N. (2017). Factores asociados a epilepsia en niños en México: un estudio caso-control. *Boletín médico del Hospital Infantil de México,*74(5), 334-340.

Frandsen, A., Quistorff, B. Schousboe, A. (1990) Phenobarbitol protects cerebral cortex neurons against toxicity induced by kainite but not by other excitatory amino acids. *Neurosci Lett.* 111 233-238. doi.org/10.1016/0304-3940(90)90374-I.

French, J. A., Dichter, M. Leepik, E. I. (1998). *Antiepileptic Drug Development* En: Lippincott –Raven, Philadelphia, New York, 161-166.

García Martín, G.,Serrano Castro, P. J. (2018). Epidemiología de la epilepsia en España y Latinoamérica. *Rev Neurol, 67*, 249. ISSN 0210-0010.

González-Maciel, A., Reynoso-Robles, R., Romero- Velázquez, R. M., Vargas L. Ayala-Guerrero, F. (2001) Effect of an anticonvuldant drug on kainic acid-induced brain damage. *Proc. West Pharmacol.* 44 121-124. PMID: 11793956.

González-Maciel, A., Reynoso-Robles, R., Romero-Velázquez, R. M., Vargas, L. Ayala-Guerrero, F. (2000). Effects of oxcarbazepine on the behavioral response and neuroanatomical alterations following administration of kainic acid. *Proc. West Pharmacol.* 43 35-37. PMID: 11056952.

Holmes, G. L. (2015). Cognitive impairment in epilepsy: the role of network abnormalities. *Epileptic Disorders,* 17(2), 101-116. doi.org/10.1684/epd.2015.0739.

Lange, C., Storkebaum, E., De Almodóvar, C. R., Dewerchin, M., Carmeliet, P. (2016). Vascular endothelial growth factor: a neurovascular target in neurological diseases. *Nature Reviews Neurology,* 12(8), 439. doi:10.1038/nrneurol.2016.88.

Leuner, B., Gould, E. (2010). Structural plasticity and hippocampal function. *Annual review of psychology,* 61, 111-140. doi.org/10.1146/annurev.psych.093008.100359.

Löscher, W. (2011). Critical review of current animal models of seizures and epilepsy used in the discovery and development of new antiepileptic drugs. *Seizure,* 20(5), 359-368. doi.org/10.1016/j.seizure.2011.01.003.

Luedke, M. W., Blalock, D. V., Goldstein, K. M., Kosinski, A. S., Sinha, S. R., Drake, C., Gierisch, J. M. (2019). Self-management of Epilepsy: A Systematic Review. *Annals of internal medicine.* doi: 10.7326/M19-0458.

Maljevic, S., Møller, R. S., Reid, C. A., Pérez-Palma, E., Lal, D., May, P., Lerche, H. (2019). Spectrum of GABAA receptor variants in epilepsy. *Current opinion in neurology,* 32(2), 183-190. doi: 10.1097/WCO.0000000000000657.

McLean, M., Schmutz, M., Wamil, A., Olpe, H., Portet, C., Feldmann, K. (1994). Oxcarbazepine : mechanisms of action. *Epilepsia* 35 S5-S9. doi.org/10.1111/j.1528-1157.1994.tb05949.x.

Niedermeyer,E. (1983) Clinical evaluation and differential diagnosis in epileptic seizure disorders. Epilepsy Guide. Diagnosis and treatment of epileptic seizure disorders. *Ernst Niedermeyer. Edit. Urban & Schwarzenberg*. Baltimore pp 90-103.

Panayiotopoulos, C. P. (2007). Epileptic syndromes and their treatment. *Neonatal seizures.* Second edition. London, 185-206. doi.org/10.1007/978-1-84628-644-5.

Roberts, E. (1978) Roles of GABA neurons in information processing in the vertebrate CNS. En: *Neuronal Information Transfer.* Eds. Karlin A, Tennyson VM, Vogel HJ. Academic Press. New York pp 213–239.

Rogawski, M. A., Cavazos, J. E. (2015). Mechanisms of action of antiepileptic drugs. *Wyllie's Treatment of Epilepsy: Principles and Practice,* 6th ed. New York, NY: Professional Communications, Inc, 522-9. ISBN (Print)9781451191523.

Rothman, S. M., Olney, J. W. (1990). Excitotoxicity and NMDA receptor. *Trend in Neurosci.* 10 299-302. doi: 10.1016/0166-2236(95)93869-y.

Rubio, D. F. (1999). *Epilepsy Clinical Manual,* JGH Editores, SALVAT Medicina, México, 114 pp.

Schmidt-Rhaesa, A., Harzsch, S., Purschke, G. (2015). *Structure and evolution of invertebrate nervous systems.* Oxford University Press.

Sitges, M. (1993) Comunicación entre las células nerviosas. Sinapsis. En: *Comunicación Neuroendocrina.* 1ª edición. Sociedad Mexicana de Ciencias Fisiológicas, México, pp. 47 – 70. [Communication between nerve cells. Synapse. In: *Neuroendocrine Communication.*]

Sitges, M., Chiu, L. M., Reed, R. C. (2016). Effects of Levetiracetam, Carbamazepine, Phenytoin, Valproate, Lamotrigine, Oxcarbazepine, Topiramate, Vinpocetine and Sertraline on Presynaptic Hippocampal Na(+) and Ca(2+) Channels Permeability. *Neurochem Res.* Apr; 41(4):758-69. doi: 10.1007/s11064-015-1749-0. Epub 2015 Nov 5.

Soares-da-Silva, P., Pires, N., Bonifácio. M. J., Loureiro, A. I., Palma, N., Wright, L. C. (2015). Eslicarbazepine acetate for the treatment of focal epilepsy: an update on its proposed mechanisms of action. *Pharmacol Res Perspect.* Mar; 3(2):e00124. doi: 10.1002/prp2.124. Epub 2015 Mar 30. Review.

Terrone, G., Frigerio, F., Balosso, S., Ravizza, T., Vezzani, A. (2019). Inflammation and reactive oxygen species in status epilepticus:

Biomarkers and implications for therapy. *Epilepsy & Behavior.* doi.org/10.1016/j.yebeh.2019.04.028.

Trimble, M,R. (2017) 4 Epilepsy – the key that unlocked neuropsychiatry *Journal of Neurology, Neurosurgery & Psychiatry* 88:A2-A3. DOI:10.1136/jnnp-2017-BNPA.4.

Vezzani, A., Fujinami, R. S., White, H. S., Preux, P. M., Blümcke, I., Sander, J. W., Löscher, W. (2016). Infections, inflammation and epilepsy. *Acta neuropathologica,* 131(2), 211-234. doi.org/10.1007/s00401-015-1481-5.

Wamil, A., Porter, C., Jensen, P., Scmutz, M., McLean, M. (1992). Oxcarbazepine and its monohydroxy metabolite limit action potential firing by mouse central neurons in cell culture. *Epilepsia* 32 S65-S66. DOI: S37-S46, 1999-05-01.

White, H. S., Wolf, H. H., Woodhead, J. H. Kupferberg, H. J. (1998). The National Institutes of Health Anticonvulsant Drug Development Program: Screening for Efficacy. En: *Antiepileptic Drug Development, Advances in Neurology,* Vol. 76, Editado por: J. French, I Leppik and MA Dichter. New York, pp. 29-39. PMID: 9408461.

In: Laboratory Animals and Neurosciences ISBN: 978-1-53618-462-4
Editors: B. Hernandez Godinez et al.© 2020 Nova Science Publishers, Inc.

*Chapter 10*

# WISTAR RATS AS A MODEL TO STUDY THE AGING PROCESS IN THE CENTRAL NERVOUS SYSTEM

***Roberto Santín Márquez*[1,2] *and Mina Königsberg*[1]**
[1]Laboratorio de Bioenergética y Envejecimiento Celular, Departamento de Ciencias de la Salud, Universidad Autónoma Metropolitana Unidad Iztapalapa, Mexico City, Mexico
[2]Posgrado en Biología Experimental, Universidad Autónoma Metropolitana Unidad Iztapalapa, Mexico City, Mexico

## ABSTRACT

Aging-research has become a rapidly-growing field because of the exponential increase of the elderly population, and therefore the search of an appropiate animal model for these studies has gained importance. Since aging is a multifactorial phenomenon, it is dificult to simulate it in *in vitro* conditions, so *in vivo* models are the most accepted to work with. However they must offer an accurately aproximation to the physiology and molecular pathways that are activated during the aging process in humans. Hence, rodent models have been widely used in this area.

Along with the growing of the elderly population, the increment of the pathologies related to the central nervous system (CNS), such as dementias, has increased too, showing a strong corretation between aging and the risk to develop a neurodegenerative disease. This has opened a new research field in order to understand the CNS natural degeneration during aging. This makes the search for a suitable model more difficult because of the complex cognitive procesess involved in human aged nervous system. Surprisingly, rats have a relative high CNS homology with humans, when compared with other animal models, making it an ideal model to study and simulate this complex process. In particular, Wistar rats are a suitable and adaptable animal model, that has been widely used in several disciplines in biomedical research due to its advantages compared with other models and much of its phisiology is alerady known. In this review, we will analize the benefits of using rats, specially the Wistar strain, as a model to study the aging process in the CNS.

**Keywords**: aging, CNS, animal modesl, rats

# INTRODUCTION

## An Overview about Aging

Aging is a multifactorial, universal, progressive and deleterious process triggered over the lifetime of living beings whose main consequence is the decline of physiologic functions, increasing their vulnerability to desease and finally, driving them to death [1, 2, 3].

Many different theories have been proposed to explain the processes that trigger aging and they can be classified into two main groups: the ones that suggest that the aging process is a programmed event; and the ones that suggest that it is caused by the accumulation of damage during lifetime [4]. One of the most recognized and controversial theories, is the "free radical theory of aging" proposed by Denham Harman [5]. It stablishes that the aging process is the result of the accumulation of damaged biomolecules during lifetime, as a consequence of endogenous reactions which involve the participation of free radicals (FR). FR are unstable molecules with an unpaired electron in their last orbital, mainly originated in the mitochondrial electron transport chain during the oxygen reduction to water. Harman hypothesized that the accumulation of oxidized molecules is correlated with the living beings lifespan [6]. Almost a decade later, transgenic animals were developed to overexpress or inhibit the expression of some antioxidant enzymes in order to demonstrate the accumulation or elimimnation of the oxidized molecules could affect animal´s lifespan. Surprisingly, no differences were found in the lifespan of transgenic animals compared with the wild type, suggesting that the reduction in FR-related damage biomolecules does not delay the aging process, but could affect the healthspan. The healthspan is a new concept that is related to the time in which the ornagism remains healthy [7, 8].

Another interesting theory is based on senescent cells accumulation in the tissues during aging, driving them to a missfunctional state and promoting the decrease of critical functions to manintain homeostasis. Cellular senescence was first described *in vitro* in 1961, and was defined as a cellular state in which the proliferation irreversibly stops after a certain number of duplications, due to the telomeres erosion or shortening [9]. This time point is often called the Hayflick limit.

Serrano et al. [10] were the first ones to show that the overexpression of the oncogene *ras* also promoted the senescence phenotype via p53 and $p16^{INK4a}$ pathway, generation a premature induced senescence. After that, more stimuli were proven to stimulate premature induced senescence, i.e., before reaching the Hayflick limit and independently of telomere shortening. Some of those stimuli are as hyperoxia, oxidative stress, proteasome inhibition, or altered autophagic process [11, 12]. Senescent cells have particular features compared with normal cells, including: 1) the incapacity to proliferate, even after mitogenic stimulation; 2) apoptosis resistance; 3) a big flat morphology; 4) epigenetic changes; 5) a particular heterochromatin structure called senescence associated heterochromatin foci (SAHF); 6) differential gene expression; and 7) the regulated secretion of different chemokines, cytokines, growth factors, matrix metaloproteases and ROS, also called senescence associated secretory phenotype (SASP) [13, 14, 15]. Initially, it was thought that the senescent phenotype was only a tumor-suppressor mechanism, in charge to stop the abnormal proliferation in response to oncogenes overexpression. However, recently senescence was shown to have an important role in other processes such as mammalian embryonic development, in which senescent cells are required for a normal morphogenesis. At the end of their role, senescent cells are cleared from tissue by macrophages, recruited by the chemoattractant molecules secreted within the SASP [16].

Curiously, the senescent cells accumulate in several tissues during aging [17, 18, 19, 20], including the nervous system [21, 22, 23], probably due to a deficient clearance response by de immune system [24] or by changes in their surface markers that avoid their immune recognition and further elimination [25].

Moreover, it has been proposed that the accumulation of dysfunctional non-degraded proteins could explain many of the features of aging process due to a gradual loss of protein homeostasis, also known as proteostasis [26]. So, the accumulation of misfolded proteins directly affects the proteostasis network, a set of different pathways that are involved in protein synthesis, maduration, and trafficking. As well as the regulation of processes such as proteins aggregation, disagreggation and degradation, resulting in loss- or gain-of-functions that could evantualy trigger several diseases and exacerbate the age phenotype [27]. Misfolded and aggregated proteins must be cleared from cells by the degradation machinery, comprised mainly by the ubiquitin-proteasome system (UPS), involved in the degradation of individual proteins through ubiquitin-conjugation as a marker for elimination; and the autophagy-lysosome system, involved in the degradation of aggregates and membrane proteins [28]. Those systems are impaired during aging, leading to an abnormal accumulation of ubiquitinated misfolded proteins, which can induce oxidative and endoplasmic reticulum stress, affecting the cell physiology [29]. It has been proven that the proteasome function (a proteic complex with a proteolytic domain capable to recognize several amino acids sequences of ubiquitinated proteins) decrease with age [30, 31, 32, 33], promoting intracellular accumulation of non-functional proteins and favoring the apparition of age related diseases. It has also been proposed that increasing the proteasome activity could ameliorate the apparition and progression of such diseases [34].

Even though several different theories were formuled trying to understand how the aging process begins, there is not a single theory capable of fully explain it without leaving aside some of the main features of aging. So, although these theories could be noted as separated postulates, it has been showen that more than two distinct theories can act at the same time, cooperating as a complex interaction net that regulate the whole aging process [35]. That is way, the aging process is viewed as a multifactorial phenomenon, regulated by intrinsic and extrinsic factors that could accelerate or slow down the biological aging progress and, thus, the age-related diseases [36].

Since aging is characterized by a decline of physiological functions, it is logic to think that every tissue and organ in an old organism is prone to deterioration, but it has been proven that some organs are more sensitive to age-associated damage than others, such as heart, liver, kidneys, lungs and brain [37]. Particularly, the nervous system is one of the most affected systems during aging, and there are a lot of different age-related diseases provoked by the neural circuit neurodegeneration, or the dysfunction of glial cells [38]. As well as the accumulation of intracellular and/or extracellular protein aggregates, also known as proteinopathies [39], contributing to the appearance of certain physiological changes that promote mental and motor alterations during natural aging, such as processes associated to memory and circadian rhythm [40].

There are some characteristic functional and structural changes in brain during aging, like lower functional connectivity, which has been linked to a decrease in cognitive processes such as memory and executive functions. In regards to the brain structure and architecture, the reduction in total brain volume is remarkable, as well as the decrease in white matter [41]. These volumetric changes occur in most brain regions, but are specially noted in specific regions, such as prefrontal cortex, putamen, hippocampus and medial lobe, affecting neural circuitry [42]. Nervous system related diseases are mainly disabling conditions that reduce patient´s ability to fend for themselves, decreasing their quality of life, due to late diagnosis, and late-appearing clinical signs [43]. Therefore the use of suitable animal models is important to understand how this phenomenon begins and progresses in order to design strategies to contend its deleterious effects.

## Wistar Rats as a Model to Study Aging

A good animal model must present the main characteristics of aging phenotype, and must allow the study of the molecular mechanisms and pathways that ocurr within the tissues and cells. Besides, it should be easy to manipulate and be able to live in laboratory conditions. It has to be small and cheap to maintain and breed [44], but also has to make sure that enough tissue could be obtained to performe the experiments or primary cultures.

So, some of the most used organisms in aging research are some non-animal organisms, like the yeast *Saccharomyces cerevisiae*, which shares many important genes with animals. Other invertebrate animal models like *Caenorhabditis elegans* and *Drosophila melanogaster* have been used to study and understand some molecular pathways involved in the aging process, taking advantage of the malleability of their genomes in order to generate transgenic strains to evaluate their lifespan and age-related modifications [44, 45]. Some non-human primates are also used, such as *Macaca mulatta*, due to to their high genomic similarity to humans [46]. Finally, the rodent models, like *Mus musculus*, *Rattus norvegicus*, and recently, *Heterocephalus glaber* [47, 48, 49]. Rodents are the main model animals used in biomedical research, and their importance in neurosciences and behavioural research has increased in the last decades because of the advantages they offer, such as its small size, handling, short lifespans and fast reproduction [50]. Moreover, many of the age-related diseases that are present in humans can be modeled in rodents, such as mouse and rats, manipulating their equivalent genes to simulate different phenotypes adquired during aging (Table 1) [51].

**Table 1. Benefits and drawbacks of model animals used in aging research**

| Animal model | Benefits | Drawbacks |
|---|---|---|
| *Saccharomyces cerevisiae* | - Conserved homology with several mammal genes involved in aging process.<br>- Easy to distinguish individual daughter cells over time.<br>- Malleable genome whose modifications impact directly in yeast´s phenotype, because of its haploidy.<br>- Numerous individual organisms per culture, favoring populational analyses.<br>- Evident metabolic, physiologic and morphologic changes while aging, like bud scars accumulation.<br>-Becomes senescent while ages. | - As long as it is an unicelullar organism, it cannot simulate the complex interaction between multicellular organism´s cells.<br>- Although conserves many genes compared with mammals, important differences can be found, as long as it is not an animal.<br>- Does not share active secretory features of senescent cells, which is very important in mammal´s aging.<br>- It cannot simulate specific-tissue/organs aging conditions, so it is not a suitable model for some disciplines, as neurosciences. |
| *Caenorhabditis elegans* | - Respond to genetical and environmental changes altering its lifespan.<br>- Its lifespan is very short, averaging 14 days, allowing studying several generations.<br>- The genes that directly affect lifespan are fully described.<br>- It is easy to maintain in laboratory conditions, and relatively cheap.<br>-It is hermaphrodite and can fertilize itself without inbreeding deleterious consequences | - It is very small, and it is quite difficult to obtain enough biological samples.<br>- Although it is an animal model, it is an invertebrate, so its physiological functions and organs are primitive, and in consequence, does not accurately simulate the aging process in superior animals.<br>- Many genes related with aging and lifespan present in this model have not homologues in vertebrates, especially in mammals. |
| *Drosophila melanogaster* | - It is easy to breed, handle and care, so it is simple to obtain numerous individuals.<br>- In spite of being an invertebrate, it has organs shared with mammals, including a well-organized nervous system.<br>Its genome is fully.<br>- Its lifespan is short, over 2-3 months.<br>-Its genome is fully characterized and it is suitable to produce mutants because of the great variety in genetical tools to modify it. | - It has not been reported senescent cells in this model, an important marker in the stablishment and development of aging process in many organisms.<br>- Although is a suitable model to induce mutations, it is complicated to administrate drugs, and doses employed, are not comparable with the doses used in other animals.<br>- It small size difficult the dissection and sample obtaining. |

**Table 1. (Continued)**

| Animal model | Benefits | Drawbacks |
|---|---|---|
| *Macaca mulatta* | -It is one of the phylogenetically closest animal models to humans, sharing about 95% of its genome.<br>- The aging process is very similar to human´s, sharing its main features and markes.<br>- There could be performed many *in vivo* clinical and behavioral trials in longitudinal studios, mimicking human aging deterioration.<br>- Larger amounts of biological samples could be obtained | - It is an aggressive specie, and its hanlding is risky.<br>-Is expensive to house and maintain until aging, and specially designed instalations must be adquired.<br>- Their lifespan is over 35 years, so it difficults short term investigations and mus wait several years until aged phenotype appears.<br>-Their breeding is complicated and they birth only one young. |
| *Heterocephalus glaber* | - They are the longest living rodents, with a lifespan of approximately 28 years.<br>-The have amazing antiaging mechanisms, like low rate metabolism, higly efficient antioxidant defenses and repair mechanisms for proteins and DNA.<br>- Posess a late-appearance of senescence.<br>- Offers an excellent model to study the anti aging mechanisms and the healthy aging. | - Special instalations adapted for simulate the complex tunnels system of *Heterocephalus glaber* is needed.<br>- It is an expensive model and they are not many colonies destined to researching.<br>-Its long lifespan could turn into a disadvantage because of the long waiting times that are required to reach an old population.<br>-It is still not a well characterized model. |
| *Mus musculus* | - It is a widely used model that is well characterized and several strains, mutans and transgenic animals have been designed to simulate many age-related processes and diseases.<br>-Its lifespan is relatively short compared with other mammals, averaging 28 months.<br>- Many of its genes related with aging have homology with human genes.<br>-It is easy to handling and breed, and it is suitable to biomedical research.<br>- Inbreed strains ares a good model to study genetics of aging | -It is small-sized, which difficults the sample collection and dissection.<br>- Its sensible to chronic handling, increasins its stress levels.<br>- Inflamatory process has disctinct features between humans and mice.<br>- It is less suitable tan rats for cognitive and behavioral trials.<br>- Inbreed strains does not represent genetical variation present in human aging. |

| Animal model | Benefits | Drawbacks |
|---|---|---|
| *Rattus norvegicus* | - It is easy to handle because of its mild nature and resistance to stress.<br>- Its lifespan is about 22-28 months depending on the strain, letting to study the aging process in a relatively rapid way.<br>- Because of its large size, it is possible to get larger amounts of biological samples.<br>- It is an ideal model for basical cognitive and behavioral tests, allowing to study the nervous system deterioring during aging.<br>- Presents classical markers of aging, like cellular senescence, low-grade chronic inflammation, increase in oxidative stress, and stem cells exhaustion.<br>- Morphologically, conserves proportions of organs and tissues similar to those found in humans. | - Develops spontaneous tumors during aging.<br>- They are pron to develop obesity during adulthood.<br>- Although are mainly outbreed strains and mimics the genetically heterogeny in human population, it difficults an appropriate genetical characterization.<br>- Although it is better model for basic cognition tests than mice, higher cognitive functions cannot being evaluated in rats.<br>- Transgenic models are difficult to obtain because of fertilized eggs sensivity to *in vitro* conditions. |

Nevertheless, rats (*Rattus norvegicus*) have gained importance as a model in aging, and especially in neuroscience research. This is mainly due to some intrinsic features that are advantageous in this particular area, such as a higher capability of learning a wide variety of tasks, along with multiple analogous pathways and physiological proportions compared to the human brain. Rats also have more cognitive and memory abilities compared with mice, making them very attractive to use in a wide variety of neuroscientific approaches [52]. Anatomically, rats have larger organs compared to mice, making easier their dissection, and allowing the acquisition of a greater amount of tissue to work with [52, 53].

Albino rats are widely used in biomedical research since the Wistar Institute, in Philadelphia, USA, developed from Norwegian rats the Wistar strain in 1906. This was the first standardized laboratory animal model [54, 55]. Wistar rats are an outbred strain, which provides them with additional advantageous features, like longer lifespans, faster growth and larger size [56]. The outbred strains present genetical heterogeneity that accurately reflects the heterogenous genetics of human populations; this is relevant to understand the diverse phenotypes shown during aging [57].

As in most mammals including humans, female Wistar rats live longer than males, with an average lifespan of 24-29 months versus 20-24 months respectively [57, 58, 59], thus allowing the study of the different aging processes related to sex [60, 61, 62].

All the above endorses that Wistar rats as a reliable model to simulate and study the aging phenotype, as well as age-related disseases. Moreover, the number of investigations using this model has increased over the last decade. In particular in the topics related with aging, such as cardiac and vascular systems [63-71], inflammation and immune system [72-80], redox state and antioxidant responses [81, 89], hepatology [90-96], senescence [97-99], and neurosciences [100-108], among others.

## WISTAR RATS IN AGING AND NEUROSCIENCES

As mentioned above, rats are an excellent model to study neurosciences, because they are easy to train in order to accomplish simple tasks that allow the evaluation of cognitive and behavioral parameters. They are also suitable to test pharmacological or surgical interventions because of their relatively larger size, fast reproduction and growth. Rats have a highly conserved homology with human physiology, and have proportional sizes and locations of important organs and regions within these, allowing to simulate several scenarios, like pathologies or physiological events. This is particularly important in the neuroscientific research, where the location, size and communication of different areas and structures are determinant for a correct function.

Therefore, many behavioral and cognitive tests were developed specifically for this animal model, taking advantage of its easiness for learning and training, and some intrinsic features of the model, like its innate curiosity for exploration, differential response to aversive and positive stimulation, and a higher resistance to stress and handling compared with mice [52].

One of the better-known cognitive test designed for rats, (that was originally developed for Wistar rats), is the Novel Object Recognition Test (NOR) designed in 1988 by Ennaceur and Delacour [109] as a rapid and relatively simple test to study short-term and working memory. This test takes advantage of the rat´s natural preference for exploring novel objects [110]. Since this test evaluates a natural-ocurred behavior, there is no need for positive or aversive stimulation [111]. The NOR can be performed, at least, in three days, in which each animal must be tested during five minutes per day. The test must be performed in an acrylic observation box, of approximately 45x45x45 cm. In day one, the habituation day, the rat is placed in the previously disinfected observation box without objects and let to explore during 5 minutes. The second day, or pretest day, two similar or identical objects, depending on the protocol, are placed in two opposite sides of the observation box and then the animal is introduced in the box to explore for five minutes. As both objects are novel for the subject of study, it explores them for a similar timelapse. The third day or test day, one of the previously used objects is changed for a different one, with disctinct texture, shape, and size (Figure 1A). If the rat´s memory pathways are intact or unharmed, the animal must explore more time the novel object compared with the previously known object, but if there is a dysfunctional memory process, it could be noted as a reduction of both, interaction time (the time in seconds the animal explore each object) and number of interactions (the numer of times each object is explored), indicating a decay in known or familiar object memory [112]. So, this test has been widely used to describe the memory process and its decaying during aging and age-related diseases in Wistar rats [112-116].

Under this same premise, Ennaceur and Meliani [117] proposed that rats were capable to discriminate between different locations of distinct objects, developing the object location memory task (OLT). This is another rapid and simple test to study spatial memory in rats, which uses a similar observation box to the one used in NOR, in which the rat is allowed to explore during 5 minutes per stage. The first day is identical to the habituation day for NOR, letting the rat to explore in the empty observation box for 5 minutes. The second day, or test day consists of two stages: the first stage or pretest, in which four objects with different shapes, but same textures and sizes are placed at equal distances in the observation box, and let the rat to explore during 5 minutes. The second stage, or test, consists in exchange the position of two random objects, letting the other two objects in their previous locations (Figure 1B). This must be performed after a short delay of time (less than 60 minutes after the pretest). If the spatial memory works appropriately, the rat will explore more time the objects with a novel location, and less time the objects with a familiar location. These two tests can be performed tougether in order to evaluate memory in a more robust way. They are usually performed to evaluate lesions or damage in memory-associated regions, such as hippocampus, prefrontal cortex, cingulate cortex and fornix, among others [118] and during the aging process [116, 119].

Another widely used test for rats is the elevated plus maze (EPM), an assay designed to evaluate the anxiety and stress responses, which was validated by Pellow, et al. in 1985 [120]. It consists of two opposite open arms of 50 x 10 cm and two opposite closed arms of 50 x 10 x 40 cm, suspended on a metallic base in an illuminated observation room. Each rat is located in the center of the maze and left to freely explore the four arms during a single five minutes session (Figure 1C). The time spent in open and closed arms must be registered, as well as the number of total enters into open and closed arms. Just like in NOR and OLT, this test was originally designed using Wistar rats. EPM is suitable to evaluate the stress and anxiety conditions during aging using the natural aversion for open spaces presented in rodents, and could be modified in order to evaluate memory as well, repeating the EPM session 24 hours after the first test [121, 122] Usually, the anxiety-related behavior is defined by the time the animal spend in the closed arms, while the more time spend in the open arms, the less anxious is its behavior [123]. It has been proposed that the anxiety levels increase with aging [124], but surprisingly, Wistar rats are less prone to develop higher levels of anxiety compared with other rat strains [125].

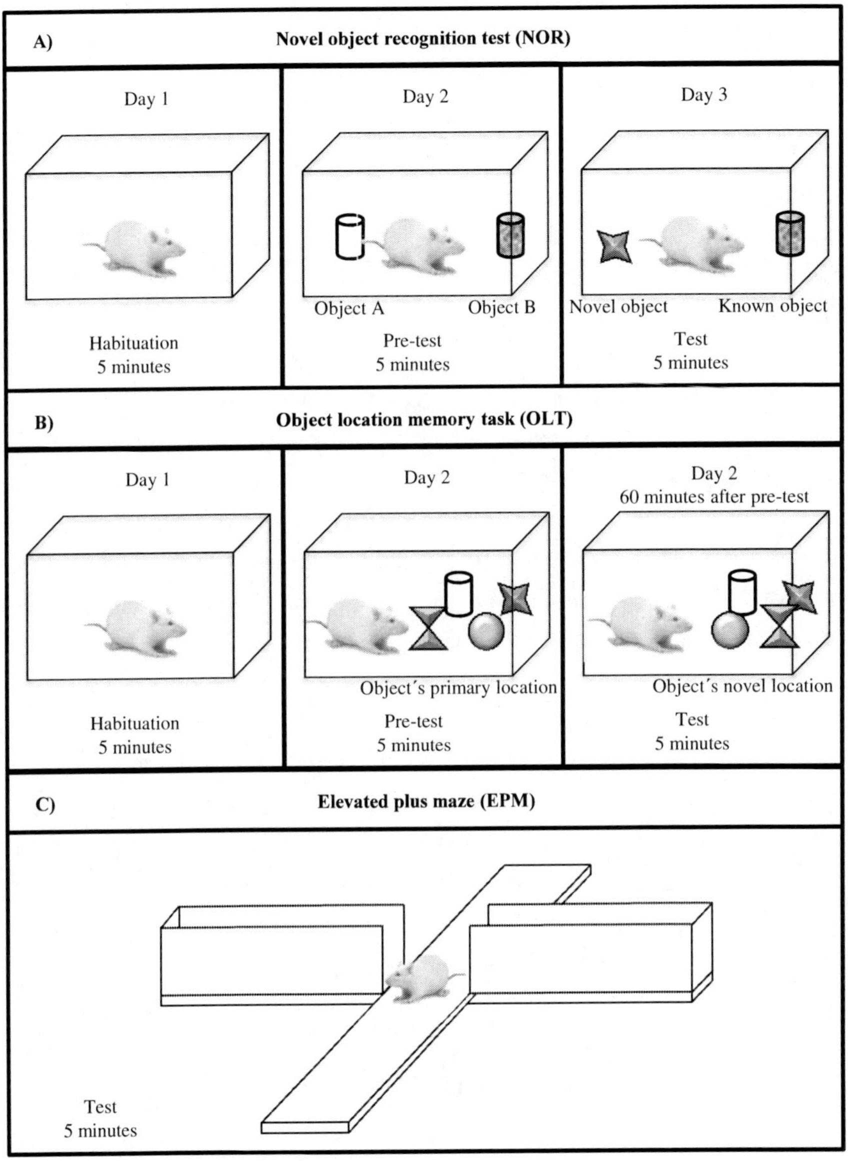


Figure 1. Cognitive tests used in Wistar rats.

## Conclusion

Both, aging and cognitive processes are complex a multifactorial phenomena which require *in vivo* models to simulate the phenotypes present in human aging, and neurodegeneration. These models allow to study the process since the beginning and stablishment of aging phenotype and deleterious neurodegeneration, up to the late stages of physiological decay. This can help to design effective strategies to contend with it and extend healthspan, and if it is possible, delay the appeareance of aging main markers. Rodents have become the most used model in biomedical research, being the rats one of the better characterized animal model. This is because of their intrinsic features that turn them into a suitable model for studying the aging process, like a relative larger size compared with mice, proportional sizes of organs and its main regions compared with human anatomy, rapid reproduction and growth and able to live in laboratory conditions. Many different rat strains have been developed according to the disctintct requirements and necessities of each research area, but one of the more importants and well characterized is the Wistar rats, an albino strain with low aggressiveness, resistance to stress and handling and a good size. With an average lifespan of 22-24 months, it is a convenient model to study the aging process in a relatively short time, and which has also been widely used in neurosciences because of its facility of training, intelligence, and cognitive complexity, making it a good choice to evaluate the progressive functional and morphological degeneration.

## Acknowledgments

This project was supported by CONACyT grants FOSSIS-272256. Santín-Márquez ia CONACyT scholarship holder.

## REFERENCES


[1] Strehler, B. L. (1962) *Time, Cells and Aging,* 1st ed., Academic Press, New York.

[2] López-Otín, C., Blasco, M. A., Partridge, L., Serrano, M., & Kroemer, G. (2013). The hallmarks of aging. *Cell,* 153(6), 1194-1217.

[3] World Health Organization. (2015). *World report on ageing and health.* Geneva: World Health Organization.

[4] Sergiev, P. V., Dontsova, O. A., & Berezkin, G. V. (2015). Theories of aging: an ever-evolving field. *Acta Naturae* (англоязычная версия), 7(1 (24)).

[5] Harman, D. (1956) Aging: a theory based on free radical and radiation chemistry, *J. Geronto L,* 11, 298-300.

[6] Harman, D. (1992). Free radical theory of aging. *Mutation Research/DNAging,* 275(3-6), 257-266.

[7] Huang, T. T., Carlson, E. J., Gillespie, A. M., Shi, Y., & Epstein, C. J. (2000). Ubiquitous overexpression of CuZn superoxide dismutase does not extend life span in mice. *Journals of Gerontology-Biological Sciences and Medical Sciences,* 55(1), B5.

[8] Pérez, V. I., Van Remmen, H., Bokov, A., Epstein, C. J., Vijg, J., & Richardson, A. (2009). The overexpression of major antioxidant enzymes does not extend the lifespan of mice. *Aging cell,* 8(1), 73-75.

[9] Hayflick, L., & Moorhead, P. S. (1961). The serial cultivation of human diploid cell strains. *Experimental cell research,* 25(3), 585-621.

[10] Serrano, M., Lin, A. W., McCurrach, M. E., Beach, D., & Lowe, S. W. (1997). Oncogenic ras provokes premature cell senescence associated with accumulation of p53 and p16INK4a. *Cell,* 88(5), 593-602.

[11] Torres C., Lewis L., Cristofalo V. J. (2006). Proteasome inhibitors shorten replicative life span and induce a senescent-like phenotype of human fibroblasts. *J Cell Physiol;* 207(3):845-53.

[12] Toussaint O., Medrano E. E., von Zglinicki T. (2000). Cellular and molecular mechanisms of stress-induced premature senescence

(SIPS) of human diploid fibroblasts and melanocytes. *Exp Gerontol.;* 35(8): 927-45.

[13] Maciel-Barón, L. Á., Morales-Rosales, S. L., Silva-Palacios, A., Rodríguez-Barrera, R. H., García-Álvarez, J. A., Luna-López, A., ... & Königsberg, M. (2018). The secretory phenotype of senescent astrocytes isolated from Wistar newborn rats changes with anti-inflammatory drugs, but does not have a short-term effect on neuronal mitochondrial potential. *Biogerontology,* 19(5), 415-433.

[14] Kuilman, T., Michaloglou, C., Mooi, W. J., & Peeper, D. S. (2010). The essence of senescence. *Genes & development,* 24(22), 2463-2479.

[15] López-Diazguerrero, N. E., Garduño, C. M. M., & Fainstein, M. K. (2005). La senescencia replicativa como una respuesta celular al estrés. *Revista de Educación Bioquímica*, 24(2), 47-53. [Replicative senescence as a cellular response to stress. *Journal of Biochemical Education*]

[16] Muñoz-Espín, D., Cañamero, M., Maraver, A., Gómez-López, G., Contreras, J., Murillo-Cuesta, S., ... & Serrano, M. (2013). Programmed cell senescence during mammalian embryonic development. *Cell,* 155(5), 1104-1118.

[17] Khapre, R. V., Kondratova, A. A., Susova, O., & Kondratov, R. V. (2011). Circadian clock protein BMAL1 regulates cellular senescence in vivo. *Cell cycle,* 10(23), 4162-4169.

[18] Tarazona, R., DelaRosa, O., Alonso, C., Ostos, B., Espejo, J., Peña, J., & Solana, R. (2001). Increased expression of NK cell markers on T lymphocytes in aging and chronic activation of the immune system reflects the accumulation of effector/senescent T cells. *Mechanisms of ageing and development,* 121(1-3), 77-88.

[19] Melk, A., Kittikowit, W., Sandhu, I., Halloran, K. M., Grimm, P., Schmidt, B. M., & Halloran, P. F. (2003). Cell senescence in rat kidneys in vivo increases with growth and age despite lack of telomere shortening. *Kidney international,* 63(6), 2134-2143.

[20] Jeyapalan, J. C., Ferreira, M., Sedivy, J. M., & Herbig, U. (2007). Accumulation of senescent cells in mitotic tissue of aging primates. *Mechanisms of ageing and development,* 128(1), 36-44.

[21] Ritzel, R. M., Crapser, J., Patel, A. R., Verma, R., Grenier, J. M., Chauhan, A., ... & McCullough, L. D. (2016). Age-associated resident memory CD8 T cells in the central nervous system are primed to potentiate inflammation after ischemic brain injury. *The Journal of Immunology*, 196(8), 3318-3330.

[22] Wu, Y., Zhang, A. Q., & Yew, D. T. (2005). Age related changes of various markers of astrocytes in senescence-accelerated mice hippocampus. *Neurochemistry international,* 46(7), 565-574.

[23] Flanary, B. E., & Streit, W. J. (2003). Telomeres shorten with age in rat cerebellum and cortex in vivo. *Journal of anti-aging medicine,* 6(4), 299-308.

[24] Freund, A., Orjalo, A. V., Desprez, P. Y., & Campisi, J. (2010). Inflammatory networks during cellular senescence: causes and consequences. *Trends in molecular medicine,* 16(5), 238-246.

[25] Pereira, B. I., Devine, O. P., Vukmanovic-Stejic, M., Chambers, E. S., Subramanian, P., Patel, N., ... & LeSaux, C. J. (2019). Senescent cells evade immune clearance via HLA-E-mediated NK and CD8+ T cell inhibition. *Nature communications,* 10(1), 2387.

[26] Vilchez, D., Saez, I., & Dillin, A. (2014). The role of protein clearance mechanisms in organismal ageing and age-related diseases. *Nature communications,* 5, 5659.

[27] Powers, E. T., Morimoto, R. I., Dillin, A., Kelly, J. W., & Balch, W. E. (2009). Biological and chemical approaches to diseases of proteostasis deficiency. *Annual review of biochemistry*, 78, 959-991.

[28] Klaips, C. L., Jayaraj, G. G., & Hartl, F. U. (2018). Pathways of cellular proteostasis in aging and disease. *J Cell Biol,* 217(1), 51-63.

[29] Ding, Q., & Zhu, H. (2015). Alteration of Proteasome System in Aging and Aging-Associated Disorders. *International Journal of Drug Development and Research.*

[30] Kastle, M., & Grune, T. (2011). Protein oxidative modification in the aging organism and the role of the ubiquitin proteasomal system. *Current pharmaceutical design,* 17(36), 4007-4022.

[31] Dasuri, K., Zhang, L., Ebenezer, P., Liu, Y., Fernandez-Kim, S. O., & Keller, J. N. (2009). Aging and dietary restriction alter proteasome biogenesis and composition in the brain and liver. *Mechanisms of ageing and development,* 130(11-12), 777-783.

[32] Gavilán, E., Pintado, C., Gavilan, M. P., Daza, P., Sánchez-Aguayo, I., Castaño, A., & Ruano, D. (2015). Age-related dysfunctions of the autophagy lysosomal pathway in hippocampal pyramidal neurons under proteasome stress. *Neurobiology of aging,* 36(5), 1953-1963.

[33] Tsakiri, E. N., & Trougakos, I. P. (2015). The amazing ubiquitin-proteasome system: structural components and implication in aging. In *International review of cell and molecular biology* (Vol. 314, pp. 171-237). Academic Press.

[34] Chondrogianni, N., Voutetakis, K., Kapetanou, M., Delitsikou, V., Papaevgeniou, N., Sakellari, M., ... & Gonos, E. S. (2015). Proteasome activation: an innovative promising approach for delaying aging and retarding age-related diseases. *Ageing Research Reviews,* 23, 37-55.

[35] Liochev, S. I. (2015). Reflections on the theories of aging, of oxidative stress, and of science in general. Is it time to abandon the free radical (oxidative stress) theory of aging?. *Antioxidants & redox signaling,* 23(3), 187-207.

[36] Jones, D. P. (2015). Redox theory of aging. *Redox biology,* 5, 71-79.

[37] Poulose, N., & Raju, R. (2014). Aging and injury: alterations in cellular energetics and organ function. *Aging and disease*, 5(2), 101.

[38] Yankner, B. A., Lu, T., & Loerch, P. (2008). The aging brain. *Annu. Rev. pathmechdis. Mech. Dis.,* 3, 41-66.

[39] Chornenkyy, Y., Fardo, D. W., & Nelson, P. T. (2019). Tau and TDP-43 proteinopathies: kindred pathologic cascades and genetic pleiotropy. *Laboratory investigation*, 1.

[40] Hung, C. W., Chen, Y. C., Hsieh, W. L., Chiou, S. H., & Kao, C. L. (2010). Ageing and neurodegenerative diseases. *Ageing research reviews,* 9, S36-S46.

[41] Damoiseaux, J. S. (2017). Effects of aging on functional and structural brain connectivity. *Neuroimage,* 160, 32-40.

[42] Carroll, M. A. (2018). Cognitive Aging and Changes in Brain Morphology. *Topics in Geriatric Rehabilitation,* 34(1), 1-7.

[43] Franceschi, C., Garagnani, P., Morsiani, C., Conte, M., Santoro, A., Grignolio, A., ... & Salvioli, S. (2018). The continuum of aging and age-related diseases: common mechanisms but different rates. *Frontiers in Medicine,* 5, 61.

[44] Lees, H., Walters, H., & Cox, L. S. (2016). Animal and human models to understand ageing. *Maturitas,* 93, 18-27.

[45] Mitchell, S. J., Scheibye-Knudsen, M., Longo, D. L., & de Cabo, R. (2015). Animal models of aging research: implications for human aging and age-related diseases. *Annu. Rev. Anim. Biosci.,* 3(1), 283-303.

[46] Chen, X., Errangi, B., Li, L., Glasser, M. F., Westlye, L. T., Fjell, A. M., ... & Rilling, J. K. (2013). Brain aging in humans, chimpanzees (*Pan troglodytes*), and rhesus macaques (*Macaca mulatta*): magnetic resonance imaging studies of macro-and microstructural changes. *Neurobiology of aging,* 34(10), 2248-2260.

[47] Bizon, J. L., Nicolle, M. M. (2006). *Handbook of Models for Human Aging.* 32 - Rat Models of Age-Related Cognitive Decline. Academic Press. 379-391. ISBN 9780123693914.

[48] Nadon, N. L., (2006). *Handbook of Models for Human Aging.* 33 - Aged Rodents for Biogerontology Research. Academic Press. 393-401, ISBN 9780123693914.

[49] Buffenstein, R. (2005). The naked mole-rat: a new long-living model for human aging research. *The Journals of Gerontology Series A: Biological Sciences and Medical Sciences,* 60(11), 1369-1377.

[50] Gorbunova, V., Bozzella, M. J., & Seluanov, A. (2008). Rodents for comparative aging studies: from mice to beavers. *Age,* 30(2-3), 111.

[51] Santulli, G., Borras, C., Bousquet, J., Calzà, L., Cano, A., Illario, M., ... & Montuori, N. (2015). *Models for preclinical studies in aging-related disorders: one is not for all.* Translational medicine@ UniSa, 13, 4.

[52] Iannaccone, P. M., & Jacob, H. J. (2009). Rats!. *Disease models & mechanisms*, 2(5-6), 206–210. doi:10.1242/dmm.002733.

[53] Ellenbroek, B., & Youn, J. (2016). Rodent models in neuroscience research: is it a rat race?. *Disease models & mechanisms,* 9(10), 1079-1087.

[54] Sengupta, P. (2013). The laboratory rat: relating its age with human's. *International journal of preventive medicine,* 4(6), 624.

[55] Foster, J. R., Frost, D. (2018). *Boorman's Pathology of the Rat* (Second Edition). 3- The History of the Rat. Academic Press. 7-12. ISBN 9780123914484.

[56] Hedrich, H. J. (2006). Taxonomy and Stocks and Strains. *The Laboratory Rat*, 71–92. doi:10.1016/b978-012074903-4/50006-6.

[57] Nadon, N. L. (2006). Gerontology and Age-Associated Lesions. *The Laboratory Rat,* 761–772. doi:10.1016/b978-012074903-4/50028-5.

[58] Austad, S. N., & Fischer, K. E. (2016). Sex differences in lifespan. *Cell metabolism,* 23(6), 1022-1033.

[59] Viña, J., Borrás, C., Gambini, J., Sastre, J., & Pallardó, F. V. (2005). Why females live longer than males? Importance of the upregulation of longevity-associated genes by oestrogenic compounds. *FEBS letters,* 579(12), 2541-2545.

[60] Borrás, C., Sastre, J., García-Sala, D., Lloret, A., Pallardó, F. V., & Viña, J. (2003). Mitochondria from females exhibit higher antioxidant gene expression and lower oxidative damage than males. *Free radical biology and medicine,* 34(5), 546-552.

[61] Kitani, K., Ohta, M., Kanai, S., & Sato, Y. (1985). Sex difference in the biliary excretion of digoxin and its metabolites in aging Wistar rats. *Archives of gerontology and geriatrics*, 4(1), 1-12.

[62] Rossetti, C. L., de Oliveira Costa, H. M., Barthem, C. S., da Silva, M. H., de Carvalho, D. P., & da-Silva, W. S. (2019). Sexual dimorphism of liver endoplasmic reticulum stress susceptibility in prepubertal rats

and the effect of sex steroid supplementation. *Experimental physiology,* 104(5), 677-690.

[63] Han, L., Li, M., Liu, Y., Han, C., & Ye, P. (2012). Atorvastatin may delay cardiac aging by upregulating peroxisome proliferator-activated receptors in rats. *Pharmacology,* 89(1-2), 74-82.

[64] Zarzuelo, M. J., López-Sepúlveda, R., Sánchez, M., Romero, M., Gómez-Guzmán, M., Ungvary, Z., ... & Duarte, J. (2013). SIRT1 inhibits NADPH oxidase activation and protects endothelial function in the rat aorta: implications for vascular aging. *Biochemical pharmacology,* 85(9), 1288-1296.

[65] Basha, D. C., Basha, S. S., & Reddy, G. R. (2012). Lead-induced cardiac and hematological alterations in aging Wistar male rats: alleviating effects of nutrient metal mixture. *Biogerontology,* 13(4), 359-368.

[66] Tezini, G. C., Dias, D. P., & Souza, H. C. (2013). Aerobic physical training has little effect on cardiovascular autonomic control in aging rats subjected to early menopause. *Experimental gerontology,* 48(2), 147-153.

[67] Rossoni, L. V., Oliveira, R. A., Caffaro, R. R., Miana, M., Sanz-Rosa, D., Koike, M. K., ... & Cachofeiro, V. (2011). Cardiac benefits of exercise training in aging spontaneously hypertensive rats. *Journal of hypertension,* 29(12), 2349-2358.

[68] Gonçalves, L., de Souza, R. R., Maifrino, L. B. M., Caperuto, É. C., Carbone, P. O., Rodrigues, B., & Gama, E. F. (2014). Resistance exercise and testosterone treatment alters the proportion of numerical density of capillaries of the left ventricle of aging Wistar rats. *The Aging Male,* 17(4), 243-247.

[69] da Luz, P. L., Tanaka, L., Brum, P. C., Dourado, P. M. M., Favarato, D., Krieger, J. E., & Laurindo, F. R. M. (2012). Red wine and equivalent oral pharmacological doses of resveratrol delay vascular aging but do not extend life span in rats. *Atherosclerosis,* 224(1), 136-142.

[70] Kim, S. Y., Park, J. T., Park, J. K., Lee, J. S., & Choi, J. C. (2011). Aging impairs vasodilatory responses in rats. *Korean journal of anesthesiology,* 61(6), 506.

[71] Machi, J. F., da Silva Dias, D., Freitas, S. C., de Moraes, O. A., da Silva, M. B., Cruz, P. L., ... & Irigoyen, M. C. (2016). Impact of aging on cardiac function in a female rat model of menopause: role of autonomic control, inflammation, and oxidative stress. *Clinical interventions in aging,* 11, 341.

[72] Sierra Rojas, J. X., García-San Frutos, M., Horrillo, D., Lauzurica, N., Oliveros, E., Carrascosa, J. M., ... & Ros, M. (2015). Differential development of inflammation and insulin resistance in different adipose tissue depots along aging in Wistar rats: effects of caloric restriction. *Journals of Gerontology Series A: Biomedical Sciences and Medical Sciences,* 71(3), 310-322.

[73] Bellaver, B., Souza, D. G., Souza, D. O., & Quincozes-Santos, A. (2014). Resveratrol increases antioxidant defenses and decreases proinflammatory cytokines in hippocampal astrocyte cultures from newborn, adult and aged Wistar rats. *Toxicology in Vitro,* 28(4), 479-484.

[74] Shailaja, M., Gowda, K. D., Vishakh, K., & Kumari, N. S. (2017). Anti-aging role of curcumin by modulating the inflammatory markers in albino wistar rats. *Journal of the National Medical Association,* 109(1), 9-13.

[75] *Melatonin Counteracts at a Transcriptional Level the Inflammatory and Apoptotic Response Secondary to Ischemic Brain Injury Induced by Middle Cerebral Artery Blockade in Aging Rats.*

[76] Costa, E., Fernandes, J., Ribeiro, S., Sereno, J., Garrido, P., Rocha-Pereira, P., ... & Vala, H. (2014). Aging is associated with impaired renal function, INF-gamma induced inflammation and with alterations in iron regulatory proteins gene expression. *Aging and disease,* 5(6), 356.

[77] Horrillo, D., Sierra, J., Arribas, C., García-San Frutos, M., Carrascosa, J. M., Lauzurica, N., ... & Ros, M. (2011). Age-associated development of inflammation in Wistar rats: Effects of caloric

restriction. *Archives of physiology and biochemistry,* 117(3), 140-150.

[78] Yuan, J., Lu, L., Zhang, Z., & Zhang, S. (2012). Dietary intake of resveratrol enhances the adaptive immunity of aged rats. *Rejuvenation research,* 15(5), 507-515.

[79] Li, M., Ouyang, W., Li, J., Si, L., Li, X., Guo, J., & Li, H. (2016). Effects of kinetin on thymus and immune function of aging rats. *Pak Vet J,* 36, 356-362.

[80] Lu, L., Yuan, J., & Zhang, S. (2013). Rejuvenating activity of salidroside (SDS): dietary intake of SDS enhances the immune response of aged rats. *Age,* 35(3), 637-646.

[81] Braidy, N., Guillemin, G. J., Mansour, H., Chan-Ling, T., Poljak, A., & Grant, R. (2011). Age related changes in NAD+ metabolism oxidative stress and Sirt1 activity in wistar rats. *PloS one,* 6(4), e19194.

[82] Zhang, Y. B., Zhong, Z. M., Hou, G., Jiang, H., & Chen, J. T. (2011). Involvement of oxidative stress in age-related bone loss. *Journal of Surgical Research,* 169(1), e37-e42.

[83] Anand, K. V., Mohamed Jaabir, M. S., Thomas, P. A., & Geraldine, P. (2012). Protective role of chrysin against oxidative stress in d-galactose-induced aging in an experimental rat model. *Geriatrics & gerontology international,* 12(4), 741-750.

[84] Avramovic, N., Dragutinovic, V., Krstic, D., Colovic, M. B., Trbovic, A., De Luka, S., ... & Popovic, T. (2012). The effects of omega 3 fatty acid supplementation on brain tissue oxidative status in aged wistar rats. *Hippokratia,* 16(3), 241.

[85] Hou, G., Lu, H., Chen, M., Yao, H., & Zhao, H. (2014). Oxidative stress participates in age-related changes in rat lumbar intervertebral discs. *Archives of gerontology and geriatrics,* 59(3), 665-669.

[86] Sharma, S., Singh, R., Kaur, M., & Kaur, G. (2010). Late-onset dietary restriction compensates for age-related increase in oxidative stress and alterations of HSP 70 and synapsin1 protein levels in male Wistar rats. *Biogerontology,* 11(2), 197-209.

[87] Devi, S. A., Chandrasekar, B. S., Manjula, K., & Ishii, N. (2011). Grape seed proanthocyanidin lowers brain oxidative stress in adult and middle-aged rats. *Experimental Gerontology,* 46(11), 958-964.

[88] Subramanian, M. V., & James, T. J. (2010). Age-related protective effect of deprenyl on changes in the levels of diagnostic marker enzymes and antioxidant defense enzymes activities in cerebellar tissue in Wistar rats. *Cell Stress and Chaperones,* 15(5), 743-751.

[89] Miler, M., Živanović, J., Ajdžanović, V., Oreščanin-Dušić, Z., Milenković, D., Konić-Ristić, A., ... & Šošić-Jurjević, B. (2016). Citrus flavanones naringenin and hesperetin improve antioxidant status and membrane lipid compositions in the liver of old-aged Wistar rats. *Experimental Gerontology,* 84, 49-60.

[90] Horrillo, D., Gallardo, N., Lauzurica, N., Barrus, M. T., San, M. F., Andres, A., ... & Fernandez-Agullo, T. (2013). Development of liver fibrosis during aging: Effects of caloric restriction. *Journal of biological regulators and homeostatic agents,* 27(2), 377-388.

[91] Mimura, S., Iwama, H., Kato, K., Nomura, K., Kobayashi, M., Yoneyama, H., ... & Deguchi, A. (2014). Profile of microRNAs associated with aging in rat liver. *International journal of molecular medicine,* 34(4), 1065-1072.

[92] Bakala, H., Ladouce, R., Baraibar, M. A., & Friguet, B. (2013). Differential expression and glycative damage affect specific mitochondrial proteins with aging in rat liver. *Biochimica et Biophysica Acta (BBA)-Molecular Basis of Disease,* 1832(12), 2057-2067.

[93] Kumar, P., Kale, R. K., & Baquer, N. Z. (2011). Estradiol modulates membrane-linked ATPases, antioxidant enzymes, membrane fluidity, lipid peroxidation, and lipofuscin in aged rat liver. *Journal of aging research,* 2011.

[94] Helmy, M. M. (2012). Potential hepato-protective effect of α-tocopherol or simvastatin in aged rats. *Pharmacological Reports,* 64(3), 698-705.

[95] Garcia-Fernandez, M., Sierra, I., Puche, J. E., Guerra, L., & Castilla-Cortazar, I. (2011). Liver mitochondrial dysfunction is reverted by

insulin-like growth factor II (IGF-II) in aging rats. *Journal of translational medicine,* 9(1), 123.

[96] Yun, K. U., Oh, S. J., Oh, J. M., Kang, K. W., Myung, C. S., Song, G. Y., ... & Kim, S. K. (2010). Age-related changes in hepatic expression and activity of cytochrome P450 in male rats. *Archives of toxicology,* 84(12), 939-946.

[97] Kumar, D., & Rizvi, S. I. (2014). Markers of oxidative stress in senescent erythrocytes obtained from young and old age rats. *Rejuvenation research,* 17(5), 446-452.

[98] Bai, X. Y., Ma, Y., Ding, R., Fu, B., Shi, S., & Chen, X. M. (2011). miR-335 and miR-34a Promote renal senescence by suppressing mitochondrial antioxidative enzymes. *Journal of the American Society of Nephrology,* 22(7), 1252-1261.

[99] Shimizu, M. H. M., Volpini, R. A., de Bragança, A. C., Campos, R., Canale, D., Sanches, T. R., ... & Seguro, A. C. (2013). N-acetylcysteine attenuates renal alterations induced by senescence in the rat. *Experimental gerontology,* 48(2), 298-303.

[100] Bellaver, B., Souza, D. G., Souza, D. O., & Quincozes-Santos, A. (2017). Hippocampal astrocyte cultures from adult and aged rats reproduce changes in glial functionality observed in the aging brain. *Molecular neurobiology,* 54(4), 2969-2985.

[101] Avramovic, N., Dragutinovic, V., Krstic, D., Colovic, M. B., Trbovic, A., De Luka, S., ... & Popovic, T. (2012). The effects of omega 3 fatty acid supplementation on brain tissue oxidative status in aged wistar rats. *Hippokratia,* 16(3), 241.

[102] Braidy, N., Poljak, A., Grant, R., Jayasena, T., Mansour, H., Chan-Ling, T., ... & Guillemin, G. J. (2015). Differential expression of sirtuins in the aging rat brain. *Frontiers in cellular neuroscience,* 9, 167.

[103] Garrido, P., de Blas, M., Del Arco, A., Segovia, G., & Mora, F. (2012). Aging increases basal but not stress-induced levels of corticosterone in the brain of the awake rat. *Neurobiology of aging,* 33(2), 375-382.

[104] Stefanova, N. A., Fursova, A. Z., & Kolosova, N. G. (2010). Behavioral effects induced by mitochondria-targeted antioxidant SkQ1 in Wistar and senescence-accelerated OXYS rats. *Journal of Alzheimer's Disease,* 21(2), 479-491.

[105] Vančová, O. G., Bačiak, L., Kašparová, S., Kucharská, J., Palacios, H. H., Horecký, J., & Aliev, G. (2010). In vivo and in vitro assessment of brain bioenergetics in aging rats. *Journal of cellular and molecular medicine,* 14(11), 2667-2674.

[106] Krištofiková, Z., Říčný, J., Ort, M., & Řípová, D. (2010). Aging and lateralization of the rat brain on a biochemical level. *Neurochemical research,* 35(8), 1138-1146.

[107] Batista-de-Oliveira, M., Lopes, A. A. C., Mendes-da-Silva, R. F., & Guedes, R. C. A. (2012). Aging-dependent brain electrophysiological effects in rats after distinct lactation conditions, and treadmill exercise: a spreading depression analysis. *Experimental gerontology,* 47(6), 452-457.

[108] Quintas, A., de Solís, A. J., Díez-Guerra, F. J., Carrascosa, J. M., & Bogónez, E. (2012). Age-associated decrease of SIRT1 expression in rat hippocampus: prevention by late onset caloric restriction. *Experimental gerontology*, 47(2), 198-201.

[109] Ennaceur, A., & Delacour, J. (1988). A new one-trial test for neurobiological studies of memory in rats. 1: Behavioral data. *Behavioural brain research,* 31(1), 47-59.

[110] Mathiasen, J. R., & DiCamillo, A. (2010). Novel object recognition in the rat: a facile assay for cognitive function. *Current protocols in pharmacology,* 49(1), 5-59.

[111] Lueptow, L. M. (2017). Novel object recognition test for the investigation of learning and memory in mice. *JoVE (Journal of Visualized Experiments),* (126), e55718.

[112] Ennaceur, A. (2010). One-trial object recognition in rats and mice: methodological and theoretical issues. *Behavioural brain research,* 215(2), 244-254.

[113] Gámiz, F., & Gallo, M. (2012). Spontaneous object recognition memory in aged rats: Complexity versus similarity. *Learning & Memory,* 19(10), 444-448.

[114] Kersten, M., Rabbe, T., Blome, R., Porath, K., Sellmann, T., Bien, C. G., ... & Kirschstein, T. (2019). Novel object recognition in rats with NMDAR dysfunction in CA1 after stereotactic injection of anti-NMDAR encephalitis cerebrospinal fluid. *Frontiers in neurology,* 10, 586.

[115] Hirst, W. D., Stean, T. O., Rogers, D. C., Sunter, D., Pugh, P., Moss, S. F., ... & Heidbreder, C. A. (2006). SB-399885 is a potent, selective 5-HT6 receptor antagonist with cognitive enhancing properties in aged rat water maze and novel object recognition models. *European journal of pharmacology*, 553(1-3), 109-119.

[116] Platano, D., Fattoretti, P., Balietti, M., Bertoni-Freddari, C., & Aicardi, G. (2008). Long-term visual object recognition memory in aged rats. *Rejuvenation research,* 11(2), 333-339.

[117] Ennaceur, A., & Meliani, K. (1992). A new one-trial test for neurobiological studies of memory in rats. III. Spatial vs. non-spatial working memory. *Behavioural brain research,* 51(1), 83-92.

[118] Ennaceur, A., Neave, N., & Aggleton, J. P. (1997). Spontaneous object recognition and object location memory in rats: the effects of lesions in the cingulate cortices, the medial prefrontal cortex, the cingulum bundle and the fornix. *Experimental brain research,* 113(3), 509-519.

[119] Cost, K. T., Williams–Yee, Z. N., Fustok, J. N., & Dohanich, G. P. (2012). Sex differences in object-in-place memory of adult rats. *Behavioral neuroscience,* 126(3), 457.

[120] Pellow, S., Chopin, P., File, S. E., & Briley, M. (1985). Validation of open: closed arm entries in an elevated plus-maze as a measure of anxiety in the rat. *Journal of neuroscience methods,* 14(3), 149-167.

[121] Morales Delgado, N., Popovic, N., De La Cruz Sanchez, E., Caballero Bleda, M., & Popovic, M. (2018). Time-of-day and age impact on memory in elevated plus-maze in rats. *Frontiers in behavioral neuroscience,* 12, 304.

[122] Walf, A. A., & Frye, C. A. (2007). The use of the elevated plus maze as an assay of anxiety-related behavior in rodents. *Nature protocols,* 2(2), 322.

[123] Leo, L. M., & Pamplona, F. A. (2014). Elevated plus maze test to assess anxiety-like behavior in the mouse. *Bio-protocol,* 4(16), e1211.

[124] Meyza, K. Z., Boguszewski, P. M., Nikolaev, E., & Zagrodzka, J. (2011). Age increases anxiety and reactivity of the fear/anxiety circuit in Lewis rats. *Behavioural brain research,* 225(1), 192-200.

[125] Ferguson, S. A., & Gray, E. P. (2005). Aging effects on elevated plus maze behavior in spontaneously hypertensive, Wistar–Kyoto and Sprague–Dawley male and female rats. *Physiology & behavior,* 85(5), 621-628.

In: Laboratory Animals and Neurosciences ISBN: 978-1-53618-462-4
Editors: B. Hernandez Godinez et al.

*Chapter 11*

# NEURAL TUBE DEFECTS: LONGITUDINAL STUDY WITH THE USE OF NON-HUMAN PRIMATES (*MACACA MULATTA*) AS AN EXPERIMENTAL ANIMAL MODEL IN THE INTRAUTERINE CORRECTION OF MYELOMENINGOCELE

***Alejandra Ibáñez-Contreras[1,2,*], Martín García-Servin[3] and Braulio Hernández-Godínez[1,2]***

[1]Non Human Unit of APREXBIO S.A.S. de C.V. Ciudad de México, México
[2]Neurophisiology Laboratory of Investigación Biomédica Aplicada (INBIOMA) S.A.S. de C.V., Ciudad de México, México
[3]Instituto de Neurobiología, Universidad Nacional Autónoma de México, Campus Juriquilla, Queretaro, México

* Corresponding Author's E-mail: Ibanez.alejandra@hotmail.com.

## Abstract

Myelomeningocele is the most common congenital malformation of the central nervous system. Experimental studies demonstrated that the neurological deficit is not a cause for a primary defect in neurulation but is probably due to the progressive mechanical and chemical damage of amniotic liquid into the nerve tissue, which remained without protection during gestation. We undertook this study to develop an animal model in myelomeningocele in *Macaca mulatta* and compare the results of prenatal management between the colocations of an impermeable silicone mesh and closed with skin. *Macaca mulatta* is an appropriate model for reproducing myelomeningocele and to evaluate the different options for prenatal management. Colocation of an impermeable silicone mesh is feasible, protecting the spine from amniotic liquid, with results similar to skin closure.

**Keywords**: neural tube defects, myelomeningocele, evoked potentials, *Macaca mulatta*

## Introduction

In the last 50 years the worldwide epidemiological transition has generated important changes, so that non transmissible diseases have replaced transmissible diseases as the main causes of mortality. Among these non transmissible diseases birth defects are recorded, it is observed that around 3-5% of infants are suffering from some major malformation, with direct functional and / or direct aesthetic.

Among the most common birth defects, there are neural tube defects (NTDs) that include a large number of congenital malformations. The neural tube begins from a flat sheet of neuroepithelial cells (the neural plate), which rolls or folds in the midline to form the neural tube. This occurs at 3–4 weeks after fertilization, a time when some women do not yet realize that they are pregnant. Closure of the neural tube begins at the cervical region and extends cranially and caudally.

However, the closure is complex, and as in other mammals, occurs in a discontinuous process (Mancebo-Hernández et al. 2008; Tauheed et al. 2017; Oliveira-Brancati et al. 2019). It's estimated that the prevalence of NTD´s is approximately 6 out of 10,000 live birds worldwide, 90% of children with NTD are born in families where this had never happened before, around 75% of affected pregnancies end up in abortion or still birth and only 25% of this children liveborn with a series of complications like paralysis, mental retardation, hydrocephalus, incontinence, etc., affecting the life of the infant and his family.

NTD´s are the leading cause of early miscarriage, stillbirth, perinatal death, and infant and child death. They are a group of conditions whose etiology is multifactorial, product of the interaction of genetic and environmental factors. They are a group of conditions whose etiology is multifactorial. Product of the interaction of genetic and enviroment factors (Vieira and Castillo Taucher, 2005; Corral et al. 2006; Oliveira-Brancati et al. 2019). Some birth defects are caused by known genetic factors, such as chromosome aberrations or genetic mutations, environmental factors, or interactions between genetic factors and environmental factors (Qu et al. 2019). For example, Zika virus infection during pregnancy has been linked to adverse congenital outcomes including microcephaly, neural tube defects, early brain malformations, structural eye abnormalities, congenital deafness, and limb contractures (Hall et al. 2017).

NTD´s contribute to 50% of neonatal deaths, besides being a leading cause of infant mortality and lifelong disabilities (Arıoğlu Aydın et al., 2015). These defects vary in severity depending on the type and level of injury. They are classified into head defects and caudal defects; in turn they are subdivided into open and closed defects. They are currently classified according to the point of closure of the affected neural tube where the cellular and tissue adhesion mechanisms failed. Based on the above, there are: spina bifida (SB), hidden spina bifida, cystic spina bifida, the latter is futher subdivided into meningocele (MC), myelomeningocele (MMC), anencephaly and rachischisis (Mancebo-Hernández 2008; Berihu et al. 2018).

**Table 1. Neural tube defect pathophysiology**

| Neural Tube Defects | Malformation |
|---|---|
| Cranial | |
| Anencephaly | Failure of fusion of cephalic portion of neural folds; absence of all or part of brain, skull and skin. |
| Exencephaly | Failure of scalp and skull formation; exteriorization of abnormally formed brain |
| Encephalocele | Failure of complete skull formation; extrusion of brain tissue into membranous sac |
| Iniencephaly | Defect of cervical and upper thoracic vertebrae; abnormally formed brain tissue and extreme retroflexion of upper spin |
| Spinal | |
| Spina bifida | Failure of fusion of caudal portion of neural tube, usually of 3–5 contiguous vertebrae; spinal cord or meninges, or both, exposed to amniotic fluid |
| Meningocele | Failure of fusion of caudal portion of neural tube; meninges exposed |
| Myelomeningocele | Failure of fusion of caudal portion of neural tube; meninges and neural tissue exposed |
| Myeloschisis | Failure of fusion of caudal portion of neural tube; flattened mass of neural tissue exposed |
| Holorachischisis | Failure of fusion of vertebral arches; entire spinal cord exposed |
| Craniorachischisis | Coexisting anencephaly and open neural tube defect, often in the cervical–thoracic region |

Note: Taken from Committee on Practice Bulletins-Obstetrics (2017).

Each year, there are about 3,000,000 pregnancies affected by NTD´s in the world. Worldwide, it is estimated that of the registered annual births, the frequency of NTD´s includes 400,000 cases of anencephaly and 300, 000 cases of spina bifida (Mancebo-Hernández 2008; Sanz – Cortez et al. 2019). Globally, more than 10% of neonatal mortality is caused by embryological malformation of the nervous system. A recent systematic review, including data from 75 countries, reported a wide-ranging prevalence; the median prevalence based on World Health Organization (WHO) region ranged from 6.9 per 10,000 births in the Western Pacific, to 21.9 per 10,000 births in the Middle East (Committee on Practice Bulletins-Obstetrics, 2017). Though the prevalence of NTDs has reduced recently in the developed world, it still remains high in the developing world with an estimated prevalence rate ranging between 1 to 11/1000 births, with almost equal frequencies between the two varieties that occur most frequently: anencephaly and spina bifida (Berihu et al. 2018).

Morbidity and mortality due to defects of the central nervous system CNS), and especially due to NTD´s, are high and vary from country to country and even in different geographical areas in the same nation (Copp et al. 2016).

An estimated 60% of the world's population lives in Asia. Worldwide NTDs, comprising anencephaly and spinal dysraphism, are estimated to occur in 15–23 per 10,000 live births, with a higher prevalence reported in Southern Asia, at an estimated 22–43 per 10,000 live births. The most common form of spinal dysraphism occurs along the dorsal spine, referred to as open spina bifida (SB). Myelomeningocele (MMC), the most common form of open SB, has long been associated with several comorbidities such as hydrocephalus, Chiari II malformation, tethered cord, scoliotic and kyphotic spinal deformities, skin injuries, as well as, neurogenic bowel and bladder (Bradko et al. 2019).

Approximately 5.6% of pregnancies in China, including both live births and pregnancy losses, are affected by birth defects. There are approximately 0.25 million births with major defects every year in China, which leads to a substantial disease burden (Qu et al. 2019).

In the United States, approximately 4000 pregnancies each year are affected by the two most common NTDs (spina bifida and anencephaly). The estimated spina bifida prevalence was reported at approximately 3.39 per 10,000 live births in the US during 2003–2004 (Au et al. 2008; Copp et al. 2016).

It is estimated that in Singapore 4% of births have NTDs, with an incidence of 0.91 per 1,000 full-term births in the period 1993-2002. The two main conditions are spina bifida and anencephaly with a percentage of 63%. While 80-90% with spina bifida survives in adulthood with varying degrees of morbidity, on the other hand anencephalic fetuses do not survive the first 24 hrs (Tan et al. 2007).

Further, in low-income countries, 17% to 70% of neonatal deaths from birth defects are attributed to NTD´s (Blencowe et al. 2010). However, scanty and fragmented surveillance information hinders the ability to adequately determine the prevalence of NTD in more than 11 million births per year in Latin America.

According to Pacheco – Santos et al. (2016), demostrated the efficiency of iron and floic acid fortification. This based on the registration of births in the center, southeast and south of Brazil. Where the prevalence of NTD´s was determined among live births and stillbirths in the period prior to the enrichment, that is, from 2001 to 2004, and in the post-enrichment period, that is, from 2005 to 2014. A distincion was made between anencephaly, encephalocele, meningocele, myelomeningocele, and other forms of SB. Their results show that were 8,554 NTD´s among the 17,925,729 live births reported between 2001 and 2014. During the same period, 2,673 NTD´s were registered among the 194,858 stillbirths. The overall prevalence of NTD´s decreased from 0.79 per 1,000 births before enrichment to 0.55 per 1,000 births after enrichment. In the case of stillbirths, the prevalence decreased from 17.74 per 1,000 stillbirths before enrichment to 11.70 per 1,000 stillbirths after enrichment.

In particular, it is know that the incidence of NTD´s in México, constitutes the third cause, in terms of frecuency of new cases, that cause neurological damage (Blanco-Muñoz et al. 2005). In Mexico, there is a prevalence of 4.9 per 10,000 of NTD's, 75% of cases correspond to SB. Mexico has one of the highest frequencies of anencephaly in the world, with a reported rate of 13.34 per 10,000 live births.

The frecuency of anencephaly cases has decreased due to spontaneous or elective abortions, influenced by prenatal diagnosis. The epidemiological registry detected a substantial reduction in the incidence of NTD's in 2002 and a second reduction in 2008; however, in 2014 a rebound was observed, mainly in anencephaly and myelomeningocele (Galván-Montaño et al. 2010).

## Mielomeningocele (MMC)

Myelomeningocele (MMC) is considered a nonlethal birth defect that affects children, causing various degrees of decline of the somatosensory system, dysfunction of the vesical and rectal sphincter, paraplegia, skeletal deformities, sexual dysfunction, hydrocephalus and mental retardation (Galván-Montaño et al. 2007; Farmer et al. 2018). The primary disorder in the pathogenesis of MMC is failed neural tube closure in the embryonic spinal region, which leads to prolonged exposure of the open neural tube to the amniotic fluid environment (Copp et al. 2016). Individuals with MMC often exhibit motor and sensory neurological deficit below the level of the lesion. There is a strong correlation between the axial level of lesion and the degree of disability experienced by individuals with MMC. This may result in lower limb weakness or paralysis. Urinary and fecal incontinence occur frequently, as does hindbrain herniation related to the Chiari II malformation of the hindbrain and associated hydrocephalus which often requires shunting. The most frequently orthopedic abnormalities are hip dislocation, contractures, scoliosis and kyphosis (Galván-Montaño et al. 2007; Copp et al. 2016).

MMC health costs are 13 times greater than those of unaffected children (Farmer et al. 2018). The lifetime cost of a child born with MMC is estimated at over €500,000 ($600,000), of which 37% comprises direct medical costs with the remainder being indirect costs including special educational and care-giver needs, and loss of employment potential (Copp et al. 2016).

In view of these life-changing health and economic consequences of MMC, it has been necessary to create experimental models that allow simulating the injuries and their possible treatments. The intrauterine surgery is an option for correction and temporary handling while the product is born. With the improvement of prenatal diagnostics and prenatal surgical techniques, surgeons began to repair the lesion before birth with the hope of preventing in utero spinal cord trauma. Preliminary studies indicated that prenatal intervention resulted in more desirable outcomes than postnatal repair (Farmer et al. 2018; Kabagambe et al. 2018; Botelho et al. 2017).

In past years several investigations have been developed in animal, establishing models that recreate congenital diseases feasible of surgical correction *in uterus (*Adzick et al. 1985, Harrison et al. 1982, Meuli et al. 1995, Michedja 1984, Olutoye and Adzick 1999, Pedreira et al. 2007, Timothy and Fuh 2003). In the last years there has been diverse research in animals, like the one performed by Heffez et al. (1990, 1993), in rats, Pedreira et al. (2002, 2003), in rabbits, Meuli et al. (1995), in sheep, Pedreira et al. 2007) in ovine fetuses and Michjeda (1984) in non-human primates *Macaca mulatta*; creating intrauterine surgical models to reproduce different diseases and perform its correction. Also, George and Fuh (2003), describe the use of non-human primates (*Macaca mulatta*), as models for the surgical correction of diseases for the neural tube. These have allowed the intrauterine correction of different pathologies in humans, such as myelomeningocele, sacrococcygeal teratoma, obstruction of the urinary tract and lung adenomatoide disease. Meuli et al. (1995, 1996), created a sheep model in fetal lambs at 75 days of gestation by excision of skin, paraspinal musculature, vertebral arches of lumbar vertebrae L1-4, and the exposed dorsal dura mater. The pregnancy was then continued to near term, and cesarean section was performed at 140 days of gestation. The lambs developed lumbar cystic sacs with abnormal spinal cord tissue on the dorsal aspect. The histology results revealed loss of neural tissue, disruption of neural bundles, and areas of cord necrosis in the exposed segments, strikingly similar to that seen in human MMC. The spinal cord and its coverings proximal to the lesion appeared normal. Clinically, the lambs demonstrated incontinence of urine and stool, flaccid paraplegia, as well as lack of sensation in the hindlimbs, which was confirmed by somatosensory evoked potentials. The first animal model was in primates (*Macaca mulatta*), in which a fetal L3–5 laminectomy was performed late in gestation. The unrepaired fetuses showed cystic MMC-like lesions at birth and had neurologic deficits. A similar group of monkeys underwent immediate repair of the laminectomy in utero using allogeneic bone paste to reconstruct the resected dorsal arches. These fetuses repaired in utero were neurologically normal at birth (Adzick 2009). In other hand, Heffez et al. (1990, 1993) used fetal rats and pigs and demonstrated the increased loss of spinal cord tissue in a group not undergoing immediate repair. Stiefel et al. (2007), studied the curly tail mouse model of exposed lumbosacral SB and demonstrated progressive deterioration of neuroanatomic appearance and neurologic function with increasing gestational age.

## METHODS

### Animals

Ten female monkeys *Macaca mulatta* between the ages of 4 and 10, weighing between 4500 grams and 7500 grams, and in week twelve of gestation were the subjects of this study. A total of nine fetuses had surgery, divided in three experimental groups, on all of them laminectomy in L5 and L6 was performed.

Monkeys were housed in captivity in the PIMVS facilities (Proyecto CAMINA A.C), registration number DGVS-PIMVS-CR-IN-1014-D.F./08 at SEMARNAT (Environmental and Natural Resources Secretary). All procedures with animals were strictly carried out according to the Mexican Official Ethics Standard NOM-062-ZOO-1999, and were also approved by the Internal Committee of Laboratory Animals Care and Use, as well as the Ethics and Research Commissions of CAMINA A.C. Research Center and APREXBIO S.A.S de C.V.

The animals were divided into four areas, each area conformed an independent social group to promote animal welfare. The rooms' building materials consisted of concrete floors. All surfaces were covered with ceramic tiles, and the outer walls were a wire mesh, firmly anchored to the walls and floors, in order to provide the animals with a natural photoperiod. The ceilings offered a secure waterproof covering, and the doors were locked to ensure the safety of both the animals and their handlers. Automatic water dispensers and feed tanks were placed outside the walls of each area to avoid food contact with feces and urine.

## Experimental Groups

The two models used in the surgical correction in order to protect the exposure of the spinal cord to the amniotic fluid were: mesh placement in three fetuses, and suture of the skin in other three fetuses. Other three fetuses exposed to the amniotic fluid were evaluated as models, simulating myelomeningocele. A tenth fetus was evaluated as a control model to compare the normal development and maturity, both intrauterine and extrauterine.

## Animal Preparation

The animals were isolated from the group in which they lived 12 hours prior surgery, they had an eight-hour fasting period, and were placed in stainless steel metabolic cages.

The cages were special for non-human primates and were in a room with controlled climate at a temperature of 23°C. They were physically restrained to administer Tiletamine-Zolazepam (Zoletil, Laboratorios Virbac S.A., Carros, France) 4mg/kg by intramuscular route, an hour before surgery (Hernández-Godínez et al. 2018, 2019). A catheter 22 (Becton Dickinson Insytec® 0.9X25 mm) was placed in the cephalic vein, and a lukewarm 5% glucosed solution, 50 ml, was administered through a venoclyisis (Flebotek®) during 30 minutes. One hundred ml of a lukewarm 0.9% sodium chlorine solution was administered during the surgical time and postoperative. Cardiac frequency, respiratory frequency, arterial pressure, oxygen saturation and temperature were monitored with an Ohmeda Cardiocap/5® monitor (Datex-Ohmeda Inc., Louisville, KY, USA). The electrodes were collocated on the thorax, to monitor the heart rate and the respiratory rate; to measure the arterial pressure we put the cuff on the inside part of the right leg thigh. Oxigen saturation was measured from the right-hand thumb with the SpO2 Sensor (Hernández-Godínez et al. 2019; Ibáñez Contreras et al. 2016, 2018).

## Animal Anestesia

Atropine, 0.02 mg/kg was administered IV, a number 3 face mask was placed, and 3 – 4 liters of oxygen with 4% of Sevoflurane was administered per minute with a vaporizer (Ohmeda®) (Galván -Montaño et al. 2010). Palpebral and deglutory reflexes were watched so intubation with and endotraqueal tube without balloon numbers 4, 4.5 or 5 could be placed when they disappeared. The size of the endotraqueal tube used depended on the individual, and a pediatric laryngoscope (Welch Allen®) with a straight blade size 2 was used to place the tube. Once the individual was intubated, the concentration of sevoflurane was reduced to 2%, staying like that for the rest of the perioperative time (Galván-Montaño et al. 2010, Hernandez-Godinez et al. 2011). Before the surgery started, 10 μg of Fentanyl were administered IV. During the surgical procedure the variables were registered every 10 minutes.

## Surgical Procedure

Once with intubation, Fentanyl 10 μcgs was supplied, by a supra-half infraumbilical incision cutting skin, aponeurosis and peritoneum. The uterus was identified and exteriorized, and the position of the fetus was determined by an ultrasound and palpation, afterwards a transverse incision was done in all layers, including the amniotic membranes, of the inferior uterus segment. The uterus was incised transversely at the level of the lumbar region of the product until the amniotic membrane opened. Amniotic fluid was withdrawn with syringes and saved for later use. At the level of the lumbar region, an incision was made and a laminectomy was performed at L5 and L6, identifying the dura, cutting and leaving the spinal cord exposed. According to the study group, at this time it was approached with skin using nylon 7-0, a silicone mesh was placed holding it around the skin with the same suture or it was left exposed. After the fetal surgery was completed, the warm amniotic fluid was reintroduced with 100 mg of cephalotin and the uterine window was sutured together with the amniotic membranes. The uterus was reintroduced into the abdominal cavity, the abdominal wall was closed by planes, and 10 mg/kg of metamizole was administered intravenously (Figure 1).

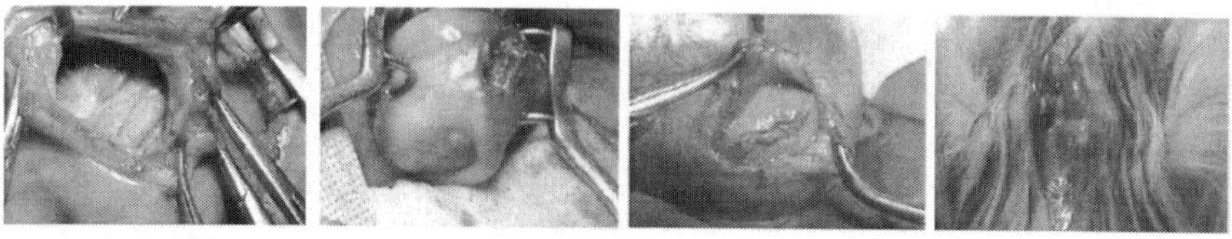

Figure 1. Surgical procedure and treatment options in intrauterine MMC repair in Rhesus monkeys.

**Table 1. Demographic dates of the mother, fetal surgey, surgery time, duration of anesthesia and relation between mother or fetal death in the immediately transoperatory**

| Case N = 9 | Weight (g) | Temperature °C | Mother age (year) | Gestation time (week) | Fetal surgery | Surgery Time (minutes) | Duration of anesthesia (minute) | Mother death | Fetal death |
|---|---|---|---|---|---|---|---|---|---|
| 1 | 6000 | 37.4 | 4 | 12 | Closing the skin | 60 | 85 | NO | NO |
| 2 | 5100 | 37.45 | 4 | 12 | Closing the skin | 80 | 91 | NO | NO |
| 3 | 7000 | 36.42 | 10 | 13 | Correction with a silicone mesh | 75 | 85 | NO | NO |
| 4 | 5735 | 37 | 10 | 13 | Exposed | 62 | 98 | NO | NO |
| 5 | 5000 | 36.75 | 10 | 14 | Exponed | 120 | 140 | NO | NO |
| 6 | 6200 | 37.76 | 8 | 13 | Correction with a silicone mesh | 72 | 64 | NO | NO |
| 7 | 5600 | 37.33 | 4 | 12 | Exponed | 62 | 72 | NO | NO |
| 8 | 6100 | 37.45 | 7 | 13 | Closing the skin | 60 | 65 | NO | NO |
| 9 | 7000 | 36.82 | 9 | 12 | Correction with a silicone mesh | 105 | 135 | NO | NO |

In this table we can observe the weight, age, temperature, from the mother and the surgical procedure that the fetus had. No reports of maternal or fetal deaths occurred during anesthetic management.

When the surgery was over 0.1 – 0.2 mg/kg of Butorfanol were administered IM (Langer et al. 1989). The extubation process started with the closure of the sevofluarane, and ended with the removal of the tube when the palpebral and deglutory reflexes were present as well as leg and arm movement. They were disconnected from the monitor until the cardiac and respiratory rates, temperature, blood pressure, and oxygen saturation, were within normal rates. The last thing to be removed was the venous catheter, corroborating that no bleeding was present in order to take the individual to its individual cage to continue with its recovery (Table 1, taken from Galván-Montaño et al. 2010).

At 23 weeks, a cesarean section was performed to extract the product, which was isolated from its mother.

## Cesarean Surgery

Fentanyl 10 μcgs was supplied, by a supra-half infraumbilical incision cutting skin, aponeurosis and peritoneum. The uterus was identified and exteriorized, and the position of the fetus was determined by an ultrasound and palpation, afterwards a transverse incision was done in all layers, including the amniotic membranes, of the inferior uterus segment. The product was extracted and the nose and mouth secretions were sucked out, a double umbilical cord campling was placed 10 cm away form the base and a cut was made between the two clamps. 0,2 mg of ergometrine melate were dispensed intravenously, the placenta and the placental remains were cleaned form the uterine cavity with sterile gases. The uterine wound was closed in two planes with Vycril 2-0 and with continous suture. The uterus was put back into place, closing the abdominal wall in two planes: aponeurosis with Vycril 2-0 and skiing with Nylon 2-0 continuous suture. Once the surgery was over butorfanol 0,1-0,2mg/Kg was supplied intramuscularly (Langer et al. 1989). The extubation started once the passage of the sevoflurane was ceased and the endotracheal cannula was removed once the palpebral and deglutory reflexes were present along with arms and legs movement. Heart and breathing rate, temperature, blood pressure and oxygen saturation were confirmed to be within normal limits before disconnecting the monitor. The last thing to be removed was the intravenous catheter taking the monkey to an individual cage. During the following three days the supply of butorphanol (0.1.0.2 mg/kg) (Galván - Montaño et al. 2010) and cephalothin continued every 12 hours (Figure 2).

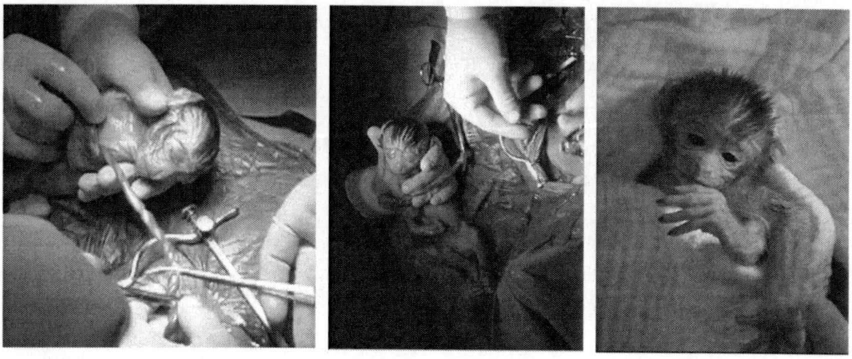

Figure 2. Cesarean surgery in Rhesus Monkeys with MMC. Fourth cesarean surgeries were done without morbidity nor mortality for the mother and products, at week 23 of gestation period.

## Care of Newborns

After the umbilical cord was severed the baby monkey was carefully cleaned and reanimated, corporal temperature was maintained placing the new born on dry-warm blankets. The remaining fluids from nose and mouth were carefully suctioned using a K-32 premature infant plastic feeding tube connected to a 10 mL syringe. Oxygen was supplied to the newborn monkeys using a pediatric mask for delivery of 3L/min simultaneous to soft chest compressions to stimulate spontaneous breathing. The remaining umbilical cord was then ligated 2-5 cm from the belly with surgical Silk 2-0. Following these steps an Apgar (Apgar 1966). Score was assessed at one minute, at three and at five minutes, and when the neonate was breathing normally on her own and a 7-minute Apgar score was reached the newborn was transferred to a pediatric heated incubator and wrapped with warm compresses. Infant feeding consisted of premature commercial formula-fed (Enfamil® Mead Johnson de Mexico, S. de R.L. de C.V Mexico, D.F. - CP – 01049) an iron-fortified milk formula for premature babies) through a hand-raised feeding schedule of 1 pre-warmed Oz each 2 hours during the first week and every 3 hours from the second week of life.

## Neurofisiological Studies

We used three nonhuman primates (*Macaca mulatta*). Two underwent an intrauterine laminectomy during the 13th week of gestation in the lumbar spine (L5 and L6) to simulate the neurological defect produced by MMC. One of the primates had the spinal cord left exposed and the other was fitted with a silicon mesh. The third monkey was used as a positive control.

Sensory pathways evoked potentials (EP) were performed in the Neurophysiology Laboratory at the APREXBIO S.A.S de C.V., using the EP special computer and software NEURONICA 5 (Neuronic; Ciudad de la Habana, Cuba), which was programed for each sensorial pathway studied. Disc electrodes were placed according to the international 10/20 systems, with impedance less than 5 kΩ. For individual handling, chemical contention was necessary, so Tiletamine-Zolacepam (Zoletil Laboratory Virbac, Carros, France) 4 mg/ kg i.m was used (Ibáñez-Contreras et al. 2018). The body temperature was kept at 38 1°C during the whole procedure using a thermostatic mattress.

To monitor medial nerve somatosensory evoked potentials (SEPMN), electrodes were placed at the cubital fossa (-), Erb point (-), 7° cervical vertebrae (C7) (-) and contralateral superior somatosensory cortex (C3 or C4) (-) to the stimulated limb, referenced to Fz (+), earth was placed in mastoid. For tibial nerve somatosensory evoked potentials (SEPNT) registration electrodes were placed in the following derivations: popliteal (-), 5° lumbar vertebrae (L5) (-), third thoracic vertebrae (T3) (-) and contralateral somatosensory cortex (C3 or C4) (-) to the stimulated limb, referenced to Fz (+), earth was placed in mastoid. The stimulus was a 100 μs monophasic electric squared pulse, at 0.5–1.1 stimulus/s frequency, which was applied behind the medial malleolus. A total of 250 stimuli were averaged. The filters used were from 5 to 2 500 Hz, at 1.5 mA intensity and the response was replicated at least once to ensure events reproducibility (Ibáñez-Contreras et al. 2018). We performed a single somatosensory evoked potential recording for each of the primates taking as individual parameters the latencies of each of the three primates undergoing surgery, classifying the surgical model as exposed, mesh and positive control. In the case of the four primates who served as negative controls, for those born via natural delivery the sample was further homogenized so that it yielded a mean and standard deviation and was subsequently compared using t test for a single sample. The parameter of each surgical case was compared against the average of the group of primates born naturally.

## RESULTS

There were no reports on maternal or fetuses deaths in the nine females that were surgically operated on. The average duration of the intrauterine surgeries was 77.3 minutes (60 to 105 minutes) and the anesthetic time varied from 64 to 140, an average of 92.7 minutes. The evaluated variable means obtained during the surgical time were as follows: heart rate of 138.9 beats per minute, respiratory rate of 34.3 breaths per minute, temperature of 34.8°C, oxygen saturation of 96.8% systolic pressure of 147.9 mmHg and of diastolic pressure of 73.6 mmHg.

In total, nine fetuses underwent surgery: three were closed with skin, three were fitted with mesh and three were exposed; surgery is carried out between 12 and 13 weeks of gestation, taking place everyone laminectomy at L5 and L6. The average time for fetal surgery was 41.22 + 12.95 minutes (30 to 69 minutes). The total time of the surgery from the time the skin was incised until the closure was an average of 70.22 + 14.8 minutes (60 to 105 minutes). The anesthesia time varied from 65 to 140 minutes, with an average 93.6 + 27 minutes. In fetuses that died in utero (22%), the time of fetal surgery was longer.

After surgery, five fetuses died (56%): three due to premature delivery at end of gestation and two in utero at 14 and 22 weeks. The deaths occurred mainly when the age and number of mother´s pregnancies was higher. Four fetuses lived (44%), two that were closed with skin, one with mesh placement and one exposed. Three of the products were born by caesarean section at 23 weeks gestation and one by vaginal delivery at 22 weeks.

The time for the extraction of the product was approximately 7 to 17 minutes with an average of 12,25 minutes, the time of the surgery was of 20 to 50 minutes with an average of 33 minutes. The anesthetic time was 30 to 54 minutes with an average of 42 minutes. The postpartum vaginal bleeding lasted 3 to 4 days. All products were born alive with an average Apgar grade of 4 after a minute of birth and 6 after three minutes of birth, obtaining an average of eight by minute five. The weight of the product was between 300 to 420g with an average of 357g, the size was 31,5 to 34,2 with an average of 33cm. All newborns began their feeding after 2 hours and 30 minutes.

In the survived newborns, the somatosensory evoked potentials show a definite wave that remained constant in the all monkeys in both anterior and posterior limbs. A recording was made of P1 in posterior limbs in both derivations. Student t-test was then used for a single sample, obtaining significant differences between the monkeys treated surgically and those who were not operated on. Significant differences were found in most of the derivations between the exposure of the medulla in comparison to the monkeys born by natural delivery except for the following derivations: right afferent T3 ($p = 0.076$) showing the latency for the monkey with the exposed medulla at 16.94 msec in relation to the average of the monkeys that were born naturally (10.8 ± 4.5 msec). In the case of the popliteal fossa, we observed a $p = 0.096$, observing that the monkey with the silicone mesh correction obtained a latency of 12 msec with an average for the monkeys that were born naturally from 5.2 ± 1.0 msec. For the two cases, we observed more elongated latencies compared with monkeys born by natural delivery. For evaluation of the usefulness of intrauterine correction of the defect through the placement of silicon mesh, it is observed in the surgical model of the silicone mesh vs. the monkeys that were born by natural delivery. The only derivations were that no significant differences were found in L5 afferent right ($p = 0.764$) with a latency of 8.23 msec for monkey with silicone mesh correction in contrast to the average of the monkeys born naturally (7.6 ± 3.8 msec). In the case of the right popliteal afferent, we observed $p = 0.851$, with a latency of 5.88 msec for the monkey with silicone mesh correction. Average for the monkeys born naturally was 5.6 ± 1.9 msec and left popliteal afferent with $p = 0.489$ with a latency for the monkey with corrected silicone mesh of 9.41 msec and average for the primates born naturally of 5.2 ± 1.08 msec. As expected, latencies in SEPNT were presented more elongated in the two monkeys that underwent intrauterine laminectomy in relation to the control monkey and the monkeys born by natural delivery. In the anterior limbs there were no significant changes (Figure 3).

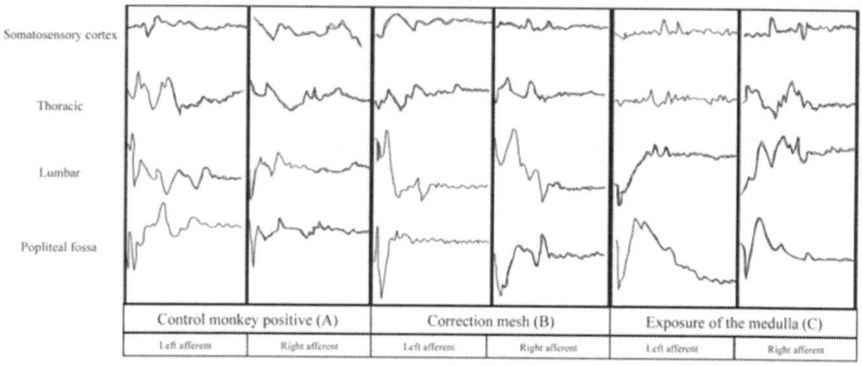


Figure 3. Morphology of the latencies obtained from the tibial nerve SEPNT. Note the lengthening of the latencies in case B and C in connection with case A. Student t test for a single sample, which compares cases A (positive control), B (mesh surgical correction) and C (exposure of medulla) against the negative control group. There was lengthening of the latencies in B and C in relation to A.

## REFERENCES

Adzick N. S. (2010). Fetal myelomeningocele: natural history, pathophysiology, and in-utero intervention. *Seminars in fetal & neonatal medicine*, *15*(1), 9–14. https://doi.org/10.1016/j.siny.2009.05.002.

Adzick, N. S., Harrison, M. R., Glick, P. L., Golbus, M. S., Anderson, R. L., Mahony, B. S., Callen, P. W., Hirsch, J. H., Luthy, D. A., & Filly, R. A. (1985). Fetal cystic adenomatoid malformation: prenatal diagnosis and natural history. *Journal of pediatric surgery*, *20*(5), 483–488. https://doi.org/10.1016/s0022-3468(85)80470-x.

Adzick, N. S., Sutton, L. N., Crombleholme, T. M., & Flake, A. W. (1998). Successful fetal surgery for spina bifida. *Lancet (London, England)*,

*352*(9141), 1675–1676. https://doi.org/10.1016/S0140-6736(98)00070-1.

Apgar, V., Stanley, J. L. (1966). *El recien nacido*. Clínicas Pediátricas de N. América. [*The newborn*. Pediatric Clinics of N. America.]

Au, K. S., Tran, P. X., Tsai, C. C., O'Byrne, M. R., Lin, J. I., Morrison, A. C., Hampson, A. W., Cirino, P., Fletcher, J. M., Ostermaier, K. K., Tyerman, G. H., Doebel, S., & Northrup, H. (2008). Characteristics of a spina bifida population including North American Caucasian and Hispanic individuals. *Birth defects research. Part A, Clinical and molecular teratology*, *82*(10), 692–700. https://doi.org/10.1002/bdra.20499.

Berihu, B. A., Welderufael, A. L., Berhe, Y., Magana, T., Mulugeta, A., Asfaw, S., & Gebreselassie, K. (2018). High burden of neural tube defects in Tigray, Northern Ethiopia: Hospital-based study. *PloS one*, *13*(11), e0206212. https://doi.org/10.1371/journal.pone.0206212.

Blanco Muñoz, J., Lacasaña, M., Borja Aburto, V. H., Torres Sánchez, L. E., García García, A. M., & López Carrillo, L. (2005). Socioeconomic factors and the risk of anencephaly in a Mexican population: a case-control study. *Public health reports (Washington, D.C.: 1974)*, *120*(1), 39–45. https://doi.org/10.1177/003335490512000108.

Blencowe, H., Cousens, S., Modell, B., & Lawn, J. (2010). Folic acid to reduce neonatal mortality from neural tube disorders. *International journal of epidemiology*, *39 Suppl 1*(Suppl 1), i110–i121. https://doi.org/10.1093/ije/dyq028.

Botelho, R. D., Imada, V., Rodrigues da Costa, K. J., Watanabe, L. C., Rossi Júnior, R., De Salles, A., Romano, E., & Peralta, C. (2017). Fetal Myelomeningocele Repair through a Mini-Hysterotomy. *Fetal diagnosis and therapy*, *42*(1), 28–34. https://doi.org/10.1159/000449382.

Bradko, V., Castillo, H., Janardhan, S., Dahl, B., Gandy, K., & Castillo, J. (2019). Towards Guideline-Based Management of Tethered Cord Syndrome in Spina Bifida: A Global Health Paradigm Shift in the Era of Prenatal Surgery. *Neurospine*, *16*(4),715–727.https://doi.org/10.14245/ns.1836342.171.

Corral S, E., Moreno S, R., Pérez G, G., Ojeda B, M. E., Valenzuela G, H., Reascos M, M., & Sepúlveda L, W. (2006). Defectos congénitos cráneo-encefálicos: variedades y respuesta a la fortificación de la harina con ácido fólico [Effect of flour folic acid fortification on the incidence of cranio encephalic congenital defects]. *Revista medica de Chile*, *134*(9), 1129–1134. https://doi.org/10.4067/s0034-98872006000900007.

Copp, A. J., Adzick, N. S., Chitty, L. S., Fletcher, J. M., Holmbeck, G. N., & Shaw, G. M. (2015). Spina bifida. *Nature reviews. Disease primers*, *1*, 15007. https://doi.org/10.1038/nrdp.2015.7.

Committee on Practice Bulletins-Obstetrics (2017). Practice Bulletin No. 187: Neural Tube Defects. *Obstetrics and gynecology*, *130*(6), e279–e290. https://doi.org/10.1097/AOG.0000000000002412.

Farmer, D. L., Thom, E. A., Brock, J. W., 3rd, Burrows, P. K., Johnson, M. P., Howell, L. J., Farrell, J. A., Gupta, N., Adzick, N. S., & Management of Myelomeningocele Study Investigators (2018). The Management of Myelomeningocele Study: full cohort 30-month pediatric outcomes. *American journal of obstetrics and gynecology*, *218*(2), 256.e1–256.e13. https://doi.org/10.1016/j.ajog.2017.12.001.

Galván-Montaño, A., Hernández-Godínez, B., Ibáñez-Contreras, A., Cárdenas-Lailson, L. E., Ramírez-Hernández, R., & Aragón-Inclán, J. (2010). Anesthetic management in intrauterine surgery to evaluate an experimental model of myelomeningocele in non human primates (*Macaca mulatta*). *Acta cirurgica brasileira*, *25*(3), 294–297. https://doi.org/10.1590/s0102-86502010000300013.

Galván-Montaño, A., Cárdenas-Lailson, E., Hernández-Godínez, B., Ibáñez-Contreras, A., Martínez-Del Olmo, A., & Aragón-Inclán, J. (2007). Desarrollo de un modelo animal de mielomeningocele y opciones de tratamiento prenatal en *Macaca mulatta* [Development of an animal model of myelomeningocele and options for prenatal treatment in *Macaca mulatta*]. *Cirugia y cirujanos*, *75*(5), 357–362.

George, T. M., & Fuh, E. (2003). Review of animal models of surgically induced spinal neural tube defects: implications for fetal surgery. *Pediatric neurosurgery*, *39*(2), 81–90. https://doi.org/10.1159/000071319.

Hall, N. B., Broussard, K., Evert, N., & Canfield, M. (2017). Notes from the Field: Zika Virus-Associated Neonatal Birth Defects Surveillance - Texas, January 2016-July 2017. *MMWR. Morbidity and mortality weekly report*, 66(31), 835–836. https://doi.org/10.15585/mmwr.mm6631a5.

Harrison, M. R., Anderson, J., Rosen, M. A., Ross, N. A., & Hendrickx, A. G. (1982). Fetal surgery in the primate I. Anesthetic, surgical, and tocolytic management to maximize fetal-neonatal survival. *Journal of pediatric surgery*, *17*(2), 115–122. https://doi.org/10.1016/s0022-3468(82)80193-0.

Heffez, D. S., Aryanpur, J., Rotellini, N. A., Hutchins, G. M., & Freeman, J. M. (1993). Intrauterine repair of experimental surgically created dysraphism. *Neurosurgery*, *32*(6), 1005–1010. https://doi.org/10.1227/00006123-199306000-00021.

Heffez, D. S., Aryanpur, J., Hutchins, G. M., & Freeman, J. M. (1990). The paralysis associated with myelomeningocele: clinical and experimental data implicating a preventable spinal cord injury. *Neurosurgery*, *26*(6), 987–992.

Hernández-Godínez, B., Ibáñez-Contreras, A., Durand-Rivera, A., Reyes-Pantoja, S. A., Ramírez-Hernández, R., Rodríguez-Guzmán, P., & Tena-Betancourt, E. (2011). Somatosensory evoked potentials of median and tibial nerves in rhesus monkeys (*Macaca mulatta*) under captivity: influence of ontogenic status in neonatal, infant, young, adult, and senile stages. *Journal of medical primatology*, *40*(2), 79–87. https://doi.org/10.1111/j.1600-0684.2010.00458.x.

Hernández-Godínez, B., Bonilla Jaime, H., Poblano, A., Arteaga-Silva, M., Medina Hernández, A., Contreras-Uribe, A., & Ibáñez-Contreras, A. (2019). Effect of different anesthetic mixtures-ketamine-xylazine, ketamine-acepromazine and tiletamine-zolazepam-on the physiological and blood biochemistry parameters of male rhesus monkeys (*Macaca mulatta*) at different ages. *Animal models and experimental medicine*, *2*(2), 83–97. https://doi.org/10.1002/ame2.12062.

Hernández-Godínez, B., Poblano, A., Bonilla-Jaime, H., Artega-Silva, M., Sánchez-Torres, S., Mondragón-Lozano, R., & Ibáñez-Contreras, A.

(2018). Effect of age on electrical nerve conduction in the somatosensory pathway and its correlation with somatometry and plasma concentrations of musculoskeletal enzymes in male rhesus monkeys (*Macaca mulatta*) held in captivity. *Journal of medical primatology*, *47*(3), 145–156. https://doi.org/10.1111/jmp.12337.

Hernández-Godínez, B., Ibáñez-Contreras, A., Durand-Rivera, A., Galván-Montaño, A., Reyes-Pantoja, S. A., & Cárdenas-Lailson, E. (2011). Latencies obtained of the somatosensory evoked potentials of the median and tibial nerve in rhesus monkey undergoing intrauterine laminectomy to simulate myelomeningocele. *Cirugia y cirujanos*, *79*(3), 237–262.

Ibáñez-Contreras, A., Hernández-Arciga, U., Poblano, A., Arteaga-Silva, M., Hernández-Godínez, B., Mendoza-Cuevas, G. I., Toledo-Pérez, R., Alarcón-Aguilar, A., González-Puertos, V. Y., & Konigsberg, M. (2018). Electrical activity of sensory pathways in female and male geriatric Rhesus monkeys (*Macaca mulatta*), and its relation to oxidative stress. *Experimental gerontology*, *101*, 80–94. https://doi.org/10.1016/j.exger.2017.11.003.

Ibáñez-Contreras, A., Poblano, A., Arteaga-Silva, M., Hernández-Godínez, B., Hernández-Arciga, U., Toledo, R., & Königsberg, M. (2016). Visual, auditive and somatosensory pathways alterations in geriatric rhesus monkeys (*Macaca mulatta*). *Journal of medical primatology*, *45*(2), 92–102. https://doi.org/10.1111/jmp.12211.

Kabagambe, S. K., Jensen, G. W., Chen, Y. J., Vanover, M. A., & Farmer, D. L. (2018). Fetal Surgery for Myelomeningocele: A Systematic Review and Meta-Analysis of Outcomes in Fetoscopic versus Open Repair. *Fetal diagnosis and therapy*, *43*(3), 161–174. https://doi.org/10.1159/000479505.

Langer, J. C., Longaker, M. T., Crombleholme, T. M., Bond, S. J., Finkbeiner, W. E., Rudolph, C. A., Verrier, E. D., & Harrison, M. R. (1989). Etiology of intestinal damage in gastroschisis. I: Effects of amniotic fluid exposure and bowel constriction in a fetal lamb model. *Journal of pediatric surgery*, *24*(10), 992–997. https://doi.org/10.1016/s0022-3468(89)80200-3.

Mancebo-Hernández, A., González-Rivera, A., Díaz-Omaña, L., LópezAlquicira, M., Domínguez-Viveros, W., Serrano-Sierra, A. (2008) Defectos del tubo neural. Panorama epidemiológico en México (I de II) *Acta Pediátrica de México*, vol. 29, núm. 1, pp. 41-47. [Neural tube defects. Epidemiological panorama in Mexico (I of II) *Acta Pediátrica de México*]

Meuli, M., Meuli-Simmen, C., Yingling, C. D., Hutchins, G. M., Hoffman, K. M., Harrison, M. R., & Adzick, N. S. (1995). Creation of myelomeningocele in utero: a model of functional damage from spinal cord exposure in fetal sheep. *Journal of pediatric surgery*, *30*(7), 1028–1033. https://doi.org/10.1016/0022-3468(95)90335-6.

Meuli, M., Meuli-Simmen, C., Hutchins, G. M., Yingling, C. D., Hoffman, K. M., Harrison, M. R., & Adzick, N. S. (1995). In utero surgery rescues neurological function at birth in sheep with spina bifida. *Nature medicine*, *1*(4), 342–347. https://doi.org/10.1038/nm0495-342 40.

Meuli, M., Meuli-Simmen, C., Yingling, C. D., Hutchins, G. M., Timmel, G. B., Harrison, M. R., & Adzick, N. S. (1996). In utero repair of experimental myelomeningocele saves neurological function at birth. *Journal of pediatric surgery*, *31*(3), 397–402. https://doi.org/10.1016/s0022-3468(96)90746-0.

Michejda M. (1984). Intrauterine treatment of spina bifida: primate model. *Zeitschrift fur Kinderchirurgie: organ der Deutschen, der Schweizerischen und der Osterreichischen Gesellschaft fur Kinderchirurgie = Surgery in infancy and childhood*, *39*(4), 259–261. https://doi.org/10.1055/s-2008-1044221. [*Journal for Pediatric Surgery: Organ of the German, Swiss and Austrian Society for Pediatric Surgery*]

Oliveira-Brancati, Camila Ive Ferreira, Ferrarese, Valéria Cristina Carvalho, Costa, Antonio Richieri, & Fett-Conte, Agnes Cristina. (2019). [PROVISIONAL] Birth defects in Brazil: Outcomes of a population-based study. *Genetics and Molecular Biology*, Epub August 12, 2019.https://dx.doi.org/10.1590/1678-4685-gmb-2018-0186.

Olutoye, O. O., & Adzick, N. S. (1999). Fetal surgery for myelomeningocele. *Seminars in perinatology*, *23*(6), 462–473. https://doi.org/10.1016/s0146-0005(99)80025-1.

Pacheco-Santos, L.M., Reyes-Lecca, R.C., Cortez-Escalante, J.J., Niskier-Sanchez, M., Rodrigues, H.G. (2016). La prevención de los efectos del tubo neural mediante el enriquecimiento de la harina con ácido fólico : un estudio poblacional retrospectivo en Brasil. *Boletín de la Organización Mundial de la Salud.* Volumen 94, Número 1, enero 2016, 1-76. [Prevention of neural tube effects by fortifying flour with folic acid: a retrospective population study in Brazil. *Bulletin of the World Health Organization.*]

Pedreira, D. A., Valente, P. R., Abou-Jamra, R. C., Pelarigo, C. L., Silva, L. M., & Goldenberg, S. (2003). Successful fetal surgery for the repair of a 'myelomeningocele-like' defect created in the fetal rabbit. *Fetal diagnosis and therapy*, *18*(3), 201–206. https://doi.org/10.1159/000069378.

Pedreira, D. A., Valente, P. R., Abou-Jamra, R. C., Pelarigo, C. L., Silva, L. M., & Goldenberg, S. (2002). A different technique to create a 'myelomeningocele-like' defect in the fetal rabbit. *Fetal diagnosis and therapy*, *17*(6), 372–376. https://doi.org/10.1159/000065388.

Pedreira, D. A., Sanchez e Oliveira, R., Valente, P. R., Abou-Jamra, R. C., Araújo, A., & Saldiva, P. H. (2007). Validation of the ovine fetus as an experimental model for the human myelomeningocele defect. *Acta cirurgica brasileira*, *22*(3), 168–173. https://doi.org/10.1590/s0102-86502007000300003.

Population Reference Bureau. *2010 World Population Data Sheet*. 2010:18. http://www.prb.org/pdf10/10wpds_eng.pdf (accessed February 2013).

Qu, P., Li, S., Liu, D., Lei, F., Zeng, L., Wang, D., Dang, S. (2019). A propensity-matched study of the association between optimal folic acid supplementation and birth defects in Shaanxi province, Northwestern China. *Scientific reports*, *9*(1), 5271. doi:10.1038/s41598-019-41584-5.

Sanz Cortes, M., Davila, I., Torres, P., Yepez, M., Lee, W., Guimaraes, C. V., Sangi-Haghpeykar, H., Whitehead, W. E., Castillo, J., Nassr, A. A., Espinoza, J., Shamshirsaz, A. A., & Belfort, M. A. (2019). Does fetoscopic or open repair for spina bifida affect fetal and postnatal growth?. *Ultrasound in obstetrics & gynecology: the official journal of the International Society of Ultrasound in Obstetrics and Gynecology*, *53*(3), 314–323. https://doi.org/10.1002/uog.20220.

Stiefel, D., Copp, A. J., & Meuli, M. (2007). Fetal spina bifida in a mouse model: loss of neural function in utero. *Journal of neurosurgery*, *106*(3 Suppl), 213–221. https://doi.org/10.3171/ped.2007.106.3.213.

Stiefel, D., & Meuli, M. (2007). Scanning electron microscopy of fetal murine myelomeningocele reveals growth and development of the spinal cord in early gestation and neural tissue destruction around birth. *Journal of pediatric surgery*, *42*(9), 1561–1565. https://doi.org/10.1016/j.jpedsurg.2007.04.019.

Tan, K. B., Tan, S. H., Tan, K. H., & Yeo, G. S. (2007). Anencephaly in Singapore: a ten-year series 1993-2002. *Singapore medical journal*, *48*(1), 12–15.

Tauheed, J., Sanchez-Guerra, M., Lee, J. J., Paul, L., Ibne Hasan, M., Quamruzzaman, Q., Selhub, J., Wright, R. O., Christiani, D. C., Coull, B. A., Baccarelli, A. A., & Mazumdar, M. (2017). Associations between post translational histone modifications, myelomeningocele risk, environmental arsenic exposure, and folate deficiency among participants in a case control study in Bangladesh. *Epigenetics*, *12*(6), 484–491. https://doi.org/10.1080/15592294.2017.1312238.

Vieira, A. R., & Castillo Taucher, S. (2005). Edad materna y defectos del tubo neural: evidencia para un efecto mayor en espina bífida que anencefalia [Maternal age and neural tube defects: evidence for a greater effect in spina bifida than in anencephaly]. *Revista medica de Chile*, *133*(1), 62–70. https://doi.org/10.4067/s0034-98872005000100008.

# ABOUT THE EDITORS

***Braulio Hernández Godínez*** - Physical Anthropologist graduated from the Escuela Nacional de Antropologia e Historia (ENAH), PhD of Biological Sciences and Health of the Universidad Autonoma Metropolitana Unidad Iztapalapa. He is a specialist in the managment of laboratory animals, with 10 yr of experience and in the case of Non-human Primates in biomedical research with more of 20 yr. He has 24 publications with an impact factor. It has been the winner of the first place in three awards given by the Academia Mexicana de Cirugía, one of the most prestigious academies in Mexico, won the National Prize for Surgery in 2006 "Académico Dr. Francisco Montes de Oca"; in 2008 he won the first place for the best publication of the oficial organ for the Academia Mexicana de Cirugía, "Académico Dr. Francisco Fonseca García" and in 2009 he won the prize for the best scientific video "Académico Dr. Manuel J. Catillejos". It also has other second and third place prizes awarded by scientific associations and national health institutes.

***Martin Garcia Servin*** - Head of the University Laboratory Of Animal House Instituto de Neurobiologia of the Universidad Nacional Autonoma de México (INB-UNAM). Diploma in Laboratory Animal Science by UNAM. Certified by the National Council of Certification in Veterinary Medicine and Zootecnia A.C. In the Area of Laboratory Animals (CONCERVET), Mexico. Responsible veterinary Physician authorized in área of bioteries by Senasica, Mexico.

Membership:

- Member of the American Association for Laboratory Animal Science (Aalas).
- Member of the Mexican Association of Laboratory Animal Science, A.C. (AMCAL).
- Member of the Federation of Hispanic Societies and Associations of North America, Central America and the Caribbean of Laboratory Animal Science (FESAHANCCCAL).

Institutional Participation:

- Member of the Bioetics Committee of Inb.Unam,
- Member of the Ethics Committee of the Faculty of Medicine, Unam
- Member of the Inb-Unam Biosecurity Committee.

Productivity:

- Co-Author of 5 Scientific Articles.
- More Than 190 Thanks in International Articles, More Than 70 in National Articles and More Than 400 In Institutional Academic Events.
- More Than 170 Acknowledgments in Doctorate, Master and Doctorate Thesis.
- 5 Collaborations In Book Chapters
- Courses, Workshops, Conferences, Seminars, Etc.

Awards and Distinctions:

- Prize Dra. Angelica Salas for the Inb-Unam
- Distinction as Professionist of the Year (2017) Awarded by the Ferederation of Colleges and Associations of the State of Queretaro.

***Alejandra Ibáñez Contreras*** is a Zootechnician veterinarian whose specialization is in the management, use and care of laboratory animals, mainly in non-human primates destined for biomedical research participating actively in the last 12 years in varios research projects National as Internacional as a Research Associate. She received her PhD in Biological and Health Sciences from Universidad Autónoma Metropolitana Unidad Iztapalapa in 2016, whose thesis work was "Relationship of oxidative stress on brain electrical activity of sensory pathways (auditive, visual and somatosensory) in geriatric Rhesus monkeys (*Macaca mulatta*). In 2018 she obteined the Medal of Academic Merit given by Universidad Autónoma Metropolitana Unidad Iztapalapa. The main lines of research are in the area of neurosciences in basic and preclinical research, mainly sensory pathways in primates whose results are reflected in 24 internacional publications with an impact factor.

# About the Contributors

***Maribel Estevez Cabrera*** - PhD student from Biological Sciences and Health, Universidad Autonoma Metropolitana in progress focused in animal health and reproduction. ORCID: 0000-0001-7913-9037.

***Tania Molina Jiménez*** - PhD. BSc in Biological and Biological and Pharmaceutical Chemistry, MSc and PhD in Neuroethology at the Universidad Veracruzana. Line of research based in the neurobiology of anxiety and depression and its impact in reproduction. ORCID: 0000-0001-5236-6838.

***Ofelia Limón Morales*** - PhD in Experimental Biology from the Universidad Autónoma Metropolitana. Postdoctoral stay at the Faculty of Chemistry of the UNAM. It has 10 articles in international magazines and 6 chapters in national books. She has taught undergraduate and postgraduate courses at the Universidad Autónoma Metropolitana, Iztapalapa Unit and participated in the direction of thesis for the Biological Pharmaceutical Chemistry career at the Faculty of Chemistry of UNAM. She is currently attached to the Universidad Autónoma Metropolitana and belongs to the

Sistema Nacional de Investigadores level I Lines of research Reproductive and neuroendocrine aspects of models of depression, behavioral effects of perinatal exposure to contaminants in the female and early manipulations in the serotonergic system and its effects on memory and learning (behavioral and molecular approaches).

***Alfonso Alfaro Rodriguez*** - Chief of Neurosciences Division, Instituto Nacional de Rehabilitación "Luis Guillermo Ibarra Ibarra". MD, Master Neurophysiological Sciences, of the Center of Neurobiology and Institute of Biomedical Research, Universidad Nacional Autónoma de México (UNAM). PhD (Neurosciences) Faculty of Sciences, Universidad Nacional Autónoma de México (UNEAM). Professor of the Subject Introduction to the Methodology of Research to Resident Physicians of the Specialty in Medicine in Human Communication, Audiology and Phoniatrics National Institute of Human Communication. Mexico City, Mexico. Professor/Tutor of master's and Doctorate, Postgraduate in Medical and Dental Health Sciences UNAM. Mexico City, Mexico. Professor/Tutor of Masters, Postgraduate in Biological Sciences, Faculty of Sciences, UNAM. Mexico City, Mexico. The research conducted by Dr. Alfonso Alfaro-Rodríguez has focused on the study of brain chemistry. He has published 103 international articles and is a member of different research committees, and editorial committees. His studies focus on the search for mechanisms of neuronal damage caused by neurodegenerative diseases such as Parkinson's, brain lesions and currently nociception. He has also ventured into the study of several antiepileptic and antidepressant medications on the central nervous system. The role of monoamines such as serotonin and acetylcholine together with several catecholamines at the neuronal and molecular level in the development of neurodegenerative diseases has been a central theme of his research. Research on the mechanisms of brain damage through different neurotoxic pathways triggered by neurodegenerative diseases has led him to successfully explore the role of neuroprotective drugs in a myriad of animal models. With his research he has allowed to assess the neuronal damage and disabilities caused by these diseases. He has currently focused on the development of new research protocols on pain mechanisms and the development of diagnostic strategies for the timely diagnosis of pain; by using new medications that could improve the quality of life of patients suffering from chronic pain.

***Herlinda Bonilla Jaime*** - PhD in Biological Sciences and Health from of Universidad Autonoma Metropolitana. Researcher of Universidad Autónoma Metropolitana-Iztapalapa. Lines of research Depresión: Behavioral, reproductive and neuroendocrine aspects. ORCID: 0000-0002-7505-0809.

***José Armando Sánchez-Salcedo*** - DVM, MSc in Clinical Ethology (Universitat Autònoma de Barcelona) and Neuroethology (Universidad Veracruzana) PhD (Biological Sciences and Health, Universidad Autonoma Metropolitana) in progress focused in animal health and reproduction. ORCID: 0000-0001-7913-9037.

***Claudia Juárez Portilla*** - BSc in Biological and Pharmaceutical Chemistry, MSc and PhD in Neuroethology at the Universidad Veracruzana. Line of research base on influence of drugs of abuse over the circadian system. ORCID: 0000- 0003-2215-058X

***Javier Morán Martínez*** - Head of the Department of Cell Biology and Ultrastructure of the Center for Biomedical Research, Coordinator of the Master's Degree in Multidisciplinary Health Research (PNPC-CONACyT), president of CICUAL, Editor of the Medicine of Torreón Journal and professor of full time at the Faculty of Medicine of the Autonomous University of Coahuila Campus Torreón. It belongs to the National System of Researchers. Professor PRODEP-SEP. Scholarship student Fogarty International Center CareerTrac, School of Public Health, University of

California at Los Angeles (Grant #D43TW623; Program Name: ITREOH). PhD in Biological Sciences, with specialization in Cell Biology and Genetics, by the Faculty of Biological Sciences of the Autonomous University of Nuevo León. Mention with the highest honor granted by the Autonomous University of Nuevo León SUMMA CUM LAUDE. Member of the Research Coordination network in the Household Water Insecurity Experiences (HWISE).

***Omar Zambrano Ortiz*** - He has a degree in Psychology from the Faculty of Health Sciences of the Juárez University of the state of Durango. He is a Master of Science in Multidisciplinary Health Research from the Faculty of Medicine of the Autonomous University of Coahuila Campus Torreón. He is currently studying doctoral studies in Biomedical Sciences at the Faculty of Medicine of the Autonomous University of Coahuila Campus Torreón. The line of research he develops is in neurology, memory and learning. Some professional activities: Evaluating psychologist at the Center for evaluation and trust control of the state of Coahuila. Coordinator of Psychology in Integral Development of the Family (DiF) Torreón.

***Alfonso Zambrano Martínez*** - Veterinary Zootechnician by the Antonio Narro Universidad Autónoma Agraria Laguna Unit. He is the founder and head of the Bioterium of the Faculty of Medicine of the Autonomous University of Coahuila Campus Torreón. Bioterist at the School of Medicine of the University Juárez of the Durango State Campus Gómez Palacio. He is a responsible physician accredited in the canine control centers of the municipalities of Francisco I. Madero in the State of Coahuila and in the Municipality of Lerdo in the State of Durango, Mexico. He is part of the Council of the Internal Committee for the Care and Use of Laboratory Animals (CICUAL) accredited by SAGARPA, of the Research Center of the Faculty of Medicine of the Autonomous University of Coahuila. Participant in the XXIII Refinement of Neurosciences Update

Conference by the Argentine Association of Science and Technology of Laboratory Animals.

***Esperanza Yasmin Calleros Rincón*** - She is a Doctor in Environmental Science and Technology from the CIMAV of Chihuahua. She is a teacher in Occupational and Environmental Health, from the Faculty of Medicine of the Universidad Juárez del Estado de Durango (UJED) of Gómez Palacio, Dgo. He is a surgeon from the Faculty of Medicine, UJED. She has conducted studies in populations on the impact of nitrates at the reproductive, endocrine, hematological and molecular levels. She belongs to the Academic group in Consolidation, Pathologies of Environmental Origin, UJED-CA-137. She has directed thesis in the career of QFB, Master of Chemical Sciences, and in the Doctorate in Biomedical Sciences, She is a full-time professor-researcher attached to the Faculty of Chemical Sciences of the UJED. She is a PRODEP professor.

***María Del Pilar Carranza Rosales*** - She is a Researcher at the Northeast Biomedical Research Center of the IMSS, Titular Researcher B, member of the National System of Researchers Level 2. She is a Chemist Bacteriologist Parasitologist from the Faculty of Biological Sciences, Autonomous University of Nuevo León (UANL), she is a Master of Science with Specialty in Cell Biology from UANL, she is a Doctor of Science with a Specialty in Morphology from UANL. He has completed two post-doctoral stays: University of Arizona, Tucson, AZ. USA and University of Groningen, Holland. He has published 49 research articles, has a patent, has published 3 book chapters. She has supervised 9 doctoral theses, 10 masters, 9 bachelor's and 4 medical specialty. She is visiting professor in postgraduate courses at the Faculty of Biological Sciences-UANL and visiting professor in postgraduate courses at the Faculties of Medicine and Chemistry of the Autonomous University of Coahuila. Other substantial activities are: Member of the CONACYT Registry of Accredited Evaluators (RCEA). Member of the evaluation committee of protocols and / or research projects of the health personnel of the Coordination of Health Research IMSS. Member of the Committee of Evaluators in the Conference of Research Seminars of Master and Doctorate Programs of the Autonomous University of Coahuila, UANL and of the Postgraduate of Medical Specialties of the High Specialty Medical Specialty Unit, Hospital # 34 of the IMSS.

***Rubén García Garza*** - Surgeon and Doctor of Science with a specialty in morphology from the Autonomous University of Nuevo León, he was a professor of histology for undergraduate, master and doctoral students at the UANL from 2008 to 2014, and professor of histology for residents of pathological anatomy 2011-2014 At the UMAE 25 of the IMSS, he graduated with honorable mention in the bachelor's degree in medicine, obtained a letter of merit for social service and Summa cum laude in the Doctorate. Head of the Department of Histology and Head of the Department of Human Anatomy and Deputy Coordinator of the basic area of the Faculty of Medicine of the UAdeC UT, is part of the academic nuclei of the Multidisciplinary Masters in Health and Clinical Research, has published 20 articles in journals indexed, he is co-author of the book "Histology and Cellular and TIsular Biology" 1st and 2nd edition (Author: Dr. Julio Sepúlveda Saavedra, McGraw Hill), as well as being the author of the "Histology Practice Manual" and the "Histology Notebook to color". Dr. García is Vice President of the Mexican Society of Hitology, member of the National System of Researchers (SNI I) and has a PRODEP Profile.

***Marisela Del Rocío González Martínez*** - She is a Chemist Pharmacobiologist at the Faculty of Chemical Sciences of the Autonomous University of Coahuila (UAdeC). She has a Specialty in Microbiology and Sub-Specialty in Clinical Mycology from the National Autonomous University of Mexico, she is a Doctor in Applied Sciences to Natural Resources at the Justo Sierra Study Center, in the state of Sinaloa. He is a Full-time Research Professor at the Faculty of Medicine of the Campus

Torreón UAdeC. He is a member of the National System of Researchers (SNI) Level I. Chemist in chief of the Microbiology Section of the UMAE 71 and she was former president of the IMSS bioethics committee. Main lines of research are focused on: Characterization of resistance genes in pathogenic bacteria; pathogenic fungi of importance in humans and description of the microbiome. Innate Immunity in Breast Cancer: The Role of Natural Killer Cell Immunoglobulin-Linked Receptors. She has published 20 articles in indexed journals, co-authored two book chapters. It works in collaboration with the International Scientific Community for Nosocomial Infection Control - INICC; with the Mexican Institute of Social Security; The National Institute of Public Health; National Autonomous University of Mexico, The School of Anthropology and History and The Max Planck Institute.

***Hector Alberto Delgado Aguirre*** - He is a Chemist Faramacobiologist from the Faculty of Chemical Sciences of the Autonomous University of Coahuila. He is a Doctor of Applied Sciences to Natural Resources at the Justo Sierra Study Center, in the state of Sinaloa. He is an associate researcher at the U.M.A.E./H.E. No. 71 of the I.M.S.S., attached to the histocompatibility laboratory of the transplant unit. Director of the Molecular Biology Laboratory and active member of the research committee number 501. He has received support from the National Research Committee of the I.M.S.S. His main lines of research focus on: HLA and KIR systems in transplant immunogenetics. He has published 13 articles in indexed journals and has been co-author of two book chapters. He works in collaboration with the International Scientific Community for Nosocomial Infection Control - INICC; The School of Anthropology and History and The Max Planck Institute.

***Natalia Belén Ortega Morales*** – She is an Environmental Process Engineer from the Universidad Autónoma Agraráia Antonio Narro Undad Laguna. She is Master in Environmental Sciences from the Autonomous

University of San Luis Potosi. She is a Doctor of Science in sustainability of Agricultural Resources from the Faculty of Agriculture and Animal Husbandry of the Juárez University of the State of Durango. Develops the Research Line in Environmental Toxicology. She is a full-time professor-researcher in the department of Biology at the Autonomous Agrarian Antonio Narro University Campus Laguna.

***Nadia Denys Betancourt Martínez*** - She is a Chemist Faramacobiologist from the Faculty of Chemical Sciences of the Juárez University of the Durango State, Campus Gómez Palacio. She is a Master of Science in Multidisciplinary Health Research from the Faculty of Medicine of the Autonomous University of Coahuila Campus Torreón. She is a Doctor of Science from the Faculty of Biological Sciences of the Autonomous University of Nuevo León. She has published 15 scientific articles, 3 book chapters, has directed 6 master's theses, 3 doctorate. She belongs to the consolidated academic body of Morphological Sciences, is a PRODEP professor and is a member of the National System of Researchers.

***Samuel Reyes-Long*** - Biologist graduated from the National Autonomous University of México, with a research field focused on neurosciences, working with nociception and epigenetics. Currently doing a master's degree in Health Sciences from the National Polytechnic Institute and the National Institute of Rehabilitation. With 12 publications in indexed scientific journals, 2 book chapters and an H-index of 3. Participated in several national and international congresses in the National Institute of Rehabilitation. Specialized in molecular biology techniques, behavioral evaluations in small animals, and clinical research with the aim of transitioning into translational research.

***Angelica Gonzalez Maciel*** - Licensed in biology, Faculty of Sciences, Universidad Nacional Autónoma de México. - Specialist in Electron

Microscopy, Applied to Biological Sciences, Universidad Nacional Autónoma de México. - Master Neurophysiological Sciences, of the Center of Neurobiology and Institutte of Biomedical Research, Universidad Nacional Autónoma de México- Doctorate in Biological Sciences, Faculty of Sciences, Universidad Nacional Autónoma de México.

***Cindy Bandala*** - Doctor of Medicine, master's degree in health sciences, PhD. In Medical Research. Currently, she is working as a medical sciences Researcher at the Luis Guillermo Ibarra Ibarra National Rehabilitation Institute. She is a member of the National Research System, level I. Co-inventor of a patent, co-author of a specialized book, author, and co-author of 71 publications in peer-reviewed / indexed journals, director of 72 thesis of health area. Winner of 32 national and international recognitions. she has been part of academic and clinical programs of the National Institute of Medical Sciences and Nutrition, Salvador Zubirán, National Rehabilitation Institute, UMAE-IMSS "Manuel Ávila Camacho", Higher School of Medicine of the National Polytechnic Institute, Naval Medical School, SEMAR, Health graduates, SEDENA, ABB Spanish Center for the Prevention and Treatment of Eating Disorders, University of Andalucía, Spain, Pablo de Olavide University, Spain.

***José Luis Cortes-Altamirano*** **-** Doctor of biological and health sciences. Professor of the State University of Valle de Ecatepec and collaborator in the National Institute of Rehabilitation, belongs to the National System of Researchers, has published research articles in internationally indexed journals, chapters of national and international books and speakers at national and international conferences.

***Jessica Vanessa Gálvez-Susano*** - An undergraduate doctor at Instituto Politecnico Nacional, she has collaborated in the research department at Universidad Anahuac México currently in the line of focal cerebral ischemia, resulting in publications at international level as well as national and international congresses; she became associate professor of the laboratory animal handling subject taught at the faculty of health sciences in Universidad Anahuac Mexico Norte. She has more than 10 years of experience in the healthcare field, started her career within the Mexican Red Cross as a medical volunteer, emergency medical technician and instructor, activities that continue to be a source of inspiration and professional accomplishment. She has more than 150 national and international courses / certifications with different organizations such as the International Federation of Red Cross and Red Crescent Societies, the Pan American Health Organization, EMS1 Academy & BoundTree University, among others. She has positioned herself as instructor for university supported courses related to medical practice, always keeping in mind that knowledge dissemination is utmost priority.

***Eduardo Vega-Sánchez*** - graduated as general practitioner from Mexico's Instituto Politecnico Nacional, he is currently a second year resident of the anesthesiology program at Hospital Regional de Tlalnepantla. He took his first steps in the field of healthcare as an emergency medical technician with the local Red Cross ambulance service which went on for 10 years of service. His interest in medical education has led him to some professional opportunities, like a position as instructor and later principal at the local Red Cross emergency medical technician school, president of the association for medicine students in prehospital medicine services (SASEMEP-IPN), and American Heart Association BLS/ACLS instructor as well as others with private companies focused on medical training and certification.

***Stella Viviana Arias-Santiago*** - a doctor from the Autonomous University of the State of Puebla. Experience in medical consultation. Teacher of medical etymologies at the Universidad Anahuac. Researcher in the area of vascular dementia, specifically in cerebral ischemia. She has published in Neural Regeneration Research also for Journal of Diabetes, Metabolic Disorders & Control; and participation in the XII and XIII Anahuac Symposium on Research in the presentation of posters.

***Yolanda Cruz*** - Doctor in biological and Health Sciences from Universidad Autonoma Metropolitana. Teacher and researcher at the Universidad Anáhuac México. Full professor of subjects such as general biochemistry, biology and laboratory animal management aimed at students from various careers in the area of health sciences. Her study area is vascular dementia, specifically cerebral ischemia, a model in which she evaluates the effect of neuroprotective and / or neuro-restorative drugs. She has published articles in magazines such as PlosOne, Elsevier and Neural Regeneration Research; and book chapters in foreign publishers such as: IntechOpen and Royal Society of Chemistry. She is currently a member of the Society for Neurosciences and is part of the Research Committee of the Universidad Anáhuac México.

***Andrea Herrera Solís*** - Andrea Herrera Solís is currently a researcher in Medical Sciences of the Biomedical Research Department in the Hospital General Dr. Manuel Gea Gonzaléz of Mexico City. Her research lines are the therapeutic effects of cannabinoids and drug addiction. She has a degree in Psychology and PhD in Biomedical Science from the National Autonomus University of Mexico and also made a postdoctoral stay in the Parç de Recerca Biomedica from Barcelona, Spain.

***Wendy Verónica Herrera-Morales*** - PhD. Wendy studied Biology at the Meritorious Autonomous University of Puebla, afterwards she obtained the degrees of Master of Sciences (Neurosciences) and PhD in Biomedical Sciences from the National Autonomous University of México. After posdoctoral work at the Neurobiology Institute of the National Autonomous University of México, she joined the Health Sciences Division of the University of Quintana Roo, where she is currently a Full Professor and develops a research line on the neurophysiological correlates of cognitive function and psychiatric conditions

***Luis Núñez-Jaramillo*** - Luis studied Biology and received his PhD in Biomedical Sciences from the National Autonomous University of México. After posdoctoral work at the Neurobiology Institute of this university, he joined the Health Sciencies Division of the University of Quintana Roo, where he is currently a tenured Full Professor and develops a research line on the neurophysiological correlates of cognitive function and psychiatric conditions.

***Mónica Méndez Díaz*** - Dr. Ciencias Biomédicas. Working in Facultad de Medicina, Departamento de Fisiología. UNAM. Grupo de Neurociencias, Laboratorio de Canabinoides. Research line: "Ontogeny of addictions." Research project: "Function of the cerebrum in self-control and alcohol consumption and its modulation by cannabinoid receptors CB1 and CB2". Recent publications: *Endocannabinoids as Therapeutic Targets*. Prospéro-García O, Ruiz Contreras AE, Ortega Gómez A, Herrera-Solís A, Méndez-Díaz M. Arch Med Res. 2019 Nov;50(8):518-526. *CB1R mediates oleamide's reward while 5HT2cR mediates aversion in the nucleus accumbens shell of rats*. Méndez-Díaz M, Amancio-Belmont O, Estrada-González V, Ruiz-Contreras AE, Prospéro-García O. Neurosci Lett. 2019 Jul 27;706:189-193. *From adolescent to elder rats: Motivation for palatable food and cannabinoids receptors*. Amancio-Belmont O, Romano-López A, Ruiz-Contreras AE, Méndez-Díaz M, Prospéro-García O. *Dev Neurobiol.* 2017 Sep;77(8):917-927.

***Oscar Prospéro García*** - PhD. Medical Doctor, Master in Psychology, PhD. in Neuroscience. Professor at the Departmento of Physiology, Faculty of Medicine, National University of Mexico (UNAM). Author of near 200

papers, including book chapters and reviews. Co-discoverer of Cortistatin and Oleamide.

***Alberto Avila Luna*** - Researcher in Medical Sciences "C", Neuroscience Division National Institute of Rehabilitation LGII. Education; 2002 Zootechnical Veterinary Doctor, Metropolitan Autonomous University, Xochimilco Unit. 2013 Master of Science, National Autonomous University of Mexico. 2019 Doctor in Biological and Health Sciences, Universidad Autónoma Metropolitana, Xochimilco Unit. Honors; (2015 to date) National Researcher, National System of Researchers, Mexico, Level 1. (2017 to date) Regular Member, Mexican Society of Physiological Sciences Mexican Academy of Sciences. Publications; A. Articles in international journals: 18 articles in indexed journals (ISI). B. Articles in journals (with arbitration): 6 C. Book chapters: 5. Conference presentations; Nationals: 12 Internationals: 7 Thesis direction; Bachelor's: 1. Projects with external financing; Conacyt: CB-2016-01-288512 (Mexico)

***Luis Enrique Ruiz Sosa*** - Biological Pharmaceutical Chemist, dedicated to developing research projects in the area of the pharmacology of epilepsy. Graduated from the National Autonomous University of Mexico. A student of the master's degree in biomedical research, she is currently working in the pharmaceutical industry developing proposals for pain medications. He has done research stays at the National Institute of Rehabilitation, the Autonomous Metropolitan University and the National Polytechnic Institute of Mexico. He has published an article and a book chapter on the pharmacology of pain.

***Verónica Salas Venegas*** - PhD student in Experimental Biology and a member of the Laboratory of Bioenergetics and Cellular Aging of the Department of Biological and Health Sciences of the Universidad Autonoma

Metropolitana (UAM) in Mexico. She has a bachelor´s degree and a master's degree in Experimental Biology from UAM.

***Norma Edith López-Díazguerrero*** - Professor at the Bioenergetics and Cellular Aging Laboratory from Universidad Autónoma Metropolitana Unidad Iztapalapa in Mexico. She is dedicated to the study of oxidative stress, cell senescence, aging, and associated diseases. She has directed bachelor's and postgraduate thesis and has publications in scientific journals. Also, Dr. López-Diazguerrero has been part of committees in the organization of different congresses and symposiums.

***Rafael Reynoso-Robles*** - Researcher in Medical Sciences. Instituto Nacional de Pediatría. Sub-Dirección de Medicina experimental. Cell and Tissue Morphology Laboratory. Title: Biologist by Universidad Nacional Autónoma de México. Field of study: Ultra cell structure, Antiepileptics, Environmental pollutants, Parasitosis by Giardia sp. Scientific publications or research activity. In the lines of Antiepileptics, Environmental Pollutants, Parasitosis by Giardia. 44 international articles have been published.

***Roberto Santín Márquez*** - Experimental biologist from the Universidad Autónoma Metropolitana Unidad Iztapalapa, Mexico City, Mexico. With a master degree in Experimental Biology. Currently, is studying the PhD in Experimental Biology in the same institution in the Department of Health Sciences, Laboratory of Bioenergetics and Cellular Aging. He is working in aging in the central nervous system of Wistar rats.

***Mina Konisberg Fainstein*** - She obtained her bachelor and master degree in Experimental Biology at the Universidad Autónoma Metropolitana and a PhD in Biological Sciences in that institution where now she is a teacher and the leader of the Laboratory of Bioenergetics and

Cellular Aging of the Department of Health Sciences. She spent one year at a research fellowship at the Barshop Institute for Aging and Longevity studies. Health Science Center University of Texas, San Antonio, with a Fulbright and CONACyT scholarship. She has published scientific and divulgation papers, and has directed undergraduate and graduate students. She is a member of the Mexican Academy of Sciences and the National System of researchers.

# INDEX

## B

## C

## D

## E



## F

## K



## L



## M

## N

## O



## P

## R

## S

## T



## U

## V



## W